THE NATURE OF THEIR BODIF

Women and Their Doctors in Victorian Can

In 1864 a woman was admitted to the Toronto asylum and diagnosed as suffering from 'mania,' a not uncommon diagnosis for women, a step beyond 'hysteria.' The cause cited by doctors for the patient's insanity was lactation.

This is one of scores of cases cited by Wendy Mitchinson in her history of the medical treatment of women in Victorian Canada. The cases, combined with the medical literature of the period, reflect the society's preoccupations, both among the general population and the medical profession. Above all, they illustrate in sharp detail the society's perceptions of women.

For most medical practitioners, the male body was taken to be the norm; women were 'other.' Doctors were uncomfortable with some of the central physiological experiences of women, such as menstruation and menopause. They often felt that healthy bodies should not undergo such stresses.

From this attitude it was a short leap to viewing the normal functions of women's bodies as illnesses to be treated by specialists. One of the most significant medical developments of this period was the rise of gynaecology and medical obstetrics as major medical specialties. Practitioners used surgical gynaecology to alleviate disorders – mental as well as physical – in women.

In documenting the changing nature of interventional medicine, Mitchinson considers the medical treatment of women within the context of what was available to physicians at the time. She also explores the kind of pressure that women themselves brought to bear. Faced with a medical profession that viewed them as creatures of weakness, women used their strength and stamina to change attitudes and treatments.

WENDY MITCHINSON is Associate Professor of History, University of Waterloo. Among her other books are *The Proper Sphere: Woman's Place in Canadian Society*, co-edited with Ramsay Cook, and *Essays in Canadian Medical History*, co-edited with Janice Dickin McGinnis.

The Nature of Their Bodies

Women and Their Doctors in Victorian Canada

Wendy Mitchinson

UNIVERSITY OF TORONTO PRESS   Toronto Buffalo London

© University of Toronto Press 1991
Toronto Buffalo London
Printed in Canada

Paperback reprinted 1994

ISBN 0-8020-5901-5 (cloth)
ISBN 0-8020-6840-5 (paper)

Printed on acid-free paper

Canadian Cataloguing in Publication Data

Mitchinson, Wendy
The nature of their bodies

Includes bibliographical references and index.
ISBN 0-8020-5901-5 (bound) ISBN 0-8020-6840-5 (pbk.)

1. Women – Health and hygiene – Canada – History –
19th century.   2. Women patients – Canada – History –
19th century.   3. Physician and patient – Canada –
History – 19th century.   4. Medicine – Canada –
History – 19th century.   I. Title.

R462.M58 1991   610'.82   C91-093376-6

This book has been published with the help of a grant from the Canadian
Federation for the Humanities using funds provided by the Social
Sciences and Humanities Research Council of Canada. Publication has
also been assisted by the Canada Council and the Ontario Arts Council
under the block grant programs.

For Rex

Contents

Preface

Research topics often emerge in unexpected ways. Indeed, the topics themselves may not be what the writer originally had envisioned. So it is with this book. In my previous work I had been struck by the ideology of domesticity that permeated discussions about women in the last half of the nineteenth century and I began to study its origins. Underlying the perception of women as wives, mothers, and homemakers was a belief in fundamental differences between the two sexes – emotional, psychological, intellectual, and physical. Most basic were the physical differences, since Victorians believed biology to be immutable. So far so good, but what were the physical differences on which Canadians focused and why did they see them as deterministic? To answer these questions, I decided that an examination of medical perceptions of women would be a good place to begin. I assumed physicians were experts on the body and if anyone were going to discuss the physical differences between the two sexes it would be members of the medical profession. This led me to a reading of Canadian medical journals and the textbooks used in Canadian medical schools in the latter half of the nineteenth century. What I discovered in these sources was a wealth of material on women – their health problems, physicians' perceptions of them, and, most significantly, physicians' treatment of them. I became fascinated by the data and lost sight of my original project. What was to be one chapter in a study of domestic ideology has become this book.

The researching and writing of this volume could not have been done without the help of many people and institutions. I would like to acknowledge funding provided by the Social Sciences and Humanities Research Council, Associated Medical Services through the Hannah Institute for the History of Medicine, and the Universities of Windsor and Waterloo. I would also like to thank the Hannah Institute for its generosity in appointing me the Hannah Visiting Professor in the History of Medicine at McMaster University for 1988–9, which allowed me the luxury of concentrating on the writing of this book. As anyone who has researched Canadian history will appreciate, little can be accomplished without the help of librarians and archivists, and I think we are fortunate in this country to have such a dedicated and enthusiastic group of professionals. Although not everyone who worked in libraries and archives can be named, I would like to acknowledge the assistance of Barbara Craig, Marcel Caya, Brian Cuthbertson, Felicity Pope, and Indiana Matters. In particular, recognition must be given to the librarians at the Academy of Medicine Library in Toronto. I would also like to express my appreciation to the officials of various hospitals who not only allowed access to their records but were willing to endure the inconvenience of having a researcher on premises not set up to accommodate one. Coping with the thousands of patient records I examined at various repositories necessitated my entry into the previously unknown world of computers. For easing this often traumatic experience I want to acknowledge staff at the University of Michigan's Inter-University Consortium for Political and Social Research Training Program in the Theory and Technology of Social Research, and in the computer division at the University of Windsor. I am especially grateful to Marg Kohli and Vic Neglia of the University of Waterloo for their patience in working with this computer neophyte.

Colleagues and friends often do not realize how important they are to your work through their interest in and encouragement of what you do. So I thank my former colleagues in the University of Windsor's history department, especially Kate McCrone and Ken Pryke, and my present colleagues in the Department of History, University of Waterloo. In addition, I owe much to the support and encouragement of Ramsay Cook over the years. Working with Alison Prentice, Beth Light, Paula Bourne, Gail Cuthbert Brandt, and Naomi Black on *Canadian Women: A History*[1] reminded me how much fun writing history could be and for that I do truly thank them. Many individuals assisted in the research of this book, especially the labour-intensive coding of patient records. Among them were Carol Cole, Susan Waterman, Marlene Epp, Megan Davies, Paul Doerr, and Peter Nunoda. I appreciate the work that Susan Johnston did on the medical glossary. Various people shared their expertise, and I would like to thank them all, in particular Dr Tony Travill. No amount of acknowledgment can express my gratitude to those who have been willing to read this manuscript in its various stages in part or in total – Charles Roland, Gail Cuthbert Brandt, James Snell, Alison Prentice, and Laura Macleod and Gerry Hallowell of the University of Toronto Press. Thanks also to Rosemary Shipton for her editing and to Gail Heideman, who so patiently typed various drafts of this manuscript. The dedication of this book reflects the obvious – throughout this project Rex was always there.

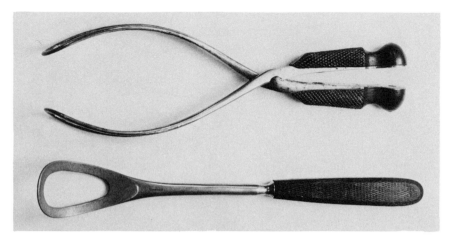

'Types of obstetrical forceps: a vectis (single-blade obstetrical forceps) and Smellie's obstetrical forceps. The use of forceps increased considerably during the nineteenth century, leading to the charge of 'meddlesome midwifery.'

Various gynaecological instruments: uterine sound, bivalve vaginal speculum with mirror, Ferguson vaginal speculum, and a pessary. Such instruments reflected the rise of gynaecology as a medical specialty and indicated the degree to which doctors were able to probe the vagina and uterine cavity.

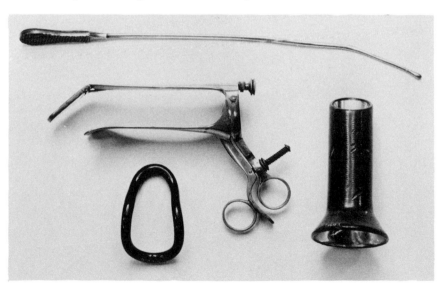

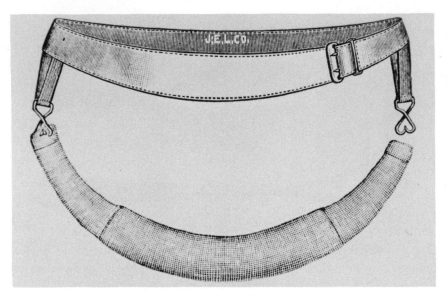

A nineteenth-century menstrual pad. Most women would not have had access to such a modern device; rather they would have used rags and reused them after washing them.

Doctors blamed the wearing of corsets for many of women's health problems; this allowed doctors to advise women on the kind of clothing they should wear and thus expand the nature of what was deemed 'medical.'

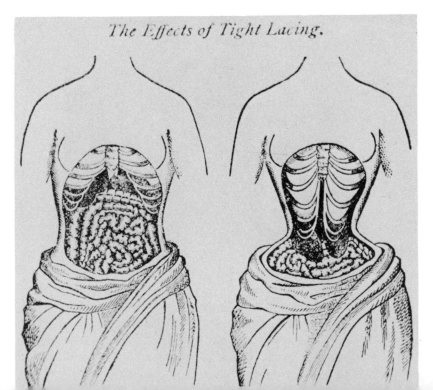

The Effects of Tight Lacing.

SEARCH ❖ON❖

LIGHTS HEALTH

Light on Dark Corners.

A COMPLETE SEXUAL SCIENCE

——AND——

A GUIDE TO PURITY AND PHYSICAL MANHOOD.

Advice to Maiden, Wife, and Mother.

LOVE, COURTSHIP AND MARRIAGE.

BY

PROF. B. G. JEFFERIS, M.D., PH.D.,

AND

J. L. NICHOLS, A.M.

SEVENTEENTH EDITION.

PUBLISHED BY

J. L. NICHOLS & CO.,

No. 33 RICHMOND STREET WEST, TORONTO, ONTARIO,

TO WHOM ALL COMMUNICATIONS MUST BE ADDRESSED.

1897.

The title page of a popular advice manual. The late nineteenth century abounded with such manuals offering guidance to readers on almost every aspect of their lives. Many were written by physicians, illustrating how doctors were seen as experts.

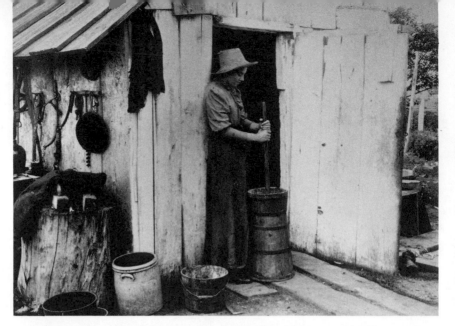

A woman with a churn near Long Branch, Ontario, 1893. Despite the very hard physical work women did in the nineteenth century, physicians tended to view them as frail.

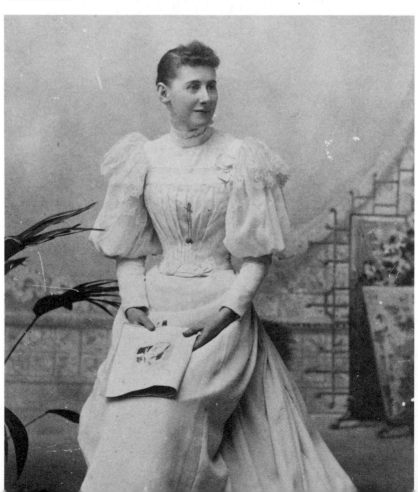

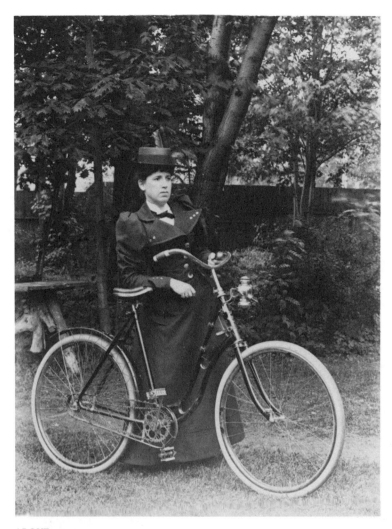

ABOVE

Mrs Albert Campbell, Ottawa East, June 1897, with a bicycle. Cycling was a new sport for women at the end of the nineteenth century and altered many people's image of them. Doctors felt obliged to advise women on the pros and cons of this new activity.

OPPOSITE

Isobel Cameron in this photo, c 1890, represents the idealized concept of womanhood that prevailed in late Victorian Canada.

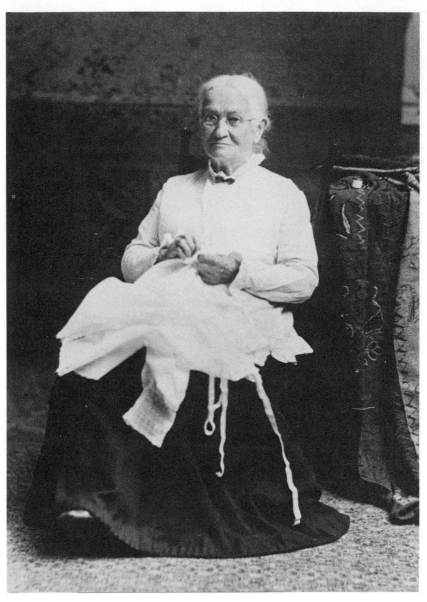

Katie Welsh was a midwife and nurse in Mrs Thomas Ewart's family in the 1880s and 1890s. Midwives were mostly older women who had borne children themselves.

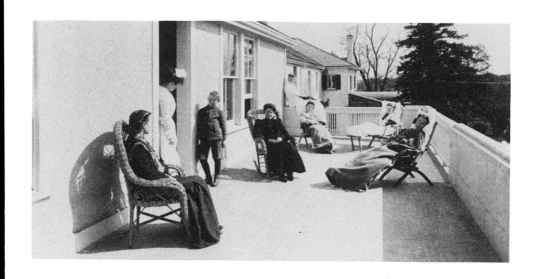

Toronto Hospital for Consumptives, porch of the new women's building, 1905. Tuberculosis was the number one killer of women in the childbearing years.

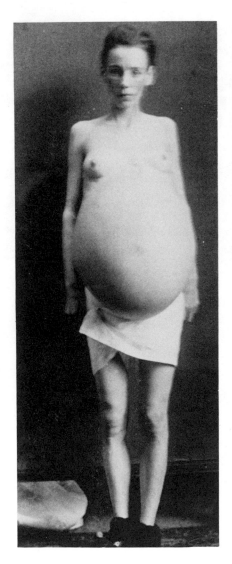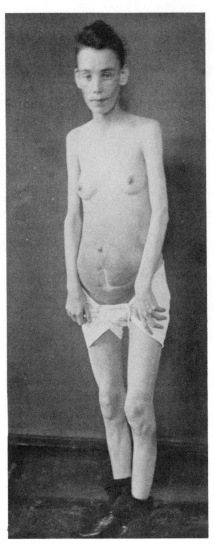

Women in the nineteenth century faced severe medical problems, as shown in these photos from an album of case studies of abnormalities, tumours, and dermatology from the Montreal General Hospital, 1884-7.

THE NATURE OF THEIR BODIES

Introduction

Underlying the work of social historians of medicine is the assumption that disease and medical care are culturally defined. The environment, the individual's pattern of eating, normative values, and the scientific perceptions of any time period influence the definition and perception of disease. 'What is sickness in one [civilization] might be chromosomal abnormality, crime, holiness, or sin in another.'[1] Medicine for social historians, then, is not totally scientific if scientific is taken to mean objective. Indeed, it is the non-scientific aspects of medicine that are its main attractions for, through a study of those aspects, the historian can come closer to understanding the society of the past. Medicine as well has its own internal dynamic. Different periods and cultures have their own favoured treatment but its perceived efficacy often lessens with time. Indeed, the power to heal is very much linked to the belief in the system being used rather than any rational underpinning for it.[2] Thus, certain therapeutics gain ascendancy and are taken up amidst great claims for their merits, but with time problems arise or they are superseded by a newer type and the older fades from memory.[3] Because medicine has extended its sway so dramatically in our society in the last two centuries, its study can tell us much about a wide variety of issues. It tells us not only what sickness existed in the past but also what sickness was thought to be. In turn, this tells us about the perception of health.[4] Health is normative and those not in conformity with it are viewed as ill or in some way deviant. Since the medical profession has had a good deal of influence in defining what is healthy and what is not, it is important to investigate medical care in the past. This is particularly true when the focus is on how the medical profession perceived and treated patients.

Patients are an integral part of the dynamic of medicine. Medicine begins with a perception of illness by the patient, or soon-to-be-patient, or those around her/him. The decision to seek medical advice is not as straightforward as it appears. People do so under a variety of circumstances: when they recognize the seriousness of the problem; when they accept the concept of personal vulnerability; when they are predisposed to act or motivated to act; when they can act; when they have knowledge of the desired action and belief in the usefulness of that action.[5] They seek medical help if they can afford it, if it is available, and if it is expected of them. Focusing on the patient forces historians to distinguish between what physicians were saying and what they were doing – that is, between medical theory and medical practice. It also encourages us to evaluate medicine's treatment not only by whether the patient's sickness is cured and the intervention such a cure necessitated but also by 'the way that care [was] provided in that intervention.'[6] Placing the patient in the centre alongside the physician does not mean, however, that the relationship between the two is equal. It is not. The patient comes to the physician because he or she feels ill and consequently vulnerable. The patient views the physician as someone who can help, who has power and expertise. This obviously gives the physician more sway in the relationship than the patient. This inequality is particularly visible when the patient is a woman.

Historians of women have in recent years become interested in the medical treatment of women.[7] The work of these historians parallels in many ways the historiography of medicine in general. Historians of women have been attracted to the concept of social control,[8] and like other historians of medicine, their own public concerns initiated their interest in the history of medicine as it related to women. Feminists raised questions about the safety of the Pill and other contraceptives; revelations about the dangers of the Dalkon Shield simply reinforced their scepticism concern-

ing medical research and practice as it applied to women. Increasing numbers of women and medical practitioners have also
questioned the rise in hysterectomies and Caesarian sections performed.[9] Such concerns motivated historians to investigate how
women patients in the past were treated. Underlying much of this
historical work is the view that women were victims of the medical profession, that when women as patients faced men as doctors
it was an uneasy meeting and certainly an unequal one. Historians
have argued that in the past, and to a certain extent in the present,
the image of the sick and the image of women were complementary. Some have argued that the Victorian period, in particular, encouraged and indeed esteemed the image of woman as
frail and sickly and that such encouragement could not help but
impinge on the way doctors looked at their female patients and
also on the way women looked at themselves. The medical profession accepted the limited public role given to women and provided a biological rationale for it. Some analysts have even gone
so far as to suggest that male Victorians and Victorian physicians
did not invent the perception of women as weaker than men but
that women themselves did so in retaliation against the limitations
of their lives; women used illness as a way of escaping the pressures placed upon them, for it allowed them 'to deviate legiti-
mately.'[10]

Not all historians who have studied the interrelationship of
women and medicine have viewed women sympathetically or as
victims of medical practice. Edward Shorter in his book *A History
of Women's Bodies* has argued that in the past women's bodies
were a burden to them, made them inferior to men, and made
women believe they were inferior to men. For this reason, women
were slow in demanding their political rights. Not until medical
science and medical practice were able to overcome some of the
deficiencies of the female body were women really able to be
independent of its demands and take their place alongside men.
For Shorter, women were victims, not of the medical profession
that wanted to help them, but of their own physiology. In addition, the physical realities of their lives compounded the weakness of their bodies. Poor nutrition led to iron deficiency anaemia,

particularly when a woman was pregnant, resulting in childbirth complications and enfeebled health.[11] He tends to be alone in this view but other historians, while not necessarily agreeing with his extreme biological perspective, have suggested that we should not view the medical profession as the villain of the piece. Such a view simplifies and distorts the past. What historians such as Gail Parsons and Regina Morantz-Sanchez have argued is for a more balanced approach.[12] They do not deny the sometimes horrendous treatment physicians meted out to their female patients but they do argue that the treatment of male patients was not much better. And they rightly point out that such treatment as did exist must be seen in the context of the time in which it was given and not from a twentieth-century perspective.

A variation on the woman as victim and physician as villain theme is the belief that female physicians were superior to male physicians in the way they treated their female patients. Some historians have suggested that women doctors intervened less than their male counterparts and that this reflected real concern for the patient.[13] This perspective is particularly strong in studies of childbirth when historians compare the work of midwives with that of physicians.[14] As in the case of the woman as victim approach, there is not total unanimity about women being better healers than men. Once again it is Morantz-Sanchez who challenged the prevailing view. In her study of two nineteenth-century American hospitals, the female-run New England Hospital and the male-run Boston Lying-In Hospital, she found there was little difference in the intervention obstetrical patients received from either male or female physicians. There were, however, minor variations. First, women doctors were much more meticulous in keeping records of their poorer patients than were men, thereby indicating greater interest in the women they were treating. Second, patients under women physicians remained in hospital after delivery approximately one week longer, suggesting that the administrators of the New England Hospital were sensitive to the needs of their largely single clientele. Third, while women physicians in fact gave more drugs to their patients than did men, this was not intervention out of control. As Morantz-Sanchez analyses it, 'the male Boston Lying-In physicians followed an objective model: drug prescription was dependent on the physical symptoms. Women physicians dispensed medication or supportive therapy for less codifiable and nonphysical reasons. Everyone received at least "beef tea," and more often a mild pharmaceutical.' In the end she concludes that the male physicians basically ignored their patients after delivery whereas the female doctors did not. Although Sanchez's study of the two hospitals reveals few differences in actual medical therapeutics between women and men physicians, it does reveal differences in the type of care they provided.[15]

What the historiography of women and medicine has suggested is that many factors motivated the medical profession – concern to help those in need, vested interest, ambition, and the values of the society in which doctors practised. While it is not always possible to determine which factor influenced physicians most in any particular situation, it is important to make the influences known. What the work of historians such as Morantz-Sanchez and others also suggests is that it is necessary to approach past medical treatment of women with care. We do not know much about the actual health of women and cannot assume it was similar to women's health today. Neither can we be so distrustful of the medical profession as to assume that its descriptions of physical manifestations in patients were imagined.

Underlying the work of this book is my belief that medicine and culture go hand in hand and that one way of discovering attitudes towards women is to examine their medical experience. Health is where the public and private worlds merge, and for women whose lives have been seen largely as private and therefore inaccessible an examination of the medical care given to them reveals an important aspect of their existence. As Margaret Conrad has pointed out, women's lives revolved around different experiences from men's. Anniversaries of marriages and deaths were ways in which women measured the passage of time. To those occasions we could add the cycle of menstruation, giving birth, and the onset of menopause.[16] Over the years, those who have wanted to keep women in the private sphere have often used science via medicine to support their stance. Doctors, as products of their own society, have done the same. As Barbara Ehrenreich has made clear: 'Medicine stands between biology and social policy, between the "mysterious" world of the laboratory and everyday life. It makes public interpretations of biological theory; it dispenses the medical fruits of scientific advances. Biology discovers hormones; doctors make public judgements on whether "hormonal imbalances" make women unfit for public office. More generally, biology traces the origins of disease; doctors pass judgement on who is sick and who is well.'[17] Doctors interpret theory into practice through the bias of their own class, ethnicity, and gender and through that of their patients. The focus of this book is on the way in which sex and gender determined the treatment women received in mid-to-late nineteenth-century English-speaking Canada.[18] Sex refers to the physiological attributes which label an individual male or female whereas gender refers to the social designation of certain characteristics and behaviour as male or female.

Sex differences are the most basic between men and women and in the late nineteenth century physicians were the individuals most familiar with those differences. By examining medical attitudes towards women and medical treatment of women, I hope to understand the perceptions of women in the wider society and the basis of discriminatory feelings about women. As the medical profession gained in stature in the last decades of the century, Canadians increasingly looked to doctors for information on the human body. Doctors' attitudes towards women were given the weight of scientific fact. Certain words in the Victorian vocabulary had symbolic meaning that the medical profession reinforced – words such as maternity, sterility, menopause. The medical world and the social world were and are interconnected. Because Canadians often looked to physicians for advice and information, doctors could influence the way in which Canadians looked at their own bodies and those of others. This could and did have repercussions in the everyday lives of people. It also affected the development of the medical profession itself. The emphasis given to the biological differences between the two sexes partially explained the emergence of gynaecology as a medical specialty during this era. Obstetrics was influenced by the emphasis that society placed on the childbearing role of women. Medicine and women interact then on two levels. The first is on the social or cultural level, for medical perceptions of the physiological nature of women reinforced and directed the non-medical perceptions of women – that is, medicine gave them a scientific rationale. The second is the actual treatment meted out to female patients. Perceptions of women's proper role in society influenced the medical care provided them.

The period under review coincides with the height of the Victorian idealization of women as wives, mothers, and homemakers and part of the motivation behind the research was to determine how influential that idealization was. The topic is a broad one and encompasses several areas each deserving its own study. Nevertheless, since there is little Canadian research in this field I decided that an overview would be more useful in stimulating research. Also, an overview provides a wider context in which to evaluate medical attitudes and treatment than a narrower focus would allow and indeed might distort. The book begins with an introduction to the popular concept of woman in Canada and how and why the medical view conformed to it. The assumption of this chapter is that the way in which doctors perceived healthy women would be instrumental in their treatment of ill women. Chapter 2 examines the perceived causes of disease in women. Essentially this chapter is the continuation of the former, for what emerges is the perception by physicians that women who deviated from their prescribed social role often caused their own illness. The next several chapters trace women through the various phases of their life cycle, puberty, menstruation, and menopause, and two issues that emerge from them which doctors medicalized – sexuality and birth control. Also medicalized was the experience of childbirth, the subject of two further chapters. Going from the experience of most women to that of a minority, the study examines the rise of gynaecology in this country and the way in which physicians combined their social perceptions of women to bolster this new specialty. Because the conventional perception of women was that they were psychologically different from men, I conclude the book with a study of the treatment of nervous disorders in women. As is evident, my central interest is in the way the medical profession treated women as patients when they were suffering from problems that were or could be related to their being female. I have not examined ailments common to both sexes, except nervous disorders for the reason already mentioned, assuming that doctors did not differentiate their treatment of them.

There are certain problems inherent in looking at the medical treatment of women. For one, it distorts the experience of women, since by examining them only as patients we do not see their activism. Those women who refused to go to doctors, treated themselves, or went to minority practitioners are lost in this record, women such as Lydia Christie who after three years of illness no longer looked to the medical profession for aid but accepted her situation as God's will.[19] The study ignores the fact that women as mothers, family members, nurses, and midwives were major providers of health care as well as consumers of that care. In doing so, it misrepresents the entire notion of medicine and who practises it. Neither are women reformers given their due. Often it was women's organizations such as the Woman's Christian Temperance Union or the National Council of Women that instigated the establishment of hospitals or special wards for women, or institutions such as the Women's Medical College in Kingston that set up a dispensary for the special treatment of women and children.[20] As with any study, there is much additional information that would have been useful to explore but was not available. Little is known about the actual health patterns of Canadians in the past and the attitudes that non-medical people had of their own bodies. Little is known about the health care that was available to Canadians outside the mainstream of regular or allopathic medicine – that is, medicine that treats disease with remedies that produce effects different from the disease symptoms. Historians have a sense that minority or alternative medicine in its various guises was important, but how important is not known. Neither do we know how often Canadians frequented any kind of health care practitioner or how many resorted to curing themselves and in what way they went about it.[21] As a result, this study is largely limited to an examination of the regular medical profession, although some homeopathic texts were consulted as were popular health manuals published at the time. The point is that, despite the emphasis on regular medicine in this book, the reader should not assume that no alternatives were available. Challenges to allopathic medicine were mounted but for the purposes of this book they are significant only in so far as they affected regular medicine and its treatment of women.

One of the problems in working in a field such as medical history is the question of whether it makes sense to examine it from a national perspective. After all, medicine as practised in nineteenth-century Canada was part of Western medicine, was it not? When the records of Canadian physicians are examined and the Canadian medical journals read, it is clear that Canadian practitioners were not isolated in a backwater or creating their own kind of medicine. They were able to keep up with the latest advances and their records abound with references to the international literature. In the 1870s Dr Hugh M. Mackay, a general practitioner in Woodstock, Ontario, made references in his medical notebook to the *New York Medical Record*, the *American Journal of Obstetrics*, and the *American Journal of Medical Sciences*.[22] Some Canadian practitioners even went beyond keeping up, they innovated. This was particularly true with respect to Richard Maurice Bucke, superintendent of the London, Ontario, Asylum, who pioneered gynaecological surgery on insane women, and Dr Charles Sheard, who when he was working at the Toronto General Hospital sponsored the use of the metrotome, a cutting instrument used in operating on the uterus.[23] This does not mean, however, that any study of Canadian medicine must only deal with the 'greats' of the field. On the contrary, for social historians it is the 'typical' practitioner who is more significant since most patients would not have been attended by the leading men in the field.[24] But will a study of them be useful or will it simply repeat another nation's experience? Needless to say this argument could be made for many other fields of Canadian history, and the reaction on the part of Canadians interested in studying those areas is to reject it. Perhaps S.F. Wise explained the rationale for what we do best: 'No doubt the stock of Canadian ideas is replenished every generation from European and American sources; and doubtless it should be an important function of the Canadian intellectual historian to perform the sort of operations that will trace Canadian ideas to their ultimate source. But [the] major task, surely, is to analyze the manner in which externally derived ideas have been adapted to a variety of local and regional environments, in such a way that a body of assumptions uniquely Canadian has been built up; and to trace the changing context of such assumptions.'[25] Because physicians in Canada practised in a different social milieu from those in Britain or the United States, their efforts are worth examining; as already argued, medical practice cannot be divorced from the society in which its practitioners lived.

In that society, Victorians revealed an ambivalence towards nature which doctors shared. At times, practitioners appealed to nature to bolster the conventional wisdom of the day regarding women, using it as a way to hold back change; at others, they pursued their urge to dominate nature in wanting to improve on its handiwork. In either case, they expanded the definition of what was medical in society. Similarly, Canadians believed in the centrality of biological sex differences as a factor in personality development and in determining an individual's social role. Doctors, too, appealed to sex to explain their positioning of men and women on the evolutionary ladder and, more significantly, in the medical care they provided to women. Perhaps because most physicians were men, they also used the male body and how it functioned as the norm by which to judge whether women were healthy or not. But using the male body as the norm went beyond what Victorians perceived as its physiological workings; it included gender expectations, what it meant to be a man in Victorian society. As is sometimes evident in this study, this did not always benefit male patients. But most often it operated against women patients. Women could not conform to the physiological norm of being male and, because of this, gender expectations for women were different as well. Indeed, the gender expectations for women in Victorian society were always more explicit than they were for men, a result of seeing women as somehow 'other' than men. Doctors shared the gender expectations respecting women and evaluated and treated their patients accordingly. Sex and gender, then, are central in understanding physicians' attitudes towards their women patients and the medical care they provided to them.

Chapter One

The Victorian World:
Doctors, Science, and 'Woman'

Referring to the physical abilities of woman, the *Globe* in 1890 reported that 'she can swim, she can dance, she can ride; all these things she can do admirably and with ease to herself. But to run, nature most surely did not construct her.' Like the domestic hen which at times attempts to fly, woman running displays 'a kind of precipitate waddle with neither grace, nor fitness nor dignity.'[1] For men, running was natural, their bodies designed in such a way as to facilitate fast and sustained movement. Running was only one of many differentiations that Canadians made between the sexes. By and large, they believed that men and women differed from one another on almost every level and, as the *Globe* quote indicates, located those differences in nature. But while Canadians had a strong sense of what was natural for women to do, they were not as clear about why this was the case. As a result, they looked to physicians, as experts on the body, for the information they needed. Doctors' perceptions of women, in turn, mirrored conventional ideology and influenced their interpretation of female physiology. By doing so, they not only bolstered their own position at a time when many doctors were feeling unsure about their status in society but also provided the scientific rationale for prevalent attitudes towards women.

Separation of spheres was a major ideological construct in the Victorian period and no woman who lived in Victorian Canada could help but be aware of it. Poems extolled its virtues, articles and books paid homage to its aesthetic balance, and sermons credited divine inspiration for its existence. Throughout the latter half of the nineteenth century, Canadians were inundated with powerful and at times maudlin descriptions of the concept of sexual separation at every level – intellectual, physical, moral, and emotional. What is fascinating about this deluge is that its real focus was not the respective characteristics of men and women but rather the proper role and place of women in society. The male role was clearly a given, the norm; few descriptions of it exist compared to those of woman's role. It was the nature of woman that fascinated and enthralled – she was a being of endless variation and Canadians did not tire of discussing her or reading about her. As it applied to woman the ideology of separation was clear cut; it revolved around her role as wife, mother, and home-maker. As the author of an article entitled 'Woman's Sphere' made clear: 'Woman's first and only place is her home. Within its sanctuary she will find her mission ... She is destined by Providence to make her home a blissful spot to those around her. It should be full of the merry sunshine of happiness – a cloister wherein one may seek calm and joyful repose from the busy, heartless world ... Her kingdom is not of this world, worldly. The land she governs is a bright oasis in the desert of the world's selfishness.' Of course the bright oasis was for her husband where he, not she, could seek 'joyful repose.' His responsibility was summed up in one sentence. 'To her lord will be left the taking part in the framing of laws and the government of the realm.'[2] Or as the author of *Domestic Sanctuary* bluntly wrote, 'It is his right to rule.'[3] The division set out by these two authors was not confined to the literary set. It permeated all classes of society and all reading material. In 1886 the Fort Macleod *Gazette* advised women: 'Don't disturb your husband while he is reading the morning or evening newspaper by asking foolish questions. Be patient and when he comes across anything he thinks you can comprehend perhaps he will read it to you.'[4] This quote suggests that the separation of spheres between men and women was a vertical delineation reflecting a hierarchy of importance. The Honourable John Dryden, minister of agriculture for Ontario in 1898, had no doubts about it. Incensed by some women's temerity at demanding the right to vote, he chastised them and their supporters: 'The man was not made for the woman, but the woman for the man.'[5]

Not all Canadians were as adamant about placing men and women in a hierarchical structure. For them a horizontal plane epitomized the relationship of the sexes. Men and women were different but equal. As the Maritime Woman's Christian Temperance Union made clear, 'A man is to a woman and a woman is to a man, a stronghold; a completeness such as no two women or two men ever can be to one another.'[6] To complete one another, the two sexes had to be different; yet when Victorian Canadians discussed men and women they focused on those differences that distinguished women from men rather than those that distinguished men from women. Woman was to be gentle, meek, patient, self-denying, tactful, devoted, tender, sympathetic, and enduring – as one commentator astutely phrased it, woman was to have 'passive virtues.'[7]

In recent years, there has been some suggestion that historians have been too willing to accept the concept of separate spheres as a reflection of reality.[8] Women were to stay home and care for the family, but during this period many women, both single and married, participated in paid employment either in the home or outside the home. Middle-class women, too, involved themselves in the public arena, using the welfare of Canadian families as their excuse. Both these examples underline the fact that the private and the public worlds were never completely separate. In addition, historians have not always been clear about whether they were discussing 'an ideology *imposed on* women, a culture *created by* women, [or] a set of boundaries *expected to be observed* by women.'[9] For the purposes of this study, differentiating among the three is not important. What is significant is recognizing the ideology's existence and the repercussions it had for the lives of women. Proof of its concreteness emerges from a study of late nineteenth-century medicine.

For most of the century, physicians had little power or prestige. At first glance, this may not seem to be the case since the move to restrict entry into the profession and thus give physicians control over the practice of medicine began very early. In 1788 'An

Ordinance to prevent persons practising Physic and Surgery within the Province of Quebec, and Midwifery in the towns of Quebec and Montreal without a licence' was implemented to impede the number of so-called quacks who were practising medicine. The law also set out the way in which inhabitants could become licensed practitioners – a five-year apprenticeship with a doctor followed by an examination. In 1795 a similar act applying to physicians in Upper Canada passed, although it only lasted until 1806. Subsequent laws in Upper Canada established medical examining boards which made clear whom they could license and thus in whose interest they were. In addition to examining those who had studied medicine through the required apprenticeship means, the 1818 legislation authorized the Medical Board of Upper Canada to grant a licence without examination to those authorized to practise medicine by any university in His Majesty's Dominions or by virtue of commissions in the military or naval services. To this were added members of the London College of Surgeons (1827), the Colleges of Surgeons of Edinburgh and Dublin, and the Faculty of Physicians and Surgeons of Glasgow (1839). The laws were to protect patients from untrained practitioners and to confine the practice of medicine to those educated in British schools rather than possible republican sympathizers trained in the United States. Similar licensing laws existed in New Brunswick (1816) and Nova Scotia (1828).[10]

Despite its intentions, the early legislation was not particularly successful in restricting access to the profession of medicine. Regulating physicians made sense if they were numerous enough to administer to the needs of British North Americans, but in the early years of the century they were not. Robert Gourlay in his 1822 *Statistical Account of Upper Canada* noted that townships in the London district had only six medical men for a population of 8907 and that the Niagara District had the same number for a population of over twelve thousand. In addition, the laws could not be enforced. As Gourlay railed, 'How absurd to think of preventing remotely scattered people from choosing whom they liked to draw their teeth, bleed or blister them – or that a woman should not have the assistance of a handy sagacious neighbour, without fear of a fine.'[11] The laws, of course, did not prevent this but rather prohibited individuals passing themselves off as trained physicians and, more significantly, charging for the services rendered. Be this as it may, the medical licensing laws, whatever their interpretation, were virtually ignored. As a result, there was little real obstacle to practising medicine and numerous groups existed who did so.

One group was composed of those who referred to themselves as doctors – the Thomsonians, Eclectics, homeopaths, and other self-styled physicians. The Thomsonians, who came to Upper Canada from the United States very early in the century, followed the principles set down in *The New Guide to Health* by Samuel Thomson (1769–1843), a New Hampshire farmer. The advantage of his system was that it used botanic or vegetable compounds only and so its impact on the patient was relatively benign. The Thomsonians had their greatest influence in the 1840s and by the 1850s had come to associate themselves and be associated with the Eclectics, practitioners who did not confine themselves to botanic or any other particular kind of therapeutics, but rather used whatever approach to specific illnesses they deemed would work. Members of both groups considered themselves qualified enough, through self-taught methods and/or formal training in their own schools, to practise medicine and to be legally recognized to do so. In 1849 alone the Eclectics unsuccessfully petitioned the Legislative Assembly of the Canadas four times for this recognition. Particularly galling to the Thomsonians and the Eclectics were the limits these refusals placed on available medical care, for they believed that the patient should have the opportunity to choose not only the doctor he/she wanted but also the kind of treatment he/she wanted.[12] Of course, they assumed that, given that choice, patients would prefer attendance by a Thomsonian or Eclectic physician. Homeopaths were another medical group that emerged at mid-century. Originating with Samuel Hahnemann (1755–1843), a German physician, homeopathy was based on the belief, in contradistinction from the allopaths, that disease was cured by drugs that produce the effects closest to the symptoms of the illness – that like cures like. In addition, homeopaths believed that the potency of the drug increased the more it was diluted,[13] with the result that their treatment allowed the patient's own body to restore itself to health. The homeopaths were a very organized and cohesive group after mid-century and determined to survive. They formed their own societies, established hospitals, and founded their own medical journal.

In addition to the Thomsonians, Eclectics, and homeopaths, other medical practitioners existed at mid-century whose involvement in medicine threatened not only the economic interests of regular physicians but also their social status. In 1863/4 the *Canada Lancet* published a letter from a Dr Granger of Dunbarton, Ontario:

Dear Sir: – I received the *Lancit* in due time, and would have written you before now, but have been disabled by a fellon on my finger, and even now can hardly hold my pen ... I noticed an attack upon me by a nabour of mine who sines his name 'live and Let Live.' Apart of his statements is true, and part is not true, but I suppose he gave them to you as he received them from others the names I have inclosed will show you what the faculty thinks of me in Whitby the most of them have none me and my practis fore more than twenty-five years.

Granger was a blacksmith who practised medicine on the side, and the purpose of the journal in publishing his letter was to bring to the attention of the regular medical profession the lack of control that existed over who could practise medicine.[14] And men such as Granger were only the tip of the iceberg.

Besides the health care providers who deemed themselves doctors, there was an assortment of others who perhaps provided most of the health care in the early period even though they were not physicians, did not consider themselves physicians, and were not considered as such. Midwives, who were chief among them, were familiar to most British North American families. Other individuals simply became noted for their medical skills and, in a society where physicians were few and far between, practised with impunity. In Portage la Prairie in the 1860s a Mrs Spence gained a reputation due to her 'simple operation' that apparently gave relief from headaches.[15] Farmer's almanacs always advertised various curing compounds and gave medical advice. For general malaise, the *Farmers' Directory* (1851) advised a change to a lighter diet and for fits recommended rubbing the patient with warm flannels.[16]

Then there were the health manuals that many families owned. One of the most popular among Methodists and others was John Wesley's *Primitive Physic or An Easy and Natural Method of Curing Most Diseases*. A wide variety of illnesses and treatments were detailed including a recipe for toothpowder consisting of ashes of burned bread, 1/2 oz of gum myrrh, 1 oz of chalk, and 1 oz of charcoal.[17] Also familiar to Canadians, especially in the latter part of the century, were patent medicines. One of the most famous was Lydia Pinkham's Vegetable Compound. Used by women to combat fatigue and a host of 'female' ailments, the compound became a familiar part of popular culture with its specialized advertisements earning recognition in song:

> Lizzie Smith had tired feelings,
> Terrible pains reduced her weight.
> She began to take the Compound,
> Now she weighs three hundred and eight.[18]

The most widespread provider of medical care, however, was the wife and mother of the family. Recipe books used by women abounded with health tips and directions for preparing remedies for various ailments. Most women probably knew about 'using Balm of Gilead for blisters, mustard plasters for colds, milk and bread poultices for boils, soda for bites, cold tea leaves for burns, salt water for sore throats, and senna tea for constipation.'[19]

Regular physicians might have been able to cope with this vast array of competitors if they had been organized and if the medicine they practised had been obviously superior to what Canadians could get elsewhere. In the early decades of the century, however, doctors' first loyalty was not to each other but to their sponsors, men of social position who could provide them with access to paying patients. 'Knowing someone' was all important

– even training depended on it in the years when apprenticeship was the only route to medical education in the various British North American colonies.[20] Despite this lack of cohesiveness, the regular physicians did share a common approach to medicine. They based their therapeutics on the concept of balance within the body and the belief, going back to the ancient Greeks, that the four elements of earth, air, water, and fire manifested themselves in constitutional body types. Each element corresponded to the qualities of dryness, coldness, moisture, or heat and, combined, they formed the humours of the body – blood, phlegm, yellow bile, and black bile. Health meant that the humours were balanced. Imbalance resulted in sickness. Because disease was the result of imbalance, efforts to cure concentrated on restoring stability through such techniques as purging and bleeding.[21] Regular practitioners also depended on an arsenal of remedies to bring about effects opposite to the symptoms of the disease being treated, and at times gave them in such large quantities that, along with purging and bleeding, their approach to medicine has been labelled by historians as 'heroic.' In his study of cholera in nineteenth-century Canada, Geoffrey Bilson detailed an example in the treatment undergone by Private Patrick Mullany of the 32nd Regiment at Quebec:

When he fell ill, he hid from the doctors until he was seen to be sick and taken to hospital on 17 July at 9 am. He was bled thirty ounces, given fifteen grains of calomel and two of opium, given a turpentine enema, rubbed with turpentine for his cramps, then given ginger tea and allowed to rest. At 2 pm he was given three grains of calomel and put on a course of one-eighth grain of opium every half-hour with calomel every third hour. In the evening he was dosed with castor oil. On 18 and 19 July he was given an enema and dosed with calomel, opium, castor oil, and port wine every two or three hours. On 20 July he was given a variety of drinks and had a blister applied to his stomach. The next day he was dosed with rhubarb, had twelve leeches applied to his stomach, followed by a second blister, and was allowed beef tea and arrowroot. On 22 July he was fit enough to eat porridge for breakfast, but the mercury had begun to blister his mouth and he was given bicarbonate of soda in addition to his beef tea and arrowroot. On 23 July the medicines were withdrawn and he began to improve slowly until on 11 August he was declared fit for duty.[22]

Such treatment was intimidating to say the least. It is also clear that the term 'heroic' medicine is apt – a patient needed to be a hero to withstand it. Some historians have argued that physicians followed heroic treatment so they could be seen to be doing something – that is, so they could impress their patient that he/she was getting something for the payment made. The irony was that because they 'did' so much, they alienated the patient who often looked elsewhere for help and thus reinforced the need of the practitioner to be seen to be doing even more. It was a cycle that doctors had difficulty breaking.[23]

At mid-century, then, Canadians enjoyed a pluralistic medical society. Each medical group had its own approach and offered the medical 'consumer' something different. What this led to was increased competition and a feeling of frustration and insecurity on the part of the regular medical profession. Many trained physicians had a difficult time making a living, particularly in poorer communities. Dr Alexander Forrest of New Glasgow, Nova Scotia, was typical in his willingness to accept payment in kind for his services.[24] Not only were physicians in precarious financial straits, but they had little influence. In Nova Scotia in the 1820s and 1830s, doctors who cared for the poor were seldom reimbursed by the government. Legislators took for granted that such 'unpaid' activity was part of any physician's normal workload.[25] The assumption that physicians were an endless source of charitable medical largesse may have been one reason why many physicians urged their respective colonial and, later, provincial governments to become more involved in providing health care to the needy. It would shift the burden from the doctors and might even be to their benefit since the government would have to hire and appoint 'experts' to help administer whatever medical care system was set up. The status of the profession was not high at mid-century and anything that acknowledged its place in society would, from the doctors' standpoint, have been seen as an improvement. Meanwhile, physicians themselves began to establish themselves as a much more unified group and to challenge their competitors on a variety of fronts.

Physicians in Canada East (Quebec) were the first to gain control of entry into the profession. As early as 1847 an act was passed that created the College of Physicians and Surgeons of Lower Canada. Composed of regular doctors, the college, through its board of directors, could certify potential candidates for licence, examine candidates (with some exceptions), and, most significantly, determine the standard of medical education or training in that province. In other words, physicians through their college controlled (in theory) who could practise medicine in the province and how they would practise it.[26] In Ontario the regulars had more difficulty controlling licensing. In 1859 the legislature passed a bill incorporating a homeopathic board for Canada West, with the power to grant licences to practise physic, surgery, and midwifery 'on homeopathic principles.' Soon after the government recognized the Eclectics.[27] In 1869 the province of Ontario went one step further and permitted the creation of the College of Physicians and Surgeons of Ontario with powers similar to those granted in the 1847 act to Quebec physicians. However, both homeopathic and Eclectic physicians had representatives in the college.[28] It would appear that a limited form of medical pluralism was, at least temporarily, firmly ensconced in the province.

Another method regular physicians used to strengthen their status and hence their influence in society was to act as a professional group, which necessitated joining and working together for a common cause. This was easier said than done. Regular physicians were often as divided among themselves as they were against alternative medical groups. Rural practitioners did not feel they had much in common with urban physicians and often envied their more lucrative practices. Where and how a physician trained created a hierarchy among those practising. University-educated physicians from Britain were not always accepting of the training many Canadian practitioners received through apprenticeship and, as we have already seen, the law gave preferential treatment to the former. Tension also existed between the francophone and anglophone medical groups in Quebec. Despite such divisions, many physicians recognized the need to join together if only to lessen their own sense of isolation in their individual practices and to keep up with the latest advances in medicine. In 1833 the Medico-Chirurgical Society of Upper Canada formed with membership restricted to regular practitioners. In Nova Scotia, doctors established the Halifax Medical Society in 1854 and began publishing a weekly column in the *Acadian Recorder* in the hope of educating readers about the benefits of scientific medicine.[29] In 1861 its successor, the Nova Scotia Medical Society, made the purpose of its existence clear in its constitution: 'It is universally admitted that *"Union is Strength"* – The Medical Profession in this Province, although numerous, are at present powerless to effect any great or important reform for their mutual benefit; hence it becomes imperative on every member to co-operate with his Brethren to exalt his Profession above the standard of Empiricism and Quackery.'[30] In 1863 a medical section of the Canadian Institute was organized which, too, was part of an effort to increase the prestige of the regular medical profession.[31] More important as a symbolic gesture of unity was the formation of the Canadian Medical Association in 1867. Although it never attracted a large membership, it attempted to speak with the authority of a nationally organized group.

Unifying the profession as well was the development of a common standard of education. This was a far cry from the earlier years of the century when the formal education of physicians was a confusing choice between apprenticeship (whatever this meant) and formal education, divided as it was among various competing proprietary schools and public institutions in Canada and medical training facilities outside the country. Nonetheless, the requirements of some of these early schools were impressive. When King's College Medical School, Toronto, opened in 1843, it insisted that, in order to graduate, students had to be over twenty-one years of age, have a degree in arts, and have a certificate of medical studies of at least four years' duration consisting of two courses of six months 'each in practical anatomy with dissection, anatomy and physiology, principles of practices of medicine and principles and practices of surgery.' One course of six months' length was required in each of materia medica and pharmacy, chemistry, midwifery and diseases of women and children, and medical jurisprudence. Students also took a three-month course in practical chemistry. Following this was eighteen months of medical and surgical practice at a hospital, including lectures for six months of that time. Lastly, a student had to write a thesis and 'to have performed upon a dead subject such capital operations as might be required by the examiners.' While the requirements of King's College Medical School were extensive, not all medical schools were equally demanding. In addition, while many of the schools provided clinical experience for their students, few if any had laboratories or research facilities.[32] Neither could medical schools provide sufficient numbers of cadavers from which their students could learn anatomy. This often resulted in the students' taking matters into their own hands and robbing graves to ensure an adequate supply. Such antics, although understandable, did not serve the profession well. Perhaps for that reason the bylaws of the Montreal General Hospital tried to instil in the medical students working there some semblance of decorum by insisting that 'every student must keep off his hat, while he is in the operating Theatre, both that he may not obstruct the view of others, and as a mark of respect, and all noise and changing of seats must be avoided, as unpleasant to the operator, and hurtful to the patient.'[33]

The major problem facing medical schools, however, was not the conduct of their students but simple survival. The smaller ones had short life spans and all faced constant financial difficulties because of the fierce competition for students they created among themselves. Despite this, allopathic medical schools survived and, by the end of the century, training in one of them, leading to a degree granted by a university, increasingly became the normative route accepted by licensing boards across the country.[34] The importance of this development should not be discounted. Even though the minority practitioners had legal recognition in some provinces, the only way of being trained in Canada was to be educated in one of the medical schools which the regular practitioners controlled. Only a strong and committed individual could go through training in allopathic medicine and still practise a form of medicine that significantly differed from it. Dr Morrison, an Eclectic member of the Ontario college, underlined this reality when writing to an American colleague in 1872. He explained that already almost one-third of the Eclectic physicians practising in Ontario had graduated from allopathic medical schools, and that to an increasing degree Eclectic physicians were following allopathic procedure.[35]

Although doctors could point to success, there were still challenges to their newly won status that made them feel uneasy. For one, not all Canadians accepted the process of medical monopolization with equanimity. In the mid-1890s, in Ontario, the Patrons of Industry, a rural populist party, challenged the College of Physicians and Surgeons and its power to restrict entry into the profession. The patrons also wanted to see the lowering of student medical fees so that more young people could enter the profession. They argued that the profession had become a monopoly of the well-to-do.[36] The profession fought back, for the last thing its members wanted to see was more physicians in a society they felt was already overcrowded with them. Using an agricultural analogy all his readers would understand, Francis W. Campbell, editor of the *Canada Medical Record*, compared the worth of a physician to a bushel of wheat: 'Just as the same wheat may be worth so much a bushel today and twice as much this day next year, so without any diminution in the intrinsic worth of the physician, his value as a necessity to the public may be very much lowered or raised, by the mere fact that the supply of doctors is greater than the demand.'[37] Restricting numbers had only been partially achieved by the creation of examining boards. By raising standards, medical societies could control the number of students entering and graduating from Canadian medical schools, but they could not regulate the number of those schools or the number of doctors entering the country. In 1895 in Nova Scotia alone, 287 out of 387 registered doctors had trained elsewhere.[38] Competition remained strong, and it was small wonder that there were ambivalent feelings when women demanded entry.

Physicians may have been concerned that women entering the profession would increase the competitive pool at a time when they felt it was already expanding. Some may also have been sensitive about maintaining the prestige they had long been struggling to attain if women were allowed to practise medicine. Still others believed that members of their sex were primarily responsible for advances in medical care and that women would not contribute much in this regard. Responding to the successful entry of women into the American medical profession, Theodore Thomas in his 1868 *Practical Treatise on the Diseases of Women*, a text used in some Canadian medical schools, made his position abundantly clear. Women, he argued, had little place in medicine and certainly not in the new specialty of gynaecology. True, in the past women had cared for other women but what they did had not really advanced that care to any degree. Only when men became involved did medical progress occur.[39] More widespread was the unease about women deviating from accepted norms by becoming physicians. Women had always been healers within the family but becoming a physician was a different matter. A physician was educated and paid for healing, two aspects that when applied to women contradicted popular conventions. Physicians were public figures, a role that many in society did not view as appropriate to women. No wonder an editorial reprinted in the 1871 *Canada Lancet* expressed ambivalence: 'As wives and mothers, sisters and dainty little housekeepers we have the utmost love and respect for them; but we do not think the profession of medicine, as a rule, a fit place for them. But if they choose to enter upon the study of the medical or any other profession which they may admire, we see no good reason why they should be denied any of the rights and privileges accorded to those of the sterner sex.'[40] The author's willingness to concede to women the right to study medicine was ahead of his time, for not until 1883 was the first woman able to graduate with a medical degree from a Canadian medical school.[41]

Making the decision to become a doctor and pursuing the required medical program was no easy task for women. Elizabeth Smith could testify to that. Just before she entered medical school her best friend pleaded with her to 'lay aside those silly thoughts and you will be a better woman.' She sympathized with Smith's desire 'to do something grand something that will carry your name on to further ages,' but felt that her first responsibility was not to herself but to her parents and their care.[42] But Smith's problems did not end with her entry into medical school at Queen's University. When only a few women students continued in the separate program for women, those who remained were integrated into the regular courses and had to face the virulent opposition of the male students. The psychological wear and tear must have been enormous for the small handful of women. Smith herself described the experience as a 'furnace fiery & severe.'[43] Even with access to education assured and a degree obtained, women who wanted to practise medicine had to face other hurdles. It was difficult for them to gain clinical experience and it was often difficult for them to gain patients. They also confronted restrictions their male colleagues did not. For example, in the province of Ontario, a woman doctor could not legally certify patients for admission into a private asylum.[44] This is possibly why so many of the early women graduates in medicine became medical missionaries. If they were not allowed to practise freely in Canada they could at least use their skills overseas where it would not be so obvious they were challenging the traditional assumptions of their own culture about women's role in society.[45] Certainly it seemed to be difficult to have one's talents accepted. On the eve of her wedding to Adam Shortt, Elizabeth Smith received a letter from Dr I.D. Macdonald congratulating her on 'the commencement of your freedom from the servitude of medical practice' which he assumed would occur now she was to be a married lady. He underlined his belief in woman's proper role, arguing 'that men and women have different spheres of labour alloted to them and that medical practice in a country town comes within the sphere of men's work.'[46]

Although the opening of faculties of medicine to women could not have occurred without the dedication and support of many male practitioners, some within the profession remained ambivalent. The editor of the *Canada Medical Record* in 1888 admitted that women should have every opportunity to pursue their studies and had no doubt they had the intellectual ability to do so. But did they have the physical stamina? About this he was not sure and he agreed with the editor of the Philadelphia *Medical Times*, who recommended that women physicians should limit themselves to the easier aspects of medicine. Two years later an editorial in the same journal suggested that if a woman doctor married a colleague she could assist him in his practice. It also recommended that women doctors take over midwifery and care of the poor, noting that male doctors were not as interested in these fields since there was not much money to be made from them. In 1890 the *Canada Medical Record*, the journal that seemed to take most interest in the subject, pointed out in an editorial that women should be accepted into medical schools not only because they were as well educated as men, but also because women in the classroom made it easier to maintain order. In addition, their presence provided an incentive for the men to work harder.[47] M.L. Holbrook, in his 'Parturition without Pain,' recognized that women patients might prefer to consult a woman doctor and to confide personal details to her that they would be unwilling to confide to a male physician.[48] Despite such support, the number of women physicians remained small. In the census of 1891 only seventy-six out of 4448 doctors listed were women.[49]

At the end of the century the regular medical profession could look back with some sense of accomplishment. Through education, its members had gained more control over who could practise medicine and who could style themselves as physicians. They were also a much more cohesive group than they had been earlier in the century. There were still areas, however, that caused physicians concern. From their perspective, the profession was overcrowded. This created financial pressures, especially for those trying to make a living in poorer communities. The American Medical Association estimated that a doctor needed 2000 patients to have an adequate living. This was going to be difficult in Canada where in 1891 the ratio of doctors to population was 1:1079.[50] Practices were expanding, especially in urban areas, but rates charged did not increase much over the years, probably because of the competition for patients.[51] The medical profession was a group on the rise but not one that had arrived. Doctors had to tread warily so as not to lose what they had so recently gained. Physicians were not about to challenge the accepted norms of society, but they did not have to. Their attitudes towards women doctors revealed the degree to which they held conventional notions about women. They, too, accepted the social division between the sexes and believed that physical differences accounted for it.

The most obvious among the differences were those related to the reproductive system. So fundamental were they, so much were they a hallmark of an individual's identity that some physicians even tried to distinguish among groups of women on the basis of variations in their reproductive organs. At the end of the century D.C. MacCallum, a leading Montreal specialist in midwifery and diseases of women, argued, for example, that pubic hair was normally short and curly but in sterile women it was straight and either shorter or longer than usual, a condition 'indicative of a feeble development.' He also maintained that the vagina was longer in virgins than in women who had borne children and longer in black women than in white.[52] While some physicians believed they could differentiate among groups of women, the real focus was on differentiating the two sexes. In 1796 a female skeleton was first reproduced in an anatomy book and, after that time, the medical emphasis was on illustrating how women differed from men.[53] As William Buchan, the author of an early self-help manual made clear: 'Women, in all civilized nations, have the management of domestic affairs, and it is very proper they should, as nature has made them less fit for the more active and laborious employments.'[54] This quote contains several themes that physicians would constantly return to throughout the century: that there was an equation between civilization and woman's domestic responsibility, that women were less capable of work outside the home than were men, and that woman's domestic role was the result of nature not society.

The appeal to nature is particularly important. As Carl Berger has illustrated, nature was a reflection to Victorians of God's design and as such directed naturalists into certain channels of sci-

entific investigation, especially 'adaptation in nature, with the
ways in which organisms had been exquisitely fitted by the skilful
contriver [God] for the places they occupied.'[55] By appealing to
nature, Buchan, and others after him, were suggesting the adaptation of women to domestic pursuits; it was part of the relentless
pressure that Darwin would later point to as natural selection.
Alexander Skene, an American gynaecologist, picked up on this
theme when he noted that woman's 'wide pelvis, large bust,
smooth, round, delicate limbs ... show a refinement of structure
adapted to her environment.'[56] While the appeal to nature was a
powerful one to which physicians resorted to explain woman's
place in society, it was not necessarily flattering to women.
Women, because of their bodies, were considered closer to nature
than men and less able to escape its thrall. Victorians extolled
the virtues of nature and the virtues of women but they also tried
to master nature through culture, both ideologically and tech-
nologically.[57]

The stress on what was natural for women stemmed from the
belief of some physicians that women's sexual organs, rather than
being a part of the whole, were virtually the whole. M.L. Holbrook
in his 1890 'Parturition without Pain' was very clear about that:
'Woman exists for the sake of the womb.' It influenced her whole
being and interconnected with other organs.[58] Compared with
men, the changes that took place in a woman's body were more
evident and made such a belief understandable.[59] Nevertheless,
the repercussions of such beliefs were significant. Holbrook made
his claim in an effort to convince women they should not practise
birth control. More disturbing, if woman was equated to her body
and, particularly, to her reproductive organs, who or what controlled them? As Elizabeth Spelman has astutely recognized:
'Woman's being or nature or sphere has been defined century
after century by men in terms of body, or "immanence," not
mind, or "transcendence." But if body is "woman's sphere," then
because women are in it, they do not have the capacity or the
right to control it – if, as so much of western philosophy has tried
to tell us, it takes mind to control body. The image of woman as
body in one fell swoop relegates woman to a certain sphere: and

undermines any claim that she should control that sphere: she would not be in that sphere if she could control it!'[60] Those knowledgeable about women's bodies (doctors) would have power over them.

In their discussions on the nature of women, physicians went further than simply suggesting that woman's body, especially her reproductive system, dominated or controlled her; it determined her function or purpose in life. In his popular *People's Common Sense Medical Adviser* published in 1882, R. Pierce insisted that the ovaries were so important to a woman that without them she became masculine and pursued masculine pursuits. The body, or at least certain parts of it, determined gender roles. Pierce insisted that simply looking at a woman and a man told the observer much about their general nature. 'Solidity and strength are represented by the organization of the male, grace and beauty by that of the female. His broad shoulders represent physical power and the right of dominion, while her bosom is the symbol of love and nutrition.'[61] The body not only reflected social roles, it somehow understood what those roles were and developed accordingly. For example, an advertisement for Dr Williams' Pink Pills claimed that they had a positive effect on the sexual organs of both sexes through the blood. This resulted in glowing cheeks, bright eyes, a 'singing laugh,' and 'the strong right arm of manhood.'[62] Somehow the bodies of women who took the pills knew enough not to develop the 'strong right arm of manhood.' What was natural for the body to do was not only the physiological response to the pills but also what was socially conventional or appropriate for it to do.[63] The bodies of women also limited how long they could actually perform their social role. At the same time that woman's body, especially her reproductive system, dominated and directed her to a specific social role, it was only able to do this for a limited time. According to Dr George Napheys's medical manual *The Physical Life of Woman*, a man was a man all his life but a woman was only a woman for a score of years.[64] By this he meant that she could only bear children for approximately half her life and a woman was a woman only when she was able to bear children. After that old age set in, a phase of life few physicians or Canadians viewed as desirable.[65]

In recent years, there has been a questioning of maternity as a normative experience for all women. Indeed, Jesse Bernard has gone so far as to challenge the existence of maternal instinct by pointing out that a society that truly believed in such an instinct would not feel the need to bring much social pressure to bear on women in order to make them mothers. Women would do it freely.[66] Such a concept was largely unheard of in the late Victorian period and certainly was not espoused by many in Canada. One woman writing in the *Canadian Magazine* made the significance of childbearing and rearing clear: 'Women who have no love for little children are women to beware of'; those who were not mothers 'have lived only a part of their women's lives.'[67] Physicians, too, saw women predominantly as childbearers or potential childbearers. In his mid-century text, *Physiological Mysteries and Revelations in Love, Courtship and Marriage*, Eugene Becklard claimed, 'I am ... convinced that there is no such thing as natural barrenness in *natural* women.' For Becklard women were baby machines whose reproductive processes dominated their lives: 'The uterus is a most important organ. Indeed, it may be said to govern the woman, for it has a place in all her thoughts, but especially in those which are occupied with love, jealousy, vanity and beauty; hence it may be said that the reproduction of the species is, in her, the most important object in life.'[68] Theodore Thomas, in his *A Practical Treatise on the Diseases of Women*, agreed: women were meant to have children and any inability to have them was a reproach to their womanhood.[69] B.G. Jefferis, in his popular manual *Searchlights on Health: Light on Dark Corners* even advised his women readers who did not want to bear children not to marry. Marriage was for the procreation of children. Pye Henry Chavasse in his advice book could not even conceive of a woman who did not want children. To any married woman, children 'are as necessary to her happiness as the food she eats and as the air she breathes,' and he warned women not to marry too early or too late or they would have difficulty in bearing children.[70] The desire to have children was also part of manhood, for some commentators believed it was not just women who naturally desired children. The love of children was innate to all true men and women and those without the desire to have children were somehow 'defective' and 'maimed.' Indeed, pregnancy was 'a needful condition to healthful and happy marriages.'[71]

Nevertheless, the emphasis was more on woman's desire for and need to have children than on man's. Perhaps this was to offset the obvious – that it was women who bore the burden of that desire in the pain of childbirth. Why else would women be willing to go through it? In his essay on childbirth, Holbrook attempted an answer by arguing that married women were healthier than unmarried. He claimed there were more single women in insane asylums than married; he argued that single women did not live as long as married, and that two-thirds to three-quarters of female suicides were single. He concluded that 'the process of child-bearing is essentially necessary to the physical health and long life, the mental happiness ... of women.'[72] As his claims make clear, he could not separate marriage from childbearing, the one naturally led to the other. He and others felt that women's bodies dictated to them the necessity of having children and, in return, they would be healthier than women who did not. For his part, George Napheys had a darker view of childbearing. He asked why the extra burden was placed on women, who obviously were the weaker sex. His answer: 'it is a wise provision that she is thus reminded of her lowly duty, lest man should make her the sole object of his worship, or lest the pride of beauty should obscure the sense of shame.'[73] Bearing children, then, kept women in their place.

Napheys believed that woman's destiny was to be married and be a mother. Women who rejected both would earn society's disdain and would live to regret their decision. While admitting that single women could be noble and unselfish, he considered that the stereotype 'of the spinster as peevish, selfish, given to queer fancies and unpleasant eccentricities' was essentially correct.[74] Others could only concur in Napheys's assumption that motherhood was woman's pre-eminent role. Dr William Goodell, a leading American gynaecologist and author of *Lessons in Gynaecology*, yearned for a time when women were like their mothers – that is, good housewives and mothers and physically capable of being so. As a physician he felt it was his mission to make women healthier so that they could give birth to healthy children.[75] He and other physicians gave advice to their women patients to ensure this would occur. Since they saw the roles of women in society as different from those of men, their advice to and treatment of women were designed to maintain that difference.

Physicians saw the body as reflecting not only explicit physiological and social differences between the two sexes but also the relationship between them. Underlying much of the medical literature was the belief that a woman's body made her inferior to man. This notion had a long history going back at least to Galen (AD 130–200). In the Galenic account, heat was a sign of perfection and men were deemed hotter than women and therefore more perfect. The difference in heat between men and women was a consequence of woman's role as childbearer. Until the nineteenth century, women were viewed as a lesser version of men, but a replica nevertheless. For example, the form of woman's reproductive system was simply a modified version of man's pushed inward. If women had been hotter than men, their reproductive organs would have descended and protruded like those of men; if women had been as hot as men, semen would have died and the nourishment needed for the fetus would have disappeared. Thus the form of woman befitted the function of woman.[76] In the nineteenth century, the Galenic sense of hierarchy did not disappear despite the shift in emphasis from woman being a lesser man to woman being different from man. Indeed, it became integrated into the separation of spheres ideology. As already seen, William Buchan in 1813 argued that nature made women less fit for active and difficult occupations than men.[77] Three decades later physicians were still arguing along these lines. Dr Becklard in his *Physiological Mysteries* stated in 1842 that 'woman has less strength but more mobility than man; less intellect, but a quicker apprehension; and her sensibility is more exquisite than that of her male companion; but she does not receive such lasting impressions.'[78] In his 1869 text *Human Physiology*, William Carpenter was equally forthright about the natural attributes of both sexes: 'For there can be no doubt that – putting aside the exceptional cases which now and then occur – the intellectual powers of Woman are inferior to those of Man. Although her perceptive faculties are more acute, her capability of sustained mental exertion is much less; and though her views are often peculiarly distinguished by clearness and decision, they are generally deficient in that comprehensiveness which is necessary for their stability.'[79] While Carpenter acknowledged that women's instinctual powers were greater than men's, it is difficult not to conclude that he believed woman was essentially inferior to man. What positive attributes she did possess paled in comparison to his.

The theme of intellectual inferiority emphasized by Carpenter is one that survived throughout the rest of the century, although increasingly couched in a semblance of scientific reasoning. In 1878 Dr Richard Maurice Bucke, superintendent of the London, Ontario, Asylum for the Insane, queried why there were no great women artists or religious leaders. He acknowledged that women more than men were capable of love and faith, but 'although the essential factor in a religious founder is faith and in a supreme artist love, yet a high grade of intellect must go along with the high moral nature if anything great in either of these lines is to be achieved. Well, we know that the average weight of a woman's brain is forty-four ounces, against forty-nine and one-half ounces for the average weight of a man's brain; but the knowledge of this fact is not necessary to assure us that woman's intellect is very much below the level of man's. Lacking, therefore, one essential factor of greatness woman can not be great ... in the same way that the greatest men are great.'[80] If women could not be as great as men, Bucke comforted them by noting they could be as morally good if not better. To Bucke's brain weight argument, other physicians added evolutionary theory by suggesting that women were lower on the evolutionary ladder than men. Henry Lyman did so in *The Practical Home Physician* (1884) when he maintained that while men and women differed physically from children, women were closer to them in nature than men were. Thus the hierarchy of development was represented by men at the top, followed by women, and then by children.[81] Alexander Skene, a leading American expert in diseases of women, also used the evolutionary rationale; he argued that the humerus (the bone in the upper arm) in women was not as well defined as in men and then observed, as an aside, that the humerus was better defined in the 'higher races.' He noted that 'women are less intellectual than men, less original in thought, less capable of continuity and logic of thought, and hence they have been called more childlike in their mental characteristics, and in this respect resemble rather the primitive races.' He further distanced women from middle-class men by aligning them with the uneducated and poorer classes, alleging that sensitivity to pain was less in such groups and that women of the better classes had learned, by reason of their femaleness, to be less sensitive to pain than men.[82] Just as scientists saw a 'chain of life,' a rank and order in the natural world, physicians in looking at the human world envisioned a similar hierarchy.[83] While the relationship between men and women that emerges from the medical understanding of the two sexes is evident, Jefferis in his popular medical book made the inequality of the relationship explicit: 'Woman naturally loves her lord and master.' As for men, 'there is nothing that affects the nature and pleasure of man so much as a proper and friendly recognition from a lady, and as women are more or less dependent upon man's good-will, either for gain or pleasure, it surely stands to their interest to be reasonably pleasant and courteous in his presence or society.'[84] Jefferis seemed oblivious to the hypocrisy to which this unequal relationship could lead and which he actually advocated.

Although women were not equal to men intellectually, they did possess characteristics that were of value. William Carpenter, who stressed the intellectual inferiority of woman, emphasized that she was man's superior in 'purity and elevation of her Feelings.'[85] He also extolled her attributes of tact, intuition, and adaptiveness. Almost fifty years after Carpenter, Skene wrote about woman's perceptive faculty, her intuition, and her adaptability.

In her ability to give birth and her mothering role in society she was also physically and mentally superior to man.[86] As seen, Richard Bucke thought woman's moral nature was higher than man's. But as in Skene's case, Bucke believed its finest expression came when she was a mother. He saw mother love as instinctual, 'largely due ... to the influence of natural selection,' and 'needful to the continuance of the life of the race.'[87] Nature, God's creation, determined woman's characteristics, not society. If anything, the moral idealization of woman was even more flowery in the popular medical literature. In his best seller, *The People's Common Sense Medical Adviser*, Pierce waxed eloquent: 'True it is, we see in her the embodiment of purity and holiness, heavenly graces, the most perfect combination of modesty, devotion, patience, affection, gratitude, and loveliness.'[88] In 1894 Jefferis referred to woman as the 'heart of humanity' and 'naturally better, purer, and more chaste in thought and language' than man.[89] Such idolatry made women into objects, separate, to be gazed on from a distance and somehow foreign to man. Women were not worshipped, but in a world in which religion was increasingly being challenged, belief in the virtue of woman became a stabilizing constant that provided security and hope for the future generations they would raise. Just as scientists of nature associated what they did with 'aesthetic appreciation and religious feelings,' so physicians could study women and appreciate what God had fashioned.[90]

What is clear about the idealization of women in which the medical profession engaged was that the characteristics attributed to women were those which made them dependent on others and responsive to others. Tact, adaptability, and intuition were traits necessary for individuals who did not have power but who had to live with those who did. They were not virtues that would guarantee worldly success.[91] Indeed they were ones that were difficult to maintain in a world where money was becoming more important as was identification with occupation. Such characteristics harkened back to a past where instinct counted more than rationality. They suggested a world that Victorians believed had been and should be but was no longer – that is, women suggested a possibility of a different kind of life if only the world was a more perfect place. That such a world had little chance of becoming reality simply reinforced its appeal. In addition, when doctors saw women as superior to men it was usually in relation to their childbearing and childrearing responsibilities. None of these perceptions of women was original. They were in keeping with the beliefs in the wider society. All physicians did was to add some vague medical support for them.

Idealization is not constructive when it applies to individuals or an entire sex. For one, idealized concepts are difficult to live up to. They are simplistic and restrictive. They also deny reality. While the characteristics attributed to women by physicians and lay people alike did not make the 'equal but different' ideology truly equitable, it would be wrong to assume that female attributes were imposed on women as part of a deliberate conspiracy to subjugate them. Women subscribed to the idealization of themselves as morally superior to men and used that idealization to extend their involvement in society in a multitude of reform causes and organizations. For Victorian men and women, form was a reflection of preordained function and, from their perspective, determined that function. As Skene made clear, woman's 'gentle, timid, affectionate expression tells the story of her mental character, disposition, and *functions* in life.'[92] Man's stronger body determined his role as protector and breadwinner. Woman's softer physique reflected her role as childbearer and childrearer. Nature was God's design and, consequently, so too were these respective social roles. They were not gender specific, they were sex specific. In some respects, Victorian Canadians were a self-satisfied lot, who feared challenges to and changes in their world. They believed in progress but their idea of progress was the same life, only better. Men would be better providers, women would be better mothers. It was incomprehensible for them to visualize anything more radical with any degree of equanimity. Gender role change suggested the decline of civilization as they knew it. Physicians played a minor but not insignificant role in hardening opposition to such change, for they provided a scientific rationale for the gender division between the sexes. What was, had to be.

Women and men were physically different in order that children could be born, and all else followed from this distinction. The balance between the sexes had to be maintained – if one sex was rational, the other must be intuitive.

Physicians helped to create the definition of a normal healthy adult woman that was different from a normal healthy adult man. The 1886 *Manual of Hygiene for Schools and Colleges* encouraged both sexes to exercise, but whereas boys were to run, leap, row, and play handball, girls were to walk, skip, play lawn tennis, and work with Indian clubs.[93] Because such a manual would have the authority of the medical profession behind it, Canadians could assume that the advice given in it was not only socially correct but also medically correct. The education of girls as well came in for some criticism. Some physicians felt that mental exertion was more debilitating for girls than for boys. If young girls ignored the 'medical advice' proffered to them, then their bodies would be sacrificed; if that occurred, their future happiness would be jeopardized, for as Dr Bayard from Saint John, New Brunswick, maintained, men were attracted to women because of their beauty.[94] And if a woman was so unfortunate as to need to work, she had to make sure she chose the right occupation. In his 'Inaugural Address' delivered on 11 December 1898 at the opening of the Training School for Nurses in Montreal, Dr D.C. MacCallum explained to his audience that certain pursuits were totally unsuitable for a woman because of 'her sex, the power and influence of her emotional nature, and the delicacy of her physical organization.' Other pursuits, however, still remained that would not be 'repugnant to her sense of womanly dignity and propriety.'[95] One can only assume, given the occasion of his speech, that the good doctor approved of nursing as an occupation for women. In the opinions expressed by physicians such as MacCallum, the medical world and the personal world of women intersected. Physicians were clearly defenders of woman's role in the home, providing scientific or medical rationales for it. Emphasis on that role increased in intensity over time. Religious doubt was on the increase, competitive business practices seemed to poison the atmosphere, and in general there was an unprecedented crassness to society. All this led to the relocation of moral values to the home and to women. But the emphasis on women often had an overtone of desperation about it, perhaps because the home and the genteel concept of woman were themselves being challenged by so many social forces. Much of the unease in society worked to the benefit of physicians. Canadians were looking for security and their search led increasingly in the direction of science and belief in its infallibility. By aligning itself with science, regular medicine could bask in reflected glory. As a result, Canadians could endow doctors' views of women, which conveniently corresponded to their own, with scientific objectivity.

The nineteenth century saw enormous shifts in medical knowledge and a quantitative leap in information about the human body. Technological innovations such as the microscope, widely available by the 1830s, aided in this expansion. From the patient's perspective, especially significant was the introduction of ether in 1846 which allowed physicians to intervene more dramatically in the body without causing the pain that so often had prevented treatment or had traumatized the patient. Chloroform quickly followed ether and in Canada became the predominant anaesthetic used until the 1870s, when ether again made a resurgence. Of benefit, too, was the acceptance of the germ theory of disease causation. Although the theory had been discussed for decades, it was not until the 1860s, with Joseph Lister's work following the path set out by Louis Pasteur, that the medical profession took any practical note. Supporters of 'Listerism' emphasized that germs outside the body threatened the health of the body and argued that the physician had to fight those germs through the use of antiseptic procedures.[96] What the introduction of anaesthesia and the eventual acceptance of germ theory did was to allow physicians to use the rhetoric of science to gain prestige and to convince Canadians that regular medicine was more scientific than other approaches. It did not matter that much of scientific medicine was of theoretical rather than practical significance. In the words of Dr Benjamin DeWolfe Fraser, president of the Nova Scotia Medical Society, what doctors *could* offer the patient was 'confidence, tranquillity and hope to the doubting and enfeebled mind, and comfort to the wasting body.'[97] The alignment of medicine with science bolstered that confidence throughout the century but especially in the latter part of the century when so many breakthroughs occurred. Nevertheless, even with the strides made in the late nineteenth century – the improvement in surgical techniques, the use of anaesthesia, and the acceptance of germ theory – the day-to-day practice of physicians did not alter significantly. Most continued to practise according to the tradition in which they had been trained and for many that predated many of the real advances within medicine. Nonetheless, what was important was 'the marketing of scientific medicine.'[98] Regular physicians offered a methodology, a spirit of investigation, and explanation, all of which connected it to the wider world of science.[99] However, the willingness on the part of the patient to accept the explanation only makes sense if the importance of science to late Victorian society is appreciated.

Science had long been popular among the educated classes but, by the mid-nineteenth century, its popularity had increased. Science bolstered the Victorian belief in progress. Canadians, among others, considered science objective and, as with nature, a reflection of God's wonder.[100] This was important because, in the mid-to-late nineteenth century, religion in its traditional guise had undergone some major challenges. The questioning of the literal interpretation of the story of Adam and Eve by evolutionists, coupled with the higher criticism of the Bible, left many of the faithful uneasy. Few stopped believing but many changed the way in which they interpreted their beliefs. If at one time they had looked to the Bible for guidance in understanding the world about them, increasingly they looked to science to do so and could comfort themselves that since science was objective, it truly reflected divine purpose. This led to much more emphasis being placed on the world of the here and now than on the afterlife, which had previously been the centre of religious belief. The churches themselves reflected this new focus in the emergence of the Social Gospel, a gospel that emphasized the creation of God's kingdom on earth in a tangible way. Indications of the esteem in which Canadians held science abound. Even the *Farm-*

er's Directory of 1851, a do-it-yourself guide if ever there was one, made a point of stating that when readers were really ill they should consult a man of science.[101] Half a century later Adelaide Hoodless, the founder of the domestic science movement in Canada, reflected how science had become the arbiter of what was of value. She could not think of a better support for domestic training than to argue that it was 'the application of scientific principles to the management of the home.'[102]

The alignment of medicine with science reinforced the interventionist side of medicine, although it did not create it. As seen in the heroic medicine practised in the early nineteenth century, intervention was already entrenched. Historians of medicine have suggested that with the introduction of anaesthesia and antisepsis, and the concomitant belief in the relationship between specific germs and specific diseases, the era of so-called heroic medicine declined.[103] Physicians now viewed disease not as a result of the body's being in a state of disequilibrium, which it was their responsibility to restore to balance, but as a consequence of some specific disease-causing agents which could be eliminated by using a particular medicinal cure. Increasingly, doctors moved away from seeing all parts of the body and person as interrelated and in need of treatment, in order to treat the diseased part, to treating the diseased part only. As we will see later, the former approach never really disappeared – the concept of reflex action was closely linked to it – but the way doctors responded to it did. Their approach to medicine had become localized and, with it, the general bleeding, purging, and induced vomiting that had characterized earlier medicine declined. Nonetheless, heroic medicine did not disappear; it only took a new tack. For example, it may be the case that once sepsis was conquered the use of forceps during childbirth increased.[104] Certainly, the resort to surgery increased. Not surprisingly, with this increase came additional status, for it placed medical practitioners in a position of greater control over their patients and emphasized their active role in medical treatment. Surgery also shifted the locale of medical treatment from the patient's home to the hospital, a physician-controlled environment.

In Canada, as elsewhere, hospitals first developed to care for those who had nowhere else to go, the poor and those without families. Hospitals also served the social pariahs of society. In 1861 most of the maternity cases in the Kingston General Hospital involved illegitimate births, and 45 per cent of admissions were a result of alcohol-induced disease.[105] Kathleen Morran, a nineteen-year-old prostitute, left the Victoria General Hospital in Halifax on 23 July 1881 and, according to the hospital, 'went to Rock Head Prison after leaving here having got in a drunk.'[106] Few hospital patients, respectable or otherwise, could afford to pay; indeed medical relief in hospital was equated with poor relief,[107] and hospitals such as the Provincial and City Hospital in Halifax provided not only bed care for the sick poor but outpatient dispensaries for them as well. Despite these limitations, the hospitals served an impressive number of people. At mid-century, the Kingston General Hospital admitted over 1700 individuals in four years.[108]

Conditions in the hospitals help to explain why patients were generally destitute and why respectable, paying patients were few. Until late in the century, hospitals were run as charitable institutions. The Kingston General Hospital was typical in having its origins in the work of the Female Benevolent Society among the sick poor in the 1820s. Hospitals were not open to the public, but tickets for entry could be obtained from members of the community elite, who decided on the worthiness of the individual and her/his need. This method of admission did decline over time. In 1853 approximately half of the patients who entered the Kingston Hospital were admitted by someone other than a physician. But by 1866 no one was so admitted, indicating the increasing control that physicians had over the hospital and its clientele. Once in the hospital, rules controlling patients were such as to alienate anyone who did not absolutely have to be there. The 1860 Annual Report of the Kingston Hospital revealed that thirteen patients had left for 'breach of rules.'[109] The Royal Columbian Hospital in New Westminster, BC, forbade patients to smoke or use foul language. The rules of the Toronto Home for Incurables insisted that all patients, who were able, help with domestic work and other patients; none could leave the premises without permission.[110] At the Victoria General Hospital, Halifax, patients could not 'play at any game of hazard.'[111] Nor did hospitals necessarily provide adequate care. Before the 1870s, because nursing staff was limited at the Montreal General, patients, if violent, might be strapped to the bed. Similarly, because of lack of nurses in the Kingston General Hospital, patients did not always receive sufficient attention. In one case, a woman who was seriously ill was left alone at night with no one to give her medicine or even a drink of water, the nurse on duty having fallen asleep from overwork.[112] The physicians who associated themselves with the early hospitals did so because, in the era before formal instruction in medical schools, medical students learned through apprenticeship. Those physicians who could offer students the most varied experience would attract the most apprentices and earn a substantial income through the fees they charged them. A hospital affiliation also brought physicians into contact with those socially prominent members of society who sat on the hospital boards as part of their charitable obligation. This could prove to be of benefit in a physician's private practice. Lastly, in hospital practice, physicians could better control their patients than they could in the patient's home.

Over time, physicians and those running the hospitals wanted to see the character of these institutions change to correspond to the image of scientific medicine emerging in the latter decades of the nineteenth century. One way to do this was to improve the conditions of hospitals and to attract paying customers – that is, to convince Canadians that when they were ill they should not be treated at home but in a hospital. This change did occur, but slowly. In 1896 the Royal Jubilee Hospital in Victoria, BC, had 22 per cent of its beds occupied by paying patients[113] and, by the end of the century, 20 per cent of the revenue of the Kingston General Hospital came from paying patients.[114] This was a start and the trend towards increasing numbers of paying patients continued. In addition to the clientele changing, the diseases treated in hospitals widened to encompass more than those associated with a loose or dissipated lifestyle. In 1858 the Montreal General

Hospital listed approximately 161 diseases or variations thereof for the patients admitted. By 1878 its records indicated well over 350 diseases.[115] Such a cornucopia would challenge physicians and offer them an opportunity for extensive experience.

By the end of the century, hospitals provided an environment in which doctors reigned supreme. Hospitals patients had limited influence but, even outside the hospitals, the patient-doctor relationship had altered in favour of the physician. Canadians' belief in the 'truth' of science and their acceptance of medicine as scientific meant they could feel confident that physicians' views on women represented scientific fact rather than an amalgam of cultural bias and what physiological information was known at the time. This would not have been all that significant, other than providing a rationale for the normative role of women in society, but the views of physicians carried over into their medical treatment of women. In the nineteenth century, and even today, the health care of women was based on three premises: that women cannot achieve the same standard of health as men; that they can remain healthy only if they remain within narrowly defined social roles; and that women are not capable of controlling their own health.[116] Nineteenth-century women often internalized these beliefs as well. Physiological differences between the two sexes did exist and had to be recognized. But as Elizabeth Spelman has pointed out, when physicians applied their *prescriptive* beliefs concerning women to their medical practice the repercussions could be serious:

The ... view of woman which defines her as in need of protection also can be used to justify practices which exploit her: on the one hand she is only a body, yet she is nevertheless somehow human and so ought to be protected by those humans better able to ascertain what is good for her; but on the other hand, since she is only body and so not fully human, she can be exploited by those superior humans ... the exploitation of woman, of her body in particular, has often been carried out in the name of protecting her from her own worst enemy, her body (and if she is nothing but her body, she is, of course, nothing but her own worst enemy).[117]

Because he believed the bodies of men and women differed owing
to the separate roles each had to play in life, and because he
believed that women were more fanciful than men, Alexander
Skene warned his young medical student readers that 'there are
psychological, moral, and mental peculiarities that modify, if indeed they do not cause, *or cure*, diseases in woman.' Women's
bodies posed greater challenges to the physician than male bodies.
'How infinitely more difficult to discover important symptoms,
to diagnosticate conditions, and to direct the great business of
cure in woman than in man!'[118] Theodore Thomas went so far as
to advocate marriage as a cure for undeveloped ovaries but did
not state whether part of the prescribed treatment was finding
husbands for such women.[119] The 1892–3 patient records for the
Victoria General Hospital in Halifax reveal that physicians focused
on women's generative system even when the illness of the patient, as in the case of gastritis and tuberculosis, was seemingly
not connected to it. The sexual system had become the mecca
for physicians in their search for disease causation in women.
Given the complexity of this system compared with men's, it
attracted much medical attention and gave rise to a vast literature
on women which reinforced Victorian Canadians in their belief
that the differences between the sexes were more significant than
the similarities. In medicine, this was reflected in the list of seemingly endless causes of disease unique to women.

Chapter Two

The Frailty of Woman

In 1895 Mary Carus-Wilson, professor of engineering at McGill University, estimated that only one out of every ten women was healthy. Of the other nine, three would seek medical help from a doctor, three would medicate themselves, and the last three would simply endure their suffering.[1] Feminist historians have been intrigued by the nineteenth-century view of women's predisposition to illness and the medical profession's focus on the diseases of women. Some have argued that this stemmed either from general hostility towards women or from the complexity of the female body, which made it more interesting for physicians to treat. While not denying that women were susceptible to a number of physical problems that men were not, these historians have been reluctant to reinforce the stereotype of female frailty. Consequently, they have focused on the psychological reasons for women's ill health rather than the physical. Understandably, the nineteenth-century medical profession was more aligned to the view of physical causation. Nonetheless, some practitioners did acknowledge that the social and cultural realities women faced contributed to their medical problems, a view which still enabled them to separate women out for special treatment.[2] By publicly discussing those causes, doctors were able to expand their area of concern, expertise, and the definition of what was deemed medical, all of which increased their control over their female patients and added to their prestige in the eyes of the public. What doctors were unable to appreciate, however, was, first, the contradiction between their image of women and the reality of women's lives and, second, the crucial distinction between sex and gender as it related to health.

The concentration on woman's health in the latter half of the century was relatively new, for earlier commentators had made little distinction between men's and women's diseases and their causes. The differences they noted seemed innocuous and non-judgmental about the qualities of either sex. For example, Edward Allen Talbot in his *Five Years' Residence in the Canadas* mentioned that women, more than men, suffered from bad teeth and neck goitres.[3] In the early 1830s an observer, writing under the nom de plume of Philanthropos, pointed out in 'A Medical Essay' that 'all disorders are caused by obstructed perspiration which may be produced by a great variety of means; that medicine, therefore, must be administered that is best calculated to remove obstructions and promote perspiration.'[4] Philanthropos clearly aligned himself with humoral theory, but the important point of his schema of disease causation was that it was general. Such a view was not to last. What replaced it was a more specific concept of disease aetiology and in many respects a more sex specific concept. Not that this was original to the Victorians; the ancients had believed in the womb as a source of disease and in fact had developed a theory where the 'wandering womb' visited havoc on a woman's body.[5] While this idea had never totally disappeared, what occurred in the late nineteenth century was an intensification of the notion of woman's vulnerability to illness because of the very nature of her body.

Increasingly, medical literature assumed that women were more susceptible to illness and disease than men. *Jayne's Medical Almanac* of 1863 provided a long list of ailments that Dr Jayne's Alternative medicine could cure – scrofula, ulcers, white swellings, cancerous and indolent tumours, mercurial and syphilitic affections, goitre, enlargement and ulcerations of the bones, joints, glands, or ligaments, skin diseases, nervous affections, epileptic fits, chorea, dropsy, and so on. In addition to these diseases, which could attack both sexes, there were 'many affections peculiar to Females, as Suppression, Irregularity, Leucorrhoea or Whites, Sterility, Ovarian, and Uterine Dropsy.'[6] The 1870 *Canada Health Journal* noted that the 'diseases of women are so prevalent in this age that the treatment of them has become a specialty with many physicians. There are journals devoted to that alone. Every college has a lecturer on that branch, distinct from other diseases.'[7] So severe were women's health problems that the *Sanitary Journal* of 1876 republished the annual address by Dr Washington Atlee before the Medical Society of the State of Pennsylvania in which he argued that women felt compelled to resort to the use of 'tonics, stimulants, nervines and opiates,' none of which could really restore health and some of which could hurt the children such women conceived.[8] By the 1880s the author of one popular health manual claimed that there were more unhealthy wives than healthy ones.[9] Hamilton Ayers in his 1881 *Everyman His Own Doctor* even went so far as to allege that 'young girls, eighteen or twenty years old, have falling of the womb. Very few entirely escape it, for very few women are entirely well.'[10] And in the 1890s Dr Edward Playter of Ottawa bemoaned the 'delicate, nervous and over-fat women,' who seemed so numerous.[11] The view that women suffered from ill health corresponded to the belief that women were physically weaker than men even when they were healthy. Because Victorians expected that those who were weaker would be more prone to disease, they would not have challenged the medical perception. In fact,the medical perception probably gained credibility because it reinforced what people already believed.

While ill health was a problem for the individual woman, it had significant repercussions for society. Pye Henry Chavasse, in his *Advice to a Wife*, believed that health was necessary for women, not just for their own sakes but so that they could bear healthy children.[12] The *Canadian Practitioner* of January 1886 went even further. Not only should women be healthy so they could give birth to healthy children, but only when women were healthy were they capable of the greater state of sexual arousal needed to conceive male offspring.[13] Unhealthy women, then, would be less able to fulfil their natural duty – bearing children, particularly male children. In order to rectify this situation, the centre of women's health problems would have to be pinpointed. Each medical specialty had its own theories but those who saw themselves as experts on the diseases of women and children were the most vocal. Gynaecologists argued that the reproductive/sexual system of women, that which distinguished them from men, was the origin of most health problems in women. As already noted, this was not a new idea. While in the nineteenth century physicians no longer believed in the actual ability of the womb to move, they did believe that a close relationship between the reproductive/sexual system and the rest of the body existed. They held that through reflex action – the ability of healthy parts of the body to sympathize with those that were diseased – gynaecological disease could show up as symptoms elsewhere and, if left untreated, become the origin of disease in any part of the body. By focusing on the very part of the body that made women female, doctors deemed the poor health of women natural and something they could not escape. In his medical recipes, Alvin Wood Chase made it clear that this condition was part of the divine plan: 'The female organism is such that what affects the general system of the male, much more frequently affects the organs peculiar to *her* system only. No reason can be given for it except the wisdom of the Creator, or the necessities of her construction. But this *debility* and *irregularity* are so interwoven together that what causes one must necessarily affect the other.'[14] Because God saw fit to design women this way, it was part of her reason for being – that is, it was related to her place and status in society. It was not society's placement but one dictated by her own body through the will of God.[15]

Although physicians could not eliminate the fundamental weakness of women's bodies, they could try to minimize it. This was going to be difficult, however, because physicians believed that a woman's reproductive system dominated her. Chavasse made it clear that in his opinion 'uterine complaints are almost always, more or less, mixed up with a woman's illness.'[16] Writing in 1882 Dr Arthur Edis agreed: 'It may be affirmed that no severe constitutional disorder can long continue in a woman during the predominance of the ovarian function without entailing disturbance in this function. And the converse is also true, that disorder of the sexual organs cannot long continue without entailing constitutional disorder, or injuriously affecting the condition of other organs.'[17] Physicians, blamed uterine disorders for insanity, sick headaches, morning sickness, neuralgia, chorea, amaurosis, asthenopia, and many other pathological conditions of the organs of vision.[18] Physicians linked the health and strength of the body to the ability of the individual to control it. As Rousseau claimed, 'the stronger the body, the more it obeys; the feebler, the more it commands.'[19] As applied to women this meant that they were dominated by their bodies, for every physician seemed to believe that women's bodies were weaker and less healthy than men's. But were they? What was it that persuaded doctors, among others, of this fantasy? It certainly was not the reality of women's lives.

Although Canada was developing into an urbanized and industrial nation, most people continued to live in rural farming areas. Farm wives were hardly ladies of leisure – they did many labour intensive tasks that were necessary for the development of a successful farm and for the well-being of their families. Those who were pioneering worked hardest, often having to go into the fields alongside their husbands to clear land and later to bring in the harvest. All farm women, except the most affluent, were responsible for keeping the clothes washed, hauling water for the use of the family, cooking on smoky and dirty wood stoves, preserving food, minding the children, making the family's clothes, tending the smaller livestock and the kitchen garden, and earning what money they could. As many farms prospered, women received help, but even those who could afford a farm servant were left with much work to do. Urban married women were not much better off. They may have had more access to ready-made goods, but access was only of use if one's family could afford to purchase them and many families could not. Working-class married women had to supplement the meagre wages their husbands and children earned in any way they could – taking in laundry, sewing, boarders – in an attempt to keep the family together and healthy. Their workday never seemed to end. Even middle-class families were not without their financial pressures, since independent businesses frequently failed during this period.[20] Although often assisted by a general servant, the women in these families still performed many household tasks so they could stretch the budget and preserve the semblance of middle-class respectability.[21]

While Canadians could perhaps ignore the work that married women did inside the home, since it was something they had always done, it was more difficult to ignore the work that increasing numbers of women were doing in paid employment outside the home. The most common job was that of domestic servant, with young girls working six to six-and-a-half or more days a week as live-in servants on call twenty-four hours a day, engaging in hard physical labour, and seldom enjoying any privacy or financial security. Women entering the factories were certainly not any better off, except that outside working hours their lives were their own. But their working conditions were generally abysmal – long hours, poor sanitary conditions, low wages, and often back-breaking work that could undermine their health. White-collar work was more appealing, but teachers and nurses had little job security, were often treated as servants, and they too worked long hours for little pay. How could Canadians confront this reality and perceive women as frail?

Although Victorians could appreciate the strength and endurance of women in their day-to-day lives, they could still argue that, relative to men, women did not work as hard or exhibit the same kind of endurance. Even assuming this was the case, it does not explain why physicians and others seldom connected the work women did in society with an image of woman as healthy. Rather, they persisted in viewing women as weak and men as strong, women as prone to ill health and men as fundamentally healthy. Part of this attitude stemmed from perceiving men as the norm and from thinking in binary terms – that is, in opposites. For example, if men were physically stronger than women, the perception of women was not that they were less strong but rather weak. The irony of this was that, contrary to conventional wisdom, life expectancy figures suggest that women were the stronger sex or at least the healthier. Some analysists have calculated that in 1851 the number of additional years a person could expect to live at the age of twenty was 41.4 for women and 39.6 for men. At the age of sixty-five women could anticipate 11.4 more years of life but men only 10.6.[22] Others suggest that men had the advantage in the younger years but agree that women had it in the older years, and that this advantage was increasing as the century progressed.[23] How aware Canadians or even physicians were of this is unknown. But what the figures do suggest is that the perception of women's frailty was not a response to biological reality. Or was it? After all, only in the older age groups did women significantly outlive men. It was certainly possible for Canadians and physicians to assume that the vulnerability of women when they were younger was somehow linked to their reproductive responsibilities, their ability to bear children – that is, to being female. Only if they survived this period of their lives would they outlive men to any extent. Being female, then, could be seen as a threat, a reason for doctors, among others, to assume that women as a sex, and because of their sex, were weaker than men.

Even assuming that women were more vulnerable during the childbearing years, was this a result of childbearing? Some women did die as a result of childbirth. In 1901 alone 699 women lost their lives. But childbirth was not the primary killer of women – tuberculosis was. Although women accounted for only 48 per cent of the population in 1901, they represented 56 per cent of those dying from TB, and most of these deaths occurred during the childbearing years. Two reasons may explain women's susceptibility to TB. The first was their predominantly indoor occupations and lack of access to fresh air and sun. They may also have been more undernourished than their fathers and brothers since in families whose budgets were limited, priority for food consumption had to be given to those members who earned the most money and these would have been the men.

A general look at mortality figures reveals other areas where cause of death between men and women was skewed. For example, in 1901 more men than women experienced diseases of the genito-urinary system despite the overwhelming perception of physicians that it was woman's system that was the weaker. If childbirth deaths are added to this category, however, women were over-represented, perhaps confirming physicians in their perception. But childbirth mortality in absolute numbers is no more significant than mortality from external causes – suicides, accidents, and the like. In this latter category men represented 78 per cent of the deaths. It would seem that in some categories women dominated and in others, men. With the exception of childbirth, no major cause of death was sex-based. However, many were gender-based. The social and cultural realities of women's lives, not their sex, accounts for their susceptibility to TB. Similarly, work expectations and consequent occupation patterns of men explain why they dominated the category of accidental deaths.[24] But accidental deaths did not represent a disease category as TB did and, as a result, would not have forced physicians to rethink their perceptions about female weakness and male strength. Neither did death from accident force doctors to face the nature of the male body as death from childbirth forced them to conceptualize the nature of woman's body. That childbed deaths may have been as socially constructed as accidental deaths was not an idea that doctors or other Victorians could have conceived.

Mortality figures, however, may not be important in accounting for why physicians viewed women as the weaker sex and why they tended to link this with their reproductive system. Hospital records and private physicians' records reveal that patients seldom came to physicians because they were dying but because they were ill and wanted to be treated. Whether the patient died after the treatment was not always known by the doctors concerned. Unfortunately, determining morbidity patterns is impossible. What follows is an examination of some hospital and private physician records to determine, not the actual pattern of disease in women, but why physicians could perceive a particular kind of pattern.

Hospital statistics indicate that for most of the nineteenth century men were the majority of patients seen by physicians in these institutions. For example, the Provincial and City Hospital in Halifax had on 31 December 1867 thirty-four patients, twenty-four men and only ten women, an accurate reflection of its patient clientele at mid-century.[25] Similarly, an examination of 1723 patients admitted to the Kingston General Hospital in the years 1853, 1856,

1861, and 1866 reveals that 60 per cent of the patients were male. This was an over-representation compared to the 48 per cent that men represented in the local population. In the Royal Jubilee Hospital in Victoria men also outnumbered women patients. In 1896, the annual report of the hospital directors listed 253 male patients and only 114 females.[26] Factors other than health can partially account for the numerical superiority of men within these institutions. As indicated earlier, conditions prevailing in mid-century and later hospitals were not such as to encourage individuals to go unless absolutely necessary. This may have been particularly true for women about whom society was more protective. Women may have consulted doctors in other ways. The records for the Halifax Dispensary Outdoor Department for 1884 reveal that almost all the patients were women. This was also true for the Montreal General Hospital from 1857 to 1873, when women outnumbered men in the outdoor department. After 1873, however, men outnumbered women.[27] For the Halifax Hospital there was another reason to account for the preponderance of male patients. Halifax was a port city and, in the 1860s and 1870s, approximately 50 per cent of the male patients admitted were seamen, many of whom were not resident in Halifax.[28] Transient male workers would also account for the predominance of men in the Kingston Hospital since Kingston, as a Great Lake port, would have attracted seasonal labourers. Similarly, Victoria attracted seamen and dock workers. The percentage of women in the Royal Jubilee reflected their smaller presence in the general population.[29] But none of these explanations takes away from the reality that doctors in these hospitals saw many more men than women patients.

What was happening in private practice is more difficult to discern. Doctors' records often separate obstetric cases from their other cases and, unless both sets of records are available, then a comparison of the numbers of men and women consulting doctors is impossible. One study of the rural Ontario practice of James Langstaff revealed that married women consulted him twice as often as what would be predicted by their proportion of the population.[30] Yet Margaret Andrews's analysis of the Vancouver practice of Dr Langis in 1890 and 1891 reveals that men consulted Dr Langis more than women relative to their population.[31] If the situation was not uniform, why was there such a consensus about attributing ill heath to women?

One reason may be that, although women were not in general hospitals in large numbers, lying-in hospitals for women existed which focused attention on the problems of women arising from their sex. The reasons for women seeking out medical aid also seems to confirm this assumption. Of the four years studied (1853, 1856, 1861, 1866) of the Kingston General Hospital records, the most frequently listed problems were ulcers (75 cases), pregnancy(96), delirium tremens (68), ophthalmia (61), diarrohea (40), bronchitis (41), rheumatism (49), and syphilis (45). Of these only one, pregnancy, was clearly a female 'problem' and one related to woman's reproductive/sexual system. What should be noted, however, is that at least two of the above were statistically linked to men – delirium tremens and syphilis. However, there was no necessary connection between these diseases and men as there was between pregnancy and women. When all the various diseases listed were collapsed into disease categories the same pattern of disease emerges. Women dominated diseases or problems of the sexual/reproductive system; whereas almost 40 per cent of the patient population was female, almost 70 per cent of patients with this kind of problem were women. For problems linked to outside causes, such as accidents or mishaps, men dominated at almost 82 per cent of the cases even though they were only 60 per cent of the patient population. This was true in private practice as well. In the late nineteenth century Toronto practice of Alexander Primrose, women were over-represented in the genito-urinary category at 67 per cent.[32] Men were approximately 75 per cent of patients whose problems could be linked to accidents, although they were only 57 per cent of his overall patient clientele. This is not surprising considering the nature of male employment during this period and the chances of being injured on the job whether that be in the field, on the wharf, or in the factory. But important from the point of view of physicians' perceptions is that these kinds of injuries were not diseases, nor were they linked to the biological fact of being male but to the social fact – that is, they were gender-based not sex-based. Just as in the case of mortality, the ease with which doctors ignored gender in favour of sex distinctions in morbidity patterns indicates more about their perceptions of gender roles than any immutable differences between the two sexes. Illness is very much socially constructed, but physicians, who were predominantly male, recognized this more with respect to men than to women. Only women seemed to have sex-based health problems to any significant extent.

What is being suggested here is not that women were physiologically weaker than men but the reasons why physicians may have thought so. The notion was not unique to them but part of the conventional wisdom of the time. Within their practice, doctors did not face a reality that would have made them change their minds, although it is true that the reality could have been interpreted differently. Women in almost all walks of life worked hard, revealing great strength and stamina. They outlived men. They may not have consulted physicians as often as men. But to conclude from this that women were as healthy as and perhaps even healthier than men would have contradicted accepted notions of gender difference. Few people would have made such an interpretation at the time. Why should doctors do so, when what they saw could also be interpreted to confirm what they believed? No matter what the reality of women's health was, the view persisted that women more than men were susceptible to disease and that the susceptibility centred on their reproductive system. Since it was dictated by nature, the cause was impossible to eradicate. Even minimizing it would be difficult, for physicians linked ill health not only to the body but also to the wider world in which women lived and the way they chose to live – to the social fabric of society itself.

The causes of disease in women seemed endless. Almost every aspect of their lives could potentially lead to ill health if they did not follow their doctor's advice. The latitude this gave the medical profession in pontificating was enormous. The list of causes, however, also provided insight into the world that many women inhabited. For example, society encouraged women to be fastidious and that was one of the benefits of modernity – the refinement of women. But this posed some real problems for women in their day-to-day lives. For those without modern water closets, normal evacuatory functions were a trial. The *Canada Lancet* of 1870 reprinted an article from the *Gynaecological Journal* on this very topic: 'As a natural consequence, delicate women soon school themselves to a postponement of the demands of nature, sometimes for days together, rather than expose themselves to the danger of taking cold and to the certainty of great annoyance. Sometimes modesty, and sometimes the dread discomfort and exposure, is the motive. In all cases the result is the same. The natural functions become disordered, the digestion is impaired, and dyspepsia, with its thousand-and-one horrors, breaks down the constitution and lays the foundation for all manner of "female complaints."'[33] While not all may have agreed upon the origins, many physicians did see constipation as a cause of women's ill health.[34] By the 1890s little had improved. Lesson 35 in William Goodell's gynaecology text was entitled 'The Relation which Faulty Closet-Accommodations Bear to the Diseases of Women.' In it he explained the importance of balance for health, that health 'denotes a state of equilibrium between wear and repair – between construction and destruction.' Any derangement of 'the nicely-balanced relation between the functions of the various organs of the body' such as that caused 'by the imperfect and unpunctual performance of the excretory functions ... begets a host of disorders,' especially in women in whom 'they are more manifest.'[35] Physicians were sympathetic. It was not women's fault that facilities were not in keeping with the refinement that women had reached. Doctors also blamed women's health problems on, among other factors, neglect of the skin, overwork, nursing the ill, and poor and insufficient food.[36] They associated neglect of the skin with infrequent bathing among the needy and immigrant groups and, while physicians acknowledged the consequences of such neglect, seldom did they admit the reasons for it – lack of access to bathing facilities. Instead, *inability* to bathe became a *refusal* to bathe among certain groups. Doctors were more sympathetic to women whose bodily weakness was due to fatigue from caring for their children or nursing the ill, perhaps because both were a result of women's meeting their expected social responsibilities within the family. Women's poor eating habits were also a consequence of their family responsibilities. Physicians, however, tended to blame the woman for not eating properly and only rarely focused on the poverty that led her to deprive herself in order that her husband, the family's major breadwinner, was fed.

While doctors could blame women for neglecting themselves and causing some of their own health problems, an examination of other perceived causes of disease suggests that the possibility of women's avoiding ill health was unlikely. Their very purpose in life assured this outcome. For example, in the pantheon of Victorian ideals, marriage was the sought-for goal of most women. It was a vehicle of upward mobility for many as well as a sign of full adulthood for all.[37] So natural was marriage and so 'right' for women that, as already mentioned, Theodore Thomas saw it as a cure for underdeveloped ovaries. George Napheys in his *Physical Life of Woman* recommended marriage as a cure for women suffering from chorea, hysteria, painful menstruation, mania, and hallucinations.[38] Unfortunately for women, marriage could also cause or exacerbate disease. The latter was particularly true for women who married while suffering from an already existing disease of the genitalia, and doctors encouraged such women not to marry.[39] More serious than intensifying an already existing condition, marriage could introduce disease to women. This was certainly the belief with respect to venereal disease. An article in the *Canadian Medical Times* in 1873 claimed that much female trouble was caused by latent gonorrhoea contracted from husbands.[40] Physicians were sensitive to the havoc that venereal disease caused to a woman's health. As Henry Jacques Garrigues in his text acknowledged, 'while a gonorrhea in a man in most cases is a trifling disorder ... in women it is one of the most serious diseases.'[41] The *Dominion Medical Monthly and Ontario Medical Journal* reprinted a lengthy article written by an American physician in 1897 in which he estimated that 15 per cent of female disease was caused by venereal disease and that in most cases innocent wives had been infected by their husbands. The author noted, however, that women were becoming more aware of the problem and insisting that the men they married be free from such infection. Modern novels, morality plays, and higher education had all played their part in alerting women. While this could only be applauded, the author was critical of the fact that the medical profession had not done more. Practitioners had been hesitant in educating the public about marriage and venereal disease and, as a consequence, had relinquished their responsibility and their position of leadership in this regard.[42]

Despite the supposed growing awareness among women of the dangers of venereal disease contracted from husbands, few women were probably willing to choose spinsterhood in an effort to protect themselves. Women were simply going to have to live with the physical problems marriage brought them. And the perception of many women must have been that it did bring problems. Time and time again the patient records of women date the beginning of their health problems to their marriage and especially the birth of their first child. When thirty-seven-year-old Emily Burgess entered the Montreal General Hospital on 25 May 1892, she linked her pelvic dorsal and lumbar pains and weakness at her menstrual periods to her marriage.[43] In the case of Madame Brunet, she had never experienced any problems until the birth of her first child in 1880. Since then she suffered pains in the iliac region and finally entered the Montreal General for treatment on 8 April 1882.[44]

Even if women deliberately chose to be celibate and avoid the health complications associated with marriage, there was no guarantee they would remain well. Celibacy entailed its own health threats. The *Practical Home Physician* made it clear that fibroid tumours occurred more frequently among women who had not borne children.[45] In his manual, Napheys linked this and other problems among celibate women to their rejection of the natural childbearing role that women were to play in society: 'Nature gave to each sex certain functions, and that the whole system is in better health when all parts and powers fulfil their destiny.'[46] If a woman rejected her maternal role then she had to expect that her health would suffer. The medical textbooks also picked up on this theme. Garrigues argued that celibacy was a predisposing cause of disease in women and, in explaining how this worked, he, too, appealed to the 'natural' role of women: 'Especially is the liability to the formation of fibromas of the uterus greater in unmarried and nulliparous women than in those who have borne children, as if the uterus, deprived of the function of building up a new being, were more liable to use the material for the formation of a tumour.'[47] The uterus had a function – to bear children; if a woman denied that function, then the uterus had no choice but to create in the best way it could. For Garrigues, a woman's purpose drove her body. At the turn of the century Dr Charles Penrose seemed to agree: 'Celibacy is an unnatural state and a common cause of disease.'[48] Considering that approximately 9 to 11 per cent of Canadian women never married, this was going to provide physicians with a good supply of patients to advise and treat.[49] Women were in a seemingly no-win situation – their health was at risk whether married or not.

More positive was physicians' advice about the benefits of exercise for women. In the latter part of the nineteenth century, women were becoming much more involved in leisure-time activities. Young women had long enjoyed walking, riding, skating, and dancing. By the end of the century, bicycling was added to the list. In addition, organized sports became more visible as teams of women curled and played tennis.[50] Not all Canadians approved of the time spent on such activities as revealed in the following verse published in the 1895 National Council of Women Yearbook:

[She] could swing a six-pound dumb-bell,
        She could fence and she could box,
She could row upon the river,
        She could clamber on the rocks.
She could do some heavy bowling,
        And play tennis all day long,
But she couldn't help her mother,
        As she wasn't very strong.[51]

While there may have been ambivalence about the degree to which some young women focused on sports to the detriment of other responsibilities, most Canadians recognized the benefits of limited exercise. This was true of doctors as well. But whereas lay people were very general in their reasoning, physicians linked their opinion to what they perceived to be the medical consequences of exercise. Whether approving or disapproving, they believed they had a medical responsibility to express an opinion.

On the whole, physicians believed in the benefits of exercise. Ira Warren, in *The Household Physician*, expressed his support for gymnastic exercises and calisthenics in order to provide women with the energy their mothers and grandmothers had. There was a sense that modern life had not benefited the health of women, so now they had to work at maintaining it. He saw the robustness of women 'dwindling away' and women 'becoming almost worthless for all the purposes for which they were made.'[52] Nature needed help. The lack of physical exercise was not totally women's fault. In the 1860s and 1870s physicians recognized that women were not encouraged to exercise, that it was considered unladylike, that their dress did not permit them to stay outdoors for very long, that the educational system emphasized the mental development of the young rather than their physical development, and that the fashions of the day idealized the delicate looking woman.[53] Some observers believed this led to some women becoming lazy. This was not a medical problem, but it did lead to the neglect of home and children. Having and raising children became a burden for such women; they complained about it and their daughters, hearing them, drew the lesson that they should rather not have children. If that was not enough to prod these women out of their lethargy, the *Sanitary Journal* made it clear that lack of exercise could lead to serious spinal problems.[54]

By the 1880s and 1890s physicians believed that some of the hostility in society towards women exercising had decreased.[55] The *Canada Lancet* in 1880 could advocate exercise for women and state that while in previous decades women had to look ill to be considered ladylike, this was no longer the case.[56] What seemed to be added to the advice in these decades was the coupling of exercise and fresh air. Women, more than men, were confined to the house and thus did not get the fresh air that they needed.[57] Without that and exercise their health would suffer[58] or, more specifically, the well-being of their reproductive system would suffer. As Alexander Skene pointed out in his 1895 gynaecology text, 'to secure normal development of the reproductive organs is to secure a uniform, harmonious development of the whole organization.'[59] Trying to appeal to women's self-interest and pride, Ottawa's Dr Playter connected exercise and good health in women to enhanced beauty.[60]

Advocating exercise for women seems common sense from our perspective and certainly the advice would appear to be harmless enough. And it was – medically. But the advice reinforced the social division between the two sexes and limited what choices women had, for doctors did not simply advocate exercise but specific forms of exercise. Of special concern was proper physical activity during the delicate time of puberty.[61] Chavasse, for example, recommended different types of exercise for girls and for boys. Those advocated for boys were the 'manly games – such as rowing, skating, cricket, quoits, football, rackets, single-stick, bandy, bowls, skittles, and all gymnastic exercises.' For girls, 'archery, skipping, horse exercise, croquet, the hand-swing, the fly-pole, skating, and dancing, are among the best.'[62] As already noted, such a division was also taken up in the 1886 *Manual of Hygiene for Schools and Colleges*.

At the end of the century when the bicycling craze was at its peak, its medical advantages and disadvantages were debated. The *Dominion Medical Monthly and Ontario Medical Journal*, the medical journal most hostile to women cycling, led the attack. An 1896 editorial argued that bicycle riding was unhealthy for women and that position was reiterated the next year: 'The best saddle does not meet the comforts or requirements of the female pelvis, that aside from the pedal motion that ever tends to provoke erethism, the jolt of the machine is not without evil effect upon the uterus and other generative organs, and is especially apt ... to induce laxity, version, prolapse, with all the concomitants of endometritis, menorrhagia, etc.'[63] Such an extreme view appears to have been a minority position. In August 1896 the lead editorial of the *Canada Medical Record* supported cycling, arguing that it would cure disease such as anaemia, constipation, amenorrhoea, and dysmenorrhoea and that it would bring about dress reform.[64] In November it was no longer as supportive.[65] The *Canadian Practitioner*, however, was convinced of cycling's benefits. In a four-page article Dr P.E. Doolittle, ex-president of the Canadian Wheelman's Association and president of the Toronto Inter-Club Association, praised the advantages of cycling for women. It maintained health and brought about health; it was of value to weak women, healthy women, and pregnant women.[66] Perhaps realizing it was going against the trend and that women were going to cycle no matter what, the editors of the *Dominion Medical Monthly and Ontario Medical Journal* published an excerpt in 1898 from *The American Year Book of Medicine and Surgery* which gave support to bicycle riding for women, although the author did see certain limits to its use: 'The bicycle is the most valuable addition to the therapeutics of women of the age. Properly utilized ... it is worth all the drugs in the pharmacopoeia together, especially in ... neurotic, anaemic women with functional heart-diseases.'[67] The telling phrase in the quote is 'properly utilized.' Who determined that? For the author the answer was obvious – the woman's physician. As advocated by him, 'no woman should ride a bicycle without first consulting her medical man.' Bicycling was a challenge to the preconceived image of woman in society. It made her much more independent, for it provided her with a means of escaping her home, her parents, and her community. It gave her the opportunity to be in control of what she did and where she went. This was heady stuff in the late nineteenth century and many women revelled in it. Cycling represented a change in woman's role that many in society did not like or feel comfortable with. What is important about the medical discussion was not whether doctors approved or disapproved, but the fact they felt the need to speak out on a topic that on the surface appears to have little to do with medicine. Both supporters and opponents agreed, however, that it did and, consequently, they spoke out and in doing so attempted to extend their influence in society and over their women patients even further.

One of the reasons many physicians supported cycling for women was that they believed it would bring about dress reform. Those who advocated other outdoor activity for women also recognized it was more difficult for women than for men to spend time outdoors in all seasons because of their dress. One of the earliest medical expressions of dismay concerning women's apparel occurred in the 1849 *Unfettered Canadian*, a Thomsonian journal:

> While thousands fall by dashing swords,
> Ten thousands fall by corset boards!
> Yet giddy females, thoughtless train,
> For sake of fashion yield to pain,
> And health and comfort sacrifice,
> To please a foolish coxcomb's eyes.[68]

Not until the 1860s and 1870s, however, did a major emphasis on dress begin. Out of the discussions emerged three themes: the problems that fashions caused to women's health; the idealization of a more natural image of woman's silhouette; and the medical profession's desire to have a say in what women should wear.

The physical ailments caused by fashion seemed to be endless. Theodore Thomas in his 1868 publication, *A Practical Treatise on the Diseases of Women*, discussed the impact of woman's dress on the uterus, on woman's breathing, and on her blood circulation. Of particular concern to him was the habit of tight waists that resulted in impressions of the ribs being left on the liver and the uterus being displaced, resulting in disease following intercourse.[69] His concern was echoed in the public health journals of the period. The *Canada Health Journal* of 1870 explained that the tight lacing used by women prevented them from breathing properly, upset their digestive organs, caused headaches, and led to bad temper and to general complaints of ill health which made them burdens to their friends and families. Their husbands in particular suffered for it.[70] The *Public Health*

Magazine also focused on the use of stays on women's health and argued that women's fashions led to weak backs and chests.[71] The *Sanitary Journal*, too, complained about the women who constricted their bodies below the waist, not allowing their lungs to expand.[72] But the concern of these authors was not just that fashions led to ill health – the dress of women was unnatural. Tight lacing was mechanical; it interfered with what God had designed a woman's body to be.[73] Many felt that women in the past had dressed more sensibly,[74] and they expressed nostalgia for the time when they assumed people had lived closer to nature.

Criticizing women's fashions was negative. Those involved in health wanted to advocate something positive and suggested that women stop using stays and allow their bodies to become self-supporting and erect.[75] In an 1879 editorial the *Canada Medical Record* endorsed the use of suspenders by women so as to take the weight of clothes off the waist and place it on the shoulders. In this way, the damage being done to women's internal organs would cease.[76] The *Sanitary Journal* went even further in involving the medical establishment with dress reform. In one of its reprinted articles the author suggested that, before dressing, ladies should submit their dress to a panel of medical women. Fortunately, those who chose to ignore such advice were not doomed. The journal comforted its readers by pointing out that 'it is fortunate for women, amidst the follies of dress and the foibles of fashionable society, that pathology and treatment have made so much progress in uterine troubles.'[77] Physicians would rescue women from themselves. In this way the balance dearly loved by Victorians was maintained. In earlier decades when women dressed more sensibly they had few physical ailments, which was just as well since the medical profession was not in any position to help them. By the 1870s, when women's dress was causing them health problems, the medical profession believed it had developed to a stage when its therapeutics were useful.

The themes of blaming fashion for women's ailments, idealizing the 'natural' woman, and giving physicians the right to advise women carried over into the 1880s and 1890s. In these decades the medical literature was much more specific about the problems fashion caused, perhaps reflecting the rise in gynaecology and increased information concerning the diseases of women. As in the earlier decades, what worried physicians most was tight lacing and the use of corsets. According to the literature, both led to miscarriages, displacement of the womb, local inflammation of the liver, gall-stones and biliary colic, wandering liver, protuberant abdomen and enteroptosis, prolapse and flexions of the womb, lateral curvatures of the spine, anaemia, chlorosis, dyspepsia, diminished lung capacity and oxygen starvation, intercostal neuralgia, weak eyes, and Bright's disease.[78] Garrigues in his text described the dress that led to such difficulties:

The mode of *dressing*, although changing under the varying caprices of fashion, is always fundamentally wrong and conducive to disease. The 'décolleté' evening dress and the bell-shaped nether garments drive the blood from the periphery to the pelvis. The lower part of the abdomen is generally insufficiently protected from cold air and blasts of wind, which become particularly dangerous to women who skate. High heels, when worn at an early age, while all articulations are yet subject to change, not only alter the shape of the foot, but are apt to cause neuralgia in the legs and a change in the inclination of the pelvis and the normal curvature of the back.

Of much greater importance yet is the use of corsets. Even a loose corset exercises a pressure of 30 pounds, which has still greater effect on the abdominal cavity than on the thoracic. The abdominal wall is thinned and weakened. In the erect posture the liver and intestines are pushed forward, driving the weakened abdominal wall in front of them, and in sitting the normal pressure backward from the abdominal wall against the spinal column is changed into one going directly down into the pelvic cavity. By tight lacing the pelvic floor is bulged down to the extent of one-third of an inch.[79]

Not as concerned about the corset, Dr Paul Mundé felt the real problem was that women did not keep warm enough and 'the immediate result of exposure ... is most commonly inflammation of the mucous membrane of the uterus.'[80] To make matters worse from the medical perspective, the desire to be fashionable permeated all classes. In his *Lessons in Gynaecology*, William Good-ell wrote a diatribe against women's fashions and the willingness of women in general to ape their betters, by which he meant to follow the style set by the upper classes. This could only lead to lower-class women wearing themselves out in an attempt to do so. Especially harmful were the long hours spent sewing garments they could not afford to buy.[81] But whatever the focus, the consensus was that women's dress presented them with medical problems.[82]

The fact that modern dress went against nature was again put forward but in a much more detailed fashion. Arnold Haultain, a writer from Peterborough, Ont., explained in the *Canada Lancet* in 1883 that one of the problems with women's fashions was that the clothing was massed around the organs of generation. As Haultain pointed out, this was opposite to what occurred in nature, for any examination of animals would reveal that around the organs of generation the hair tended to be sparse. The result of so much clothing centred on one place more than another led to an unequal distribution of temperature. This in turn created problems of blood circulation.[83] The use of the animal analogy is quite interesting. It perhaps reflects the work done by Darwin and others and how quickly it had permeated mainstream thought. It underscores, once again, how important the example of nature was for Victorians as a guide to their own behaviour. What is also intriguing is that, while Victorians may have been willing to see in the animal world a model for their own physical being, they were unwilling, as we will later note, to do so in the moral realm. Nature was not always an unquestioned guide.

While physicians in the later decades of the century were more specific in their concerns about the ill effects of fashions, they, as their predecessors had, felt that the situation had been better in the past. Perhaps no one was more vehement about this than Chase: 'In the good old *grandmother-days*, of girls helping with the work of the household; warm but loose clothing, plain food, good thick-soled shoes, and absence of novels to excite sexual thoughts ... such a thing as a feeble, debilitated woman or girl was hardly known, but now sedentary habits, stimulating food, every conceivable unphysiological style of dress, paper-soled shoes, checking perspiration, excitable reading, repeated colds by exposure going to and from parties thinly clad, standing out talking with supposed friends (real enemies) when they ought to be by the fire or in bed, masturbation, excessive co-habitation, miscarriages ... all tend to general debility; and the real wonder is that there are so few cases.'[84] Such an overt outpouring of resentment against the modern woman was rare, but the constant yearning for a past that no longer existed and probably never had was not. Of course, doctors were not alone in their uneasiness about modern society or even about fashions. In Canada, the Ontario Woman's Christian Temperance Union was on record as seeing women's fashions as unhealthy.[85] In the United States in the 1840s and 1850s, feminists had attempted to reject fashion's dictates and to wear the bloomer costume popularized by Amelia Bloomer. And at the turn of the century, German dress reform advocates were partially motivated by hatred of 'decadent and artificial accretions of the urban and industrial society.' They favoured a return to nature, a return to health, and a return to what they saw as a strictly Aryan past.[86]

Because doctors could explain the repercussions of following fashion's dictates they had a duty 'to show, on scientific principles, where lie the violations of the rules of health and to combat any arguments that may be raised in their defence.'[87] They did not underestimate the enormity of their task. They knew that convincing women to alter their way of dressing was not going to be easy. Women were accustomed to their tight lacing and, because they had started it at such a young age, many did not really believe they were tight. The author of one article reprinted in the *Canada Medical Record* also claimed that corsets were held in high regard because of the warmth they provided.[88] So accustomed were women to tight stays that Alexander Skene felt that, for some, they were now necessary – their bodies had become dependent on them for support.[89] Doctors did not simply concentrate on trying to convince women that their dress was foolish. They realized that women were encouraged to dress the way they did because men expected it of them. As Thorstein

Veblen has described it, fashion was a symbol of conspicuous consumption and very much linked to class.[90] Consequently, doctors tailored some of their arguments to male readers. They pointed out to men that while a small waist might be all very attractive in the woman a man courted, they had to realize that a small waist in a wife usually meant a sickly and hence a costly one.[91] Chavasse in his medical manual went one step further and proclaimed that 'a fashionable wife and happy mother are incompatibilities.'[92] Despite these efforts, physicians' endeavours went unrewarded. Most women were unwilling to change their fashions and, when some did, they were greeted with dismay. One school trustee in Toronto responded to women teachers wearing the bloomer costume by insisting that the inspector should find out which women were doing so and instruct them to stop, since he considered the costume immoral.[93]

While some women's fashions probably did lead to health problems for women, the arguments used to criticize them revealed concerns other than medical.[94] They revealed an unease with modern society and the role of women in it. Doctors perceived that the traditional role was changing, and many wanted to return to a time when they believed women had concentrated their activities on having and raising children. There is no denying the hostility exhibited towards the fashionable woman who emphasized her sexuality through the pushing up of her breasts above a small waist and the spread of her hips below; she was seen as rebelling against woman's ordained place in society. Focusing on dress as a cause of ill health was also a way doctors and other Victorians had of ignoring more serious issues. Many women did experience ill health, but more often from malnutrition than from fashion. As we have seen, some physicians acknowledged malnourishment as a problem, but it was not a cause of disease on which many focused. And when they did, the tendency was to see the malnourishment as a consequence of poor eating habits rather than lack of food.[95] The latter was simply too difficult to accept for a people who believed they lived in a civilized and prosperous society. More comfortable was the concentration upon the dangers of corseting and other aspects of modern life.[96]

Many doctors were not enamoured with the world of the late nineteenth century. They saw women as unhealthy and, unsure of what to blame, they fell back on a vague form of environmentalism. Civilization itself was at fault. This perception of civilization as causing disease was not unique to the medical profession. Although Victorians had a strong belief in progress, it was balanced by a sense of unease with some aspects of modern society. According to novelist Grant Allen, writing in the *Canada Lancet* of 1894, civilization had led to a decline in marriage and the birth rate: 'Wild animals in confinement seldom propagate their kind ... Civilization and its works have come too quickly upon us. The strain and stress of correlating and co-ordinating the world we live in are getting too much for us.'[97] The repercussions on women were especially severe. Dr Emily Howard Stowe argued that 'as man has been remote from Truth or remained in the realm of negative darkness – has his activities introduced confusion and chaos, into the social and economic world,' but more than this he has 'rendered its atmosphere unwholesome – filled it with vapors of disease and decay.' That this was the situation in late nineteenth-century society she could only lament.[98] For Theodore Thomas, civilized life made women inferior to men. It also made them inferior to their mothers and their grandmothers. Women who had lived and still lived working the land were strong; they conceived and had their babies easily. Women in the urban society that was beginning to dominate modern life had lost that ability. For them childbirth had become a trial, one their bodies could not cope with easily.[99] Others could only concur. Modern life accentuated the development of woman's spiritual life to the detriment of her physical. The result may have been a greater mental refinement, but in return woman had given up her physical health. She had become more susceptible to bodily disorders and disease and often could cope only through the use of sedatives.[100] This weakness was not natural. Some physicians, although not most, believed that if women were not interfered with, they could compete in endurance and strength with men. It was the customs and habits of civilized life that undermined women and made them more susceptible to ill health. Their bodies already made them more prone than men were to problems, and modern life accentuated this vulnerability by removing the conditions in which women could live a more natural way of life. This evolutionary development was going to be difficult to overcome, but the attempt had to be made. Some doctors argued they should not encourage women to accept their illnesses.[101] Rather, women had to fight against them, although how they were to do this was never described. How does one fight against the inevitability of evolution? To become peasant women once again was hardly a solution.

In their discussion of civilization, doctors contrasted the natural life of the past to the unnatural life of the present. They compared modern women with peasant women who, many felt, were equal in strength to men and had fewer health problems.[102] Of course they were comparing two different classes of women. They seldom talked about the farm women who still laboured in the home and field, or the women who worked long hours in factories or as domestic servants. William Goodell had some sympathy with those women forced to work on a treadle sewing machine all day, since he believed such activity could only result in uterine derangement.[103] Dr D.C. MacCallum, who between 1867 and 1875 had been in charge of the University Lying-in Hospital in Montreal, also worried about female workers. In reviewing his years there, he noted the rarity of pelvic deformity among the women he saw but wondered whether that would continue: 'Of late years ... cotton, tobacco and india-rubber factories have ben established in this city, giving employment to numerous young girls, and it remains to be seen if in the future we may not meet with obstructed labour from distorted pelvis more frequently than we do at present.'[104] However, MacCallum's concern was rare and perhaps reflected his years of association with a charity hospital. Most doctors in their writings concentrated not on working-class women but on those more fortunate. Their dismay about modern women came from the middle- and upper-class women who were their clientele and whom they considered selfish and no longer willing to work as their mothers had.[105] This emerges very strongly in the popular health manuals. Chase blamed the ill health of women on their spending too many late nights partying.[106] Chavasse and R. Pierce believed that luxurious living, idleness, and stimulants resulted in suppression of the menses or amenorrhoea and other forms of uterine disease. Indeed, Chavasse associated barrenness with the 'pampered, the luxurious, the indolent, the fashionable wife.' Pierce described what he referred to as 'a type of this class': 'The patient is an only daughter, the idol of her parents, who, in mistaken kindness, have stimulated her with every facility for mental improvement and graceful accomplishments. Her physical powers are exhausted by mental effort; she becomes pale and feeble, discouraged and heart-weary, and finds solace in the old arm-chair which now rocks in rhythm with her own sluggish feelings. Rich food does not excite the appetite, but her disordered stomach loathes it. She has lost relish for intellectual efforts and enjoys the sensation of a yellow-covered pamphlet of fiction. The effort to entertain company only exhausts, and she thinks she is rather *too delicate* to ride out. She does not like to incur the *risk* of exposure to the open air.'[107] Medical texts and journals echoed the same refrain. A life of luxury and late hours led to dysmenorrhoea and other forms of ill health in women.[108] So did reading novels, overdoing the honeymoon trip, over-indulgence, emotional excitement, and an improper mode of life.[109] Skene, in his text, made it clear that the real problem was lack of self-control leading to frustration and ultimately to disease. Parents, he wrote, should stop indulging their children, for this could only result in selfishness and a constant focus on themselves. Imaginary ailments would be the outcome.[110] Women especially were at risk; since their bodies already dominated them, anything that focused attention on them would likely result in perceived illness.

Doctors' focus on civilization and modern life as underlying causes of disease in women is not surprising but, rather, a consequence of a society that was increasingly becoming urbanized and industrialized. In such a society, everything seemed to impinge on everything else. Family, home, work, education, politics, and health were no longer separate and self-contained, if indeed they ever had been. But what the modern society of the late nineteenth century did was to make it impossible to *believe* that they were.[111] Doctors were responding to a reality they and other Canadians could no longer avoid. And in certain respects this benefited physicians. The focus on civilization as a cause of disease in women guaranteed a permanent roster of patients. Women could not avoid civilization and, in order to cope with the physical repercussions on their bodies, they would have to look to the medical profession. Civilization as a cause of disease also provided doctors with a reason if they failed to cure – who could expect one man to offset generations of development? Physicians also extended their area of influence. What topic could not be subsumed under the general rubric of civilization? If civilization caused disease in women, then physicians had the right to speak out on all aspects of it.

The causes of ill health in women seemed endless – the way they ate, the way they dressed, their lack of exercise, marriage, celibacy, civilization itself. All conspired against them. Many were causes that could not be eliminated, for they were part of the social fabric of society. The way in which modern women lived placed their bodies at risk. Even worse, from the perspective of evolution, their bodies were letting them down. Victorian Canadians believed in progress, but the medical perception of female health was clearly that it was one area where it did not seem to be occurring – women needed help, they no longer could assure their own health. Although evolution suggested a 'natural' development, physicians did not necessarily view it this way. They saw evolution as effected by both nature and human endeavour. Increasingly, however, the natural world was associated with the past. Physicians viewed it with nostalgia but did not really believe it was possible to return to it; nature had to be modified and was modified by evolutionary adaptation to modern society. Unfortunately that adaptation was not perfect and caused serious health problems for women. To rectify this situation, doctors proffered advice to women on how to live, advice which corresponded to their view of woman's proper role. Women were to get married and have children, they were to spend their time raising those children and taking care of the family. Celibacy was dangerous for them as were late hours, reading novels, or focusing on their appearance. Unfortunately, marriage had its own dangers and, as we will see in chapter 7, so did childbirth. But fortunately for women, physicians were there to assist them. Despite the belief in evolution and the sense it had decreased women's physical fitness, physicians still held that women, if not totally to blame for their ill health, were certainly culpable. It was the responsibility, then, of the physician to point out where women had gone wrong and, in those areas where women were not to blame, physicians had a responsibility to mitigate the consequences of ill health. As Skene pointed out, the job of a doctor was not just to give drugs but to try to improve the environment that caused the illness.[112] By examining the causes of ailments in women, particularly those connected to their way of life, physicians were entering the realm of preventive medicine, an area in which the boundary between medical and non-medical was hazy. Doctors were becoming 'the priests of the body.'[113] As such, they oversaw almost all aspects of a woman's life. Their belief in her body's inherent inferiority and weakness compared to man's justified this intervention. But the causes of disease examined in this chapter were only the tip of the iceberg, focusing as they did on social factors. Almost everything about woman's body, especially those areas which distinguished her from man, could be problematic. It all began with puberty.

Three Mysteries: Puberty, Menstruation, and Menopause

'In a perfectly healthy woman, with the organs of generation in a normal condition, the function of menstruation is painlessly performed or, at most, is attended by slight symptoms of discomfort.'[1] With these words, Dr D.C. MacCallum of Montreal described how women should experience what was a normal physiological function. But how many 'perfectly healthy' women were there? From the last chapter, it would appear not very many. As we have seen, doctors proffered advice on the relative benefits of marriage versus celibacy, exercise, fashions, and general way of life in an effort to maintain women's health. They were fighting a losing battle, however, for not only did medical practitioners believe that social factors were working against them but they were convinced that women, by the fact of being female, were predisposed to illness. Women's problems emerged with puberty, followed them through menstruation, and continued throughout the climacteric. The reality of some of these ailments and the fact they were clearly specific to women meant that physicians tended to interpret what was physiologically normal in women as somehow intrinsically problematical and, at times, even pathological. Being female, in and of itself, created a predisposition to illness. Physicians were uneasy about puberty, menstruation, and menopause. They were somehow 'strange' phenomena that the male body did not undergo, or in the case of puberty not in the same way. All three emphasized women's difference from men, not only physically but also, as doctors argued, psychologically and intellectually.

Since puberty in women was much more visible and complex than it was in men, physicians, not surprisingly, focused on it. They viewed the reproductive system in women as their dominating physiological characteristic and the source of most of their health problems. Before puberty the system was quiescent. Puberty, however, signalled its awakening and with it the fundamental differences between the two sexes came into play. To understand it better doctors gathered as much information on puberty as they could, believing, as did those studying nature, that all observations were of equal value and that science advanced as a result of the accumulation of such data. Only when they knew all the facts on a subject could scientists (doctors) determine which ones, if any, were of value.[2] After much gathering of statistics, physicians agreed that puberty began somewhere between the ages of thirteen and sixteen.[3] Less clear were the conditions that brought about menstruation. In his 1858 *Course of Lectures on Obstetrics*, William Tyler Smith stressed climate, class, and locale. According to him, puberty came earlier to women in warmer than in colder climates. For example, statistics indicated that girls began menstruating at the age of thirteen in southern regions such as Africa compared with the age of fifteen in England. Apparently rich women reached puberty earlier, as did women living in towns.[4] Thus, for him, and others writing at the time, modern civilization affected the biological development of women.[5] As doctors continued to gather data they added other factors to the list. Arthur Edis made it clear to medical students and practitioners that race was influential, as was hair colour, with menstruation occurring earlier in brunettes than in blondes, and Alfred Galabin, in his text, argued that early stimulation of the mental faculties and premature sexual stimulus brought about early menarche.[6]

While some of the conditions listed appear to be historical curiosities and harmless enough, the writers who connected the onset of puberty with high living often went beyond description. They associated puberty with some sort of moral stigma. In *The*

Household Physician, Ira Warren argued that women who menstruated later were healthier, and he castigated modern life, and indirectly the women who enjoyed it, for hurrying the process: 'Under the hot-house culture of modern society, and especially among the wealthy classes, where indolence, luxury, and excitement, unite to weaken the constitution, this change is constantly occurring at a more tender age.'[7] In an address given in 1870 Professor Agnew, lecturer on the diseases of women and children at Victoria Medical School, Toronto, discussed whether climate influenced the female constitution. Taking his text from Robertson's *Physiology and Diseases of Women*, he argued that the association between warm climate and early puberty was a notion that supported the racial superiority of those living in the colder regions. Most pundits agreed that reasoning power came to both sexes relatively late in their youth. If in colder climates puberty, and the female beauty that was associated with it, came later as well, then the development of reason and beauty coincided to create a superior woman. Where puberty came at a young age, as in a warmer climate, beauty was already fading before reason matured. Agnew maintained that such logic was faulty, for, unlike many of his colleagues, he maintained there was no scientific basis for the popular assumption that a warm climate brought about early menstruation. Just because plants were stunted in their growth as one moved further north did not mean the development of human growth (puberty) was as well.[8] His voice, however, was in a minority, and most physicians who wrote on the subject continued to make the association between climate and age of puberty.

Whereas age of puberty suggested divisions between women according to where and how they lived, puberty also separated young people psychologically (both male and female) from adults. In his *Physiology of Man*, Austin Flint divided the early stages of life into three phases: from birth to the age of two was infancy; from two to fourteen was childhood; and from fourteen to seventeen puberty reigned.[9] Thus he acknowledged a separate stage in life that we refer to as adolescence. Dr Richard Maurice Bucke recognized that this stage was an emotional one in which the moral sense of the young was more active compared with that of adults and the intellectual nature not as developed.[10] Although this was true for both sexes, each experienced puberty differently and, because the indices of puberty in women were so graphic, doctors focused their description of puberty on them.

Puberty in girls occurred when the feminine characteristics became visible. It was a milestone in a woman's life – almost all peoples and cultures agreed on that – but reaction to it varied. The Kwakiutl Indians on the west coast of Canada acknowledged the onset of puberty with four days' seclusion in a menstrual hut during which time the young girl was forbidden to eat most foods except smoked salmon. Other taboos were placed on her as well but at the end of the four days she underwent a purifying bath and a public and symbolic cleansing, received new clothes, and joined in a public feast. The tribe celebrated her entry into womanhood.[11] European-based Canadian society did not celebrate pubescent girls. Indeed, one young British Columbia girl referred to her first menstruation as an 'attack.'[12] That she did not have a positive view is not surprising. Doctors treated girls' entry into womanhood as something to be wary of and an event that signalled the need to restrict their activities. Up until that point, physicians saw few differences between the two sexes and made little distinction between the kind of activities in which each should engage. The child was a sexless being with only the 'rudiments of sexual organs.'[13] With puberty this changed. In the young woman the ovaries began to dominate and 'mould her character.'[14] As Theophilus Parvin detailed, the changes were both physical and emotional:

The circumference of the neck is greater, and the voice changes; the body is fuller and more gracefully rounded, sharp irregular and angular outlines are replaced by symmetrical curves, and new beauty of form and general expression is manifested – it is the springtime of female life, the bud unfolding into the flower. The girl passing into womanhood puts away childish things, turning from frivolous amusements, from the toys and plays, or from rude sports in which she has found pleasure, she enters a new life, has new thoughts, desires, and emotions. Hitherto she has been living solely in and for the present; but now the future with its lights and shadows, its hopes and fears, makes a large part of her life. She is more sensitive and reserved, and manifests a modest dignity, giving and expecting respect; her individuality becomes more manifest, her sense of duty stronger, and her ambition greater.[15]

The emotional or psychological changes were thought to be as important in defining a woman as the physical manifestations. Women who lacked them were somehow deficient, not quite normal or healthy.

As noted in chapter 1, many physicians believed that women were intellectually inferior to men and some linked this imbalance to the menarche. Alexander Skene described how the two sexes were equal to each other until puberty. At that point they diverged. Because her sex function dominated woman, all her energies had to focus on the development of her reproductive system. Bodies only had a finite amount of energy and, as a result of the demands of her body, Skene believed that a woman's 'mental growth becomes slower and more limited' compared to man's.[16] He was not alone. According to Herbert Spencer, the father of sociology, evolutionary development (or progress) slowed, if not ceased, at puberty and, because women reached puberty at a younger age than men, woman's position on the evolutionary ladder was lower than man's. When it is remembered that the intellect was the last to evolve, the relative intellectual inferiority of women to men appeared to have a scientific basis.[17] But perhaps nature knew best for, as George Napheys made clear, at puberty a young girl's focus shifted from concern about herself as an individual to her 'peculiar obligations ... to the whole race.'[18] She, as an individual, ceased to be important; rather, her destiny as a childbearer became paramount.

Puberty not only accounted for women being intellectually inferior to men and having a limited role in society, but it also made them physically weaker than men. Women, therefore, were to be removed from active participation in the outside world and sheltered. Very early on medical pundits described the physical ail-

ments that often accompanied puberty. William Buchan, in his
Domestic Medicine, advised keeping young women cheerful since
any emotional upset could 'occasion obstructions of the menstrual flux' which could prove to be incurable.[19] Ira Warren concurred. Ill health could easily begin at puberty and it was
imperative to establish good habits. Especially at risk were women
during their first menstruation, which Warren saw as accompanied by 'headache, dizziness, sluggishness of thought, and disposition to sleep.'[20] Such descriptions acknowledged the extra
stress that women's bodies underwent as a consequence of puberty but also reflected a deep-seated belief that women's bodies
could not carry out what was essentially a normal physiological
function without exhibiting pathological symptoms. Because of
the added stress concomitant with puberty, physicians advised
those caring for young pubescent girls to treat them as convalescent patients, to provide them with good food, and to discourage
the wearing of tight clothing.[21] Activity was healthy but, as already
noted, it should be different from that engaged in by boys.[22] And
to give their bodies time to develop they advised young women
not to bear children until at least the age of twenty.[23] If young
women followed this advice they would stand a better chance of
avoiding ill health. They would also be relatively passive, home
oriented, and not intellectually inclined. They would be waiting
for their bodies to develop to the point where they could accept
the role destined for them – motherhood. The coincidence between the medical advice given to young women and the values
that Canadian society encouraged in women in the latter part of
the nineteenth century is not surprising. Physicians supported the
perceived social role of women with medical reasoning. Indeed,
they tended to interpret the workings of the female body from
that role. They saw what could go wrong and did go wrong for
some women and generalized that condition to all women. They
argued that society did not limit women, their own bodies did.

One of the reasons doctors considered puberty to be a time
when the physical health of young women was at risk was that it
coincided with other demands being placed on women. In particular, many physicians viewed education with a jaundiced eye.

This was at a time when young women were increasingly attending school and at rates that often exceeded that of young men at the primary and secondary levels. Nonetheless, doctors argued that education prevented young women from getting the kind of rest they needed during the delicate years of puberty. Referring to the situation in the United States, but which his student readers could equally apply to Canada, Theodore Thomas complained that 'girls of tender age are required to apply their minds too constantly, to master studies which are too difficult, and to tax their intellects by efforts of thought and memory which are too prolonged and laborious. The results are, rapid development of brain and nervous system, precocious talent, refined and cultivated taste, and a fascinating vivacity on the one hand; a morbid impressibility, great feebleness of muscular system, and marked tendency to disease in the generative organs, on the other.'[24] Henry Lyman in *The Practical Home Physician* concurred – the mind and the genital function were closely aligned and strain on the former could affect the latter.[25] Such attitudes followed the arguments set out by Edward H. Clarke, a professor of medicine at Harvard University. In 1874 Clarke published *Sex in Education; or a Fair Chance for Girls*, a diatribe against higher education for women. In it he argued that while boys developed steadily throughout their lives, at puberty girls experienced a sudden and unique period of growth when their complex reproductive system formed. Because the energy needed for the formation and operation of the female reproductive system was so great, it was difficult for young girls to have any surplus energy with which to engage in other activities such as education. If they tried, they could face faulty development of the reproductive system and the possibility of not having children or of bearing them with difficulty. Clarke explained the dilemma facing women as stemming from the body's inability to do 'two things well at the same time' – that is, to develop both physically and mentally. While Clarke concluded that women could not engage in higher education during the years between twelve and twenty, he felt they could labour in a factory. For him, brain work was more liable to destroy feminine capabilities than physical work.[26]

Clarke's arguments found a ready audience among medical practitioners. In the year his book was published, an article in the *Sanitary Journal* asserted that co-education after the age of thirteen or fourteen occasioned 'constant and inordinate excitement' in both sexes but particularly in young women. Young girls' brains must not be crowded or 'proper and complete sexual development will be seriously interfered with and actual disease will be likely to follow; and the fresh blooming, and promising girl will be blighted at the very threshold of womanhood.'[27] The *Canada Lancet* followed suit and in an editorial quoted Clarke in support of its views. It even advocated a regime whereby girls at the age of puberty were removed from schools and tutored at home. These girls were to rest more frequently and not attend parties.[28] Two decades later, Henry Garrigues was still blaming education for the gynaecological woes of women: '*Education* has great influence in the development of gynecological diseases. Too great assiduity in study in early youth concentrates the nerve-energy on the brain, and deprives the uterus and ovaries of their share at a time when these organs are undergoing an enormous development, and preparing for the important functions of womanhood and motherhood.'[29] As already seen, some physicians felt that women did not have the physical stamina to pursue medical education. Young women furthered their education at their own peril. Doctors warned that in the eventuality of physical breakdown, women could face sterility.[30] Considering doctors' views of woman's proper role in society, this was the ultimate threat. In 1879 the *Canada Medical Record* republished excerpts from William Goodell's presidential address before the American Gynecological Society in which he explained how this could happen. Mental exhaustion weakened the nerve centres of the body, which in turn resulted in a poor blood supply. Because the sexual system dominated women, its organs bore the full weight of this depletion. To illustrate his point, Goodell described what he considered a typical case. A young girl enters puberty 'in blooming health' and begins to be over-taxed at school. 'She looses [sic] her appetite and becomes pale and weak. She has cold feet, blue finger-nails, and complains of an inframammary pain. Headache, and back-ache and spineache, and an oppressive sense of exhaustion distress her.' Her periods begin to trouble her and become painful. She develops leucorrhoea and this is followed by bladder problems. She becomes exhausted and hysterical. Eventually she goes to consult with a physician and has to undergo the 'moral rape' of a vaginal examination. The physician, no doubt blaming her womb for all her problems, begins to treat her – with no success. 'Unimproved, she drags herself from one consulting-room to another, until finally, in despair, she settles down to a sofa in a darkened room and relapses into hopeless invalidism.'[31] Hopeless, because the real cause of her problems was never appreciated and mitigated before it was too late.

Not all physicians were diametrically opposed to education for girls, but what support did exist was often grudging and ambivalent. The editors of the *Canada Medical Record* of 1890, perhaps recognizing the reality of increasing numbers of women going to school, published a piece endorsing co-education, although their approval was somehow muted when they admitted they really believed woman's proper place was in the home.[32] Many physicians particularly opposed education that would change the role of women (such as medical education) and challenge the status quo of gender roles in society. They transformed higher education for women into a medical issue just as they had done with bicycle riding for women. But furthering women's education represented a more fundamental change than cycling. Higher education for women offered women a future other than marriage. This is what Clarke and others in the United States feared and it was not an unwarranted fear in Canada. University-trained women did not marry as often as their uneducated sisters. Of the women attending Dalhousie University between 1885 and 1900, for example, 41 to 55 per cent remained single.[33] And when such women did marry, they gave birth to fewer children. That it was the challenge to the status quo which dismayed doctors is evidenced in the kind of education they supported. Learning music, art, and languages was fine, even the rudiments of hygiene were safe to know, although any understanding of anatomy and physiology would just concentrate women's attention on their bodies and lead to ill health.[34] The real danger was when women competed with men 'for place, for honors, for power,' for then the evolutionary history of the sexes was disrupted. Place, honour, and power for women could be gained, not from women's participation in the world with men, but through allowing men to plead women's cause for them and through women's life in the home.[35] Goodell in his text was even more honest than most about what bothered him in modern education: 'Too much brain-work, too little housework.'[36]

The influence of those physicians who argued against education for women should not be underestimated. They came out against it at a time when increasing numbers of Canadian women were attempting to gain entry to the universities of this country. Opponents of education for women used the arguments provided by physicians, and those arguments were powerful. Opponents did not engage in philosophic discussions about gender roles but rather concentrated on what appeared to lay Canadians to be scientific facts – the capabilities of women's bodies.[37] Women might be able to compete intellectually with men but the price of that competition was too great a price to pay. It would unsex women. Only very strong women would be able to withstand that kind of rhetoric. Certainly supporters of higher education of women had to take the argument of woman's frailty seriously and try to respond to it. Most advocates of higher education for women did not deny the physical weakness of women vis-à-vis men and some acknowledged a mental inferiority as well. To do otherwise would have embroiled them in a controversy over the broader issue of women's rights and alienated much of their support. By agreeing with the prevailing ideology concerning women, they disarmed their critics. For some this was a tactical consideration, for others a sincere belief. Women were weaker than men. Instead of eliminating women from universities, however, they argued that their physical and mental weakness served to underline their need of further training. Higher education would give women that strength of mind, without which they would indeed be feeble. By denying them access to universities, Canadians were compounding women's inferiority to men.[38]

Some even tried to offset opposition to education for women by arguing that it actually improved the physical health of women. J.W. Dawson, principal of McGill University, made it clear that physical education was to be an important component of women's education at his institution. Supporters also attempted to assuage the fears of those, like Goodell, who predicted that education for women would result in rejection or neglect of the home. Writer Agnes Machar suggested that higher education would prevent the young woman with energy, intelligence, and time to spare from developing frivolous habits of mind and body.[39] Perhaps even more comforting was the idea that education would make women more womanly. Insisting that the characteristics that made women feminine were inherent and hence natural, supporters of education concluded they could not be unlearned. 'I should rather be inclined to suppose,' maintained one observer, 'that the evolution of faculties not peculiar to either sex can only result in making women more womanly, as in making men more manly.'[40] Education would make women better wives and mothers. Fortunately for Canadian women, the opponents of education did not win. If they had, the dreams young girls such as Maude Abbott confided to their diaries would never have come true: 'One of my day-dreams, which I feel to be selfish, is that of going to school ... I do so *long* to go. And here I go again; once begin dreaming of the possibilities and I become half daft over what I know will never come to pass.'[41]

Once young women were past the years of puberty, their bodies still did not give them any relief. Menstruation itself could be problematic and the arguments used to limit women's activities during puberty carried through the menstrual years. Perhaps this was to be expected. Uneasiness about menstruating women has a long history. Aristotle believed that menstruation revealed woman's inferiority to man: 'The colder female ... is a case of arrested development. She cannot go beyond menstrual blood to produce semen.' Others viewed a menstruating woman as unclean and a source of uncleanness, as evidenced in Leviticus, chapter 15, verses 19 and 24, and chapter 20, verse 18:[42]

And if a woman have an issue, *and* her issue in her flesh be blood, she shall be put apart seven days: and whosoever toucheth her shall be unclean until the even.

And if any man lie with her at all, and her flowers be upon him, he shall be unclean seven days; and all the bed whereon he lieth shall be unclean.

And if a man shall lie with a woman having her sickness, and shall uncover her nakedness; he hath discovered her fountain, and she hath uncovered the fountain of her blood; and both of them shall be cut off from among their people.

In the nineteenth century, too, some doctors associated the theme of inferiority and distaste with menstruation. At mid-century Tyler Smith viewed women as more hysterical during menstruation and more liable to emotional breakdown.[43] Women could not be blamed for this since it was God's design and something over which they had no control. As noted by Alvin Wood Chase in his popular manual:

It is a self-evident fact that the finer the work, and the more complicated a piece of machinery, the more liable is it to become deranged or out of order; and the more skilful must be the mechanic who undertakes to make any necessary repairs.

Upon this consideration I argue that the system of the female is the finer and more complicated, having to perform a double work (childbearing), yet confined to the same or less dimensions than the male. And to perform this double function of sustaining her own life, and giving life to her species, it becomes necessary, in the wisdom of God, to give her such a peculiar formation, that between the ages of fourteen and forty-five, or the child-bearing period, she should have a sanguineous (blood-like) monthly discharge.[44]

Several themes in this quote characterized physicians' attitudes towards women. Chase paid passing homage to the fineness of women's bodies, remarking on how delicate they were compared to men's. Of course this meant that when the female body broke down a very skilful mechanic (physician) was needed, a nice little aside that ensured the centrality of the profession. His uneasiness with the function of menstruation is revealed by his reference to 'a peculiar formation,' although he acknowledged it was linked to a woman's childbearing abilities and had been determined by 'the wisdom of God.' Women, then, were constrained by their bodies. The belief that women's bodies during menstruation placed them in physical jeopardy existed throughout the century but was based on little understanding of the female cycle. Realizing their limited knowledge, physicians often looked to the animal kingdom for analogies to further their understanding.

From the 1860s through the 1880s there was a strong belief within the medical community that menstruation placed women at some physical disadvantage. So vital a process was it that any attempt to suppress it, such as dipping feet in cold water, could lead to death within hours.[45] Theodore Thomas warned that women needed to be kept warm, for cold taken during this period might result in eventual insanity.[46] Women believed these warnings. Amelia Ferris entered the Victoria General Hospital, Halifax, on 12 February 1900 complaining of a dragging pain in her back and along her legs which became worse at the menstrual cycle. According to her case history, she blamed the pain on 'the sudden cessation of her period 3 years ago, consequent to exposure to wet & cold.' After that time, menstruation stopped for five months and had never been normal since.[47] But taking precautions was not enough. Women were advised to rest because menstruation signalled a different physiological state than usual.[48] The fact that a monthly discharge was normal for most adult women apparently did not take away from the danger it posed. Even when physicians recognized the normalcy of it, they associated it with discomfort.[49] So did many women. The *Canada Medical and Surgical Journal* of 1877 reported an American study of 1000 women in which they were asked to what degree menstruation interfered with their lives. Of the 268 who responded, only 35 per cent claimed they were free from any pain during menstruation. The article argued there was nothing intrinsically distressful about menstruation but, because of 'existing social conditions,' discomfort did occur and necessitated rest for women.[50] Of course it is difficult to know how to interpret the results of such a survey. We do not really know the kind of women who were questioned or even the details of the questions. Such a questionnaire might elicit more responses from women who had something to complain about than those who did not. Most likely menstruation during these years did generate some distress, if only from the fact that sanitary arrangements surrounding it were rudimentary. No sanitary napkins were available, so women had to use cloths, wash them, and reuse them. The sometimes tight and heavy clothing women wore during these decades would also be conducive to painful menstruation. In addition, the secrecy surrounding menstruation and the fact that many young girls experienced their first period without knowing what was happening could leave an indelible mark on them throughout life. Society was not comfortable with such bodily processes and this unease would be passed on and internalized by women themselves. Doctors, too, were not comfortable with menstruation. In May 1888 when a patient came to see Dr Gardner of the Montreal General Hospital, he noted she was menstruating and referred to her euphemistically as being 'unwell.'[51]

That physicians used the term 'unwell' to describe menstruating women should not be surprising when it is remembered that no one knew much about the monthly cycle. Throughout this period, different theories emerged to try to explain the importance of menstruation and the actual reasons for it. In 1851 F.K. Kiwisch posited that excitement of the nervous and vascular system created changes in the ovary and increased the quantity of blood in the genitalia. This in turn caused a rupture in the ovarian follicle and uterine bleeding. In 1863 E. Pflüger provided some support for this theory by maintaining that ovulation and menstruation occurred at the same time from the same cause – increased quantity of blood due to nerve impulses.[52] In the mid-1890s research on transplanted ovaries effectively established the link between ovaries and menstruation – that is, without ovaries women did not menstruate. Nevertheless, the exact nature of the process and how it was connected to a woman's fertile period remained unknown until well into the twentieth century.[53] Because there was so little understanding of the monthly cycle in women, physicians looked to the world of nature in an attempt to understand what was happening. They deemed menstruation to be the equivalent of being in heat in the lower animals and, as a result, physicians predicted that women would be most fertile at or around menstruation.[54] Not only did such an analogy demean women – since men were not compared to the lower animals – but the deduction taken from the analogy was incorrect. Women were not at their most fertile during this time, they were at their least fertile. Yet the association of menstruating women with animals in heat may not be as bizarre as it sounds. Discharge from animals in heat does occur and, because they are also ovulating at the same time, they are most fertile at that time. In women, however, ovulation and menstruation are separate acts.[55] Not realizing this distinction, doctors continued to use the animal analogy. In 1884, in an article quoted from the *British Medical Journal*, the *Canadian Practitioner* was drawing the same erroneous conclusions, although it did recognize some differences between women and animals: 'As sexual aptitude is not confined in women solely to the period of heat, and intercourse may be indulged in at any time, it is obvious that a disturbing element is introduced, and that, under artificial conditions ova may be matured through sexual stimulation, or follicles ruptured under sexual excitement which, but for such intervention, would have remained quiescent or dormant until the next normal oestruation.'[56] But the differences noted placed women in an unnatural position, for the underlying suggestion of the quote was that, except for 'artificial conditions,' women's bodies would have acted more like those of animals and would have remained 'dormant' until the next 'normal oestruation.' What women were experiencing was not normal and signalled a disruption within their bodies from that dictated by nature.

The idea that menstruating women were at risk, the lack of understanding of female physiology, and the use of animal imagery continued well into the 1890s. Physicians continued to see women who menstruated as unwell.[57] Too much activity or imprudence during menstruation led to illness, particularly to gynaecological diseases.[58] Henry Garrigues complained that 'women not only move about, but dance and skate, at a time when a process is going on that is so easily turned in an abnormal direction.'[59] Women were urged to rest, to think of themselves as fragile, and to avoid a life of luxury.[60] Dr John Hett, in a book he published himself in Berlin, Ont., entitled *The Sexual Organs: Their Use and Abuse*, was blunt about the limitations this placed on women: 'A woman, when she is menstruating, is very often physically unfitted for the active pursuits followed by men.'[61] How accurate were doctors' perceptions of the experience of menstruation? Patient records at the Victoria General Hospital in Halifax in the early 1890s do indicate that many women suffered from irregularities in menstruation. However, by the fact of their being in a hospital, such women were a pre-selected group.[62] Their experiences may or may not reflect the vast majority of women outside the hospital. In addition, it is difficult to know how to interpret irregularities of menstruation. Since little was known about what constituted normal menstruation, any deviation may have been interpreted as pathological, whereas in actuality it may have fallen within an average deviation among any group of women. At this stage it is impossible to know what women's menstrual experience was in these years. But patient records in hospitals such as the Victoria General indicate that whether women were admitted for menstrual disorders or not, their case files invariably mention their menstrual history, reflecting the central place doctors believed it had in a woman's health experience. And as in the earlier decades, we do know that physicians in the 1890s evaluated menstruating women on a faulty understanding of their monthly cycles.

Physicians continued to give out incorrect information about a woman's fertile period.[63] In addition, the myth that menstruating women were a danger, with its origins in prehistory, still found some support. In 1891 the editor of the *Canada Lancet* pointed out that, owing to the introduction of aseptic surgery, some people were concerned that menstruating nurses were allowed in the surgical room since menstrual blood, as partially disintegrated matter, presented a potential septic danger. While acknowledging that such blood could be a threat, the editor pointed out that this was true of any bodily excretions and, if that kind of logic were used, perspiring surgeons should be banned as well.[64] Even though the author rejected the idea of prohibiting menstruating nurses from the operating room, the fact that it could even be raised and considered reflected a continuation of the age-old distrust and fear of menstruating women. About the only change that did occur in the 1890s was the profession's penchant for quantifying, as with the age of puberty. In this case, doctors associated the quantity of menstrual discharge with the kind of life a woman led and where she lived; rich and indolent women who ate well would be more likely to have a heavy discharge, as would those women in warmer climates.[65]

Analogies with the animal kingdom also continued to be the favoured way of understanding menstruation. Despite the fact that physicians knew that menstruation was not equivalent to heat in animals, it was as close a comparison as they could find.[66] While in and of itself this did not pose a problem, the tone with which they made the comparisons still revealed uneasiness with menstruation and a sense that in higher beings such a state would not occur. For example, Dr Gardner, professor of gynaecology at McGill University and gynaecologist to the Royal Victoria Hospital as well as consulting gynaecologist to the Montreal General Hospital, published an article in March 1897 that referred to the function of menstruation as 'one of the most remarkable in the animal economy' and 'confined to the human female and certain monkeys.'[67] Considering that physicians and most lay people in the 1890s were quite familiar with evolutionary theory, any reader could not help but draw the inference that women occupied a lower rung of the evolutionary ladder than men for whom few animal analogies were made.

Late nineteenth-century theories about menstruation in women cannot be dismissed simply as curiosities, for they reflected deep-seated attitudes towards women. The emphasis given to the medical problems that could accompany menstruation reinforced the image of women being less strong than men. Doctors revealed a certain degree of unease with the process of menstruation and a sense that it was not a particularly efficient way of having a body work. Recent critics of medicine's treatment of women have attempted to explain this attitude by arguing that physicians generally use a male model of health. When the male body is taken to be the norm, deviation from it is often interpreted as sickness or weakness. As one perceptive modern critic has noted, this applies in particular to menstruation: 'Bleeding is a sign of injury in men's bodies, rather than evidence of fecundity or the natural accomplishment of birth, as it commonly is in women's. Once a man's body is taken as the standard and blood seen as a sign of injury, the *normal* events of menstruation and birth are likely to be viewed as alarming and interpreted on the model of disease or injury.'[68] Instead of comparing menstruating women with men whose bodies could not menstruate, physicians would have done better to compare them with other menstruating women. This would have revealed the real problems that some women had with menstruation.

If women's medical problems began with puberty and lasted throughout menstruation, they did not end with menopause. Physicians viewed the end of the childbearing cycle in a way similar to the beginning – as a shock to the physical system that could result in ill health. They also viewed such women as old, the description given to Mrs Halloran when she entered the Victoria General Hospital in August 1900 at the age of fifty.[69] The assumption in society that women were less strong than men and that their *raison d'être* was to have children was reflected in medical perceptions that menopausal women were delicate and that menopause signalled a decline in a woman's femininity. William Buchan in his *Domestic Medicine* argued that menopause was a dangerous and critical time for women, for any 'stoppage of ... habitual evacuation, however small, is sufficient to disorder the whole frame, and often to destroy life itself!'[70] The 1866–7 annual report of the Provincial and City Hospital, Halifax, listed one woman who had died from climacteric disease.[71] Jayne's *Medical Almanac* of 1863 agreed that menopause was a threat to health by referring to it as a 'decline.'[72] The negative connotation of the word 'decline' was also picked up in Archy McCurdy's lecture notes from Trinity Medical College in 1873: 'After the menstrual period ceases, the genitals loose [sic] their size and become atrophied, hairs make their appearance on the face, the voice changes, the breasts dry up and the whole body assumes the masculine form.'[73]

The 1880s simply brought out these themes in more detail. In his *People's Common Sense Medical Adviser*, R. Pierce viewed menopause as 'the critical age.' He described the changes that occurred in the body when it no longer evacuated blood through menstruation. He envisioned the blood trying to find some other outlet and failing, forming tumours in the breast or uterus.[74] The symptoms doctors associated with menopause would make anyone view it with dismay. When Miss Hamilton came to the Montreal General Hospital on 17 June 1882 complaining of nausea and vomiting after eating, her physician put it down to 'approaching menopause.'[75] According to medical texts and popular manuals alike, menopause could also bring about swelling of the breasts, hot flashes, pains, wind, nosebleeds, skin eruption, flooding, a sense of choking, faintness, and general ill health.[76] In some women menopause returned them to the poor health they had experienced before puberty.[77] For sterile and single women womb disease became likely.[78] Also rife at this time was neurasthenia, neuralgia, hysteria, convulsive disease, melancholia, and other mental affections. Because of all these dangers, John Thorburn advised his student readers that menopausal women were to be guarded like young girls in puberty. If not, society would lose the social and philanthropic contributions that such women were still capable of making.[79] In addition, most physicians suggested that menopause somehow made a woman less a woman. According to Napheys, menopausal women were less womanly and less attractive. They became fretful, grew stout, accumulated fat at the base of the neck, their breasts became hard and flat, their abdomen enlarged, hair grew on their face, and their voice grew harder. Essentially 'the characteristics of the female sex bec[a]me less and less distinct.'[80] Hamilton Ayers associated it with death: 'The process of death is the reverse of the process of development. The generative functions fail first, the animal next, and the organic becomes impotent last.'[81] It was a concrete sign of the beginning of the end, a sign that men did not have.

Of course, not all menopausal women were doomed. Some physicians even suggested that 'the change of life' was not a negative occurrence. Dr William Playfair, for example, felt that the dangers of menopause had been greatly exaggerated. For hysterical women he even considered menopause a real boon. Because hysteria was often associated with the onset of puberty, menopause was seen as a potential cure.[82] Hamilton Ayers, in his 1881 *Everyman His Own Doctor*, reported that many women considered menopause in a positive light. It is understandable why this was the case. Menopause ended a woman's childbearing years and the demands that childbearing placed on her body. It also meant that women could engage in sexual intercourse without worrying about the possibilities of conception. Ayers, himself, although associating menopause with decline or death, did not believe that menopause in itself was either good or bad. He claimed it neither built you up nor weakened you.[83] While this was hardly an overwhelming endorsement, it was optimistic compared with other medical writers.

The 1890s saw no diminution of the idea that menopause led to ill health and that menopausal women had lost their attractiveness. In his *American Text-book of Gynaecology*, John Baldy emphasized, as others had before him, that menopause was a dangerous period, a time when malignant disease of the uterus could emerge, when women could experience vertigo, fainting, flushes, cold hands and feet, constipation, diarrhoea, palpitations, sweatings, loss of memory, irritability, fear, melancholia, hysteria, facial hair, and flaccidity of the breasts. All this was the result of congestion in specific areas of the nervous system due to the 'nonescape of the customary monthly bloody discharge.' About the only consolation Baldy seemed able to give North American women was that menopause came later in colder climates than in warmer.[84] The problem with the long list of menopausal symptoms was that while some were accurate, many more were not. Unfortunately, the former provided credibility to the latter. Not that all practitioners in the 1890s imagined menopause to be the dire phenomenon that Baldy envisioned. For the author of an article in the *Canadian Practitioner* of 1898, menopause was of concern only if a woman had ignored her health when she was younger. In that case, such women were to rest, take moderate exercise, and avoid stimulants.[85] D.C. MacCallum of the Montreal General Hospital noted that, although menopause was a critical period, its symptoms were slight for most women. But even he warned that 'in some instances, diseases before latent, then declare themselves.'[86] More positive, in a backhanded way, was Skene in his *Medical Gynecology*, when he pointed out that whereas women's mental development had stopped at puberty so that all her energies could be focused on the development of her reproductive system, at menopause it resumed again and her mental abilities became more like a man's.[87] Of course this was a two-edged sword. What woman gained mentally she lost physically. Some physicians believed that women's sexual appetite declined and in some cases disappeared in these last years of her life. For William Goodell this only made sense. What was the point of a woman feeling sexual desire if she could no longer have children?[88] This view hinted at the underlying cause of the distaste for menopausal women exhibited by these physicians – such women no longer could perform the duties for which their bodies had been destined. Their usefulness was over.

Medical attitudes towards puberty, menstruation, and menopause reveal a deep-seated belief that women's bodies placed them at a disadvantage compared to men's. But it was more than simply their bodies, it was the reproductive organs of their bodies that did so. They dominated women to such a degree that they determined woman's social role and, from the medical perspective, made her less than equal to man. Since physicians believed women were at medical risk because of the complications attending the three physiological processes, physicians felt an understandable obligation to help them and to give advice. However, their understanding of the female body was limited by what medical science knew at the time. As a result, doctors drew on the world of nature for analogies to explain the workings of women's bodies. But nature did not provide woman with any comfort;

rather, it reinforced the concept of her inferiority, both physical and intellectual, compared with man. Underlying all the descriptions of pubescent, menstruating, and menopausal women was the sense that these people were not like men and that men's bodies were somehow the way bodies should be. Women deviated from men, men did not deviate from women. This was a situation from which women could not escape. Their bodies were their destiny and, from the medical descriptions, it was a destiny few physicians envied. Discussions of female sexuality made this even more evident.

Chapter Four

Sexuality in Women

In her diary entry of Friday, 8 April 1898, Lucy Montgomery recalled a passionate love affair she had had with a young man. She remembered the need she had felt to consummate their relationship and, even after the passage of time, what she wrote in her journal made the intensity of her desire unmistakable:

The most horrible temptation swept over me – I remember to this minute its awful power – to *yield* – to let him stay where he was – to be his body and soul if that one night at least!

What saved me? What held me back. No consideration of right and wrong. I was past caring for *that*. No tradition or training – that had all gone down before the mad sweep of instinctive passion. Not even fear of the price the woman pays. No, that which saved me from Herman Leard's dishonoring love was *the fear of Herman Leard's contempt*. If I yielded – he might despise me![1]

With these words Montgomery revealed the tension between natural feeling and social expectation, the reality of physical desire and the need to control it. Her experience of sexuality, like that of many others, was a blend of nature and nurture and, because of the latter, sexuality has become a topic of interest to historians.

More than physiological changes within the body, culture defines sexual behaviour. Historians have noted that, with industrialization, the timing of births spread more evenly over the year, a development which suggests that intercourse was becoming more frequent and regular.[2] The gap between the age of marriage for men and for women began to close, transforming the way in which individuals looked at the bodies of their spouses, with the result that sexual attractiveness became a more important component of the marital relationship.[3] Historians have also argued that by the end of the nineteenth century, a restrictive model of sexual behaviour was in place which contrasted to an earlier openness about human sexuality. The transition, however, was not uniform and could cause consternation when those espousing one view came into contact with those espousing the other. This was certainly the experience of one visitor to Canada West in 1842. He was at a loss to understand the disregard with which some respectable young women viewed illegitimacy. He recalled one 'lady who volunteered the information, that "her Betty" had been two years old at her marriage.' Rather than being ashamed of her sexual transgression, she was proud of it. Children were useful in a pioneer, farming society, and proof that a woman was fruitful did not harm her marriage prospects in the least. As a result, the 'corrector feeling on this subject, of females from the old country [were] condemmed as ridiculous.'[4] If true, this did not remain the case for long; by the end of the century, while some Canadian women might find the 'corrector feeling' confining, few would challenge it. Even if they had, doctors were there to assure them that passions outside the respectable bounds of marriage would lead to disease. Most physicians were uncomfortable with the idea of women experiencing strong sexual feelings and used what influence they had to create a model of how a 'normal' (healthy) woman should behave.

At first glance, Victorian attitudes towards sexuality appeared repressive. According to conventional wisdom, Victorians were distressed by sexual matters, even to the point of supposedly covering piano 'legs' with skirts. They refused to acknowledge their sexual feelings and, as a result, led very controlled public lives, although their private lives may have been much different. But if Victorians adopted a more restrictive sexual ideology than their predecessors, historians have not been able to agree on how to explain why. Freud in his work associated sexual repression with capitalism, and historians, when they first focused on sexuality as a topic worthy of investigation, expanded and developed this idea. Peter Cominos, in an early article, described how middle-class Victorians' concern with saving money and delaying gratification so they could get ahead professionally complemented their attitudes towards sexuality. They restrained their sexual needs so they would not waste energy, and delayed marriage until they could comfortably support a family. Nineteenth-century sexual restraint, then, was compatible with the values of thrift and abstinence demanded by a capitalist society.[5]

Closely linked to the economic theory of repression was one of class. Cominos argued that Victorian morality helped the middle classes maintain their standard of living by limiting the size of their families and thereby decreasing or at least not increasing the cost of maintaining them. The higher birth rate of the working classes fit the needs of the economy by ensuring an endless supply of children, who became cheap labourers in the factories of industrializing England and, at the same time, confirmed the middle classes in their perception that workers were lacking in sexual restraint.[6] Stephen Kern, in his pioneering book *Anatomy and Destiny*, described how the increasing density of European cities resulted in and/or coincided with the desire to have privacy. In the erotic sphere, this was reflected by 'the relegation of sexuality to the bedroom and its restriction by conventions requiring that it be kept under the covers and in the dark.' The middle classes especially adopted this attitude and interpreted such restrictions as a virtue, a sign of respectability, and a way of separating themselves from the lower orders.[7]

A third explanation for Victorian sexual restraint was social. In the nineteenth century, increasing numbers of young people were on their own as they left the countryside, attracted to the cities by the job opportunities there. Since external control over their actions, as represented by family and community, no longer existed, internal or self-control became necessary to curb sexual activity and limit illegitimacy rates.[8] The ideology of sexual repression provided that control. Religion also played a part. In the United States the trend towards sexual restraint emerged with

the Second Great Awakening in the 1830s.[9] Not to be ignored either
was the influence of Pope Pius IX's 1854 proclamation of the doctrine of the Immaculate Conception, which rendered the virgin
mother as an impossible ideal for Catholic women.[10] In Canada,
Carol Bacchi has linked restrictive attitudes towards sexuality to
the concern of Canadians about racial degeneration. Social purity
(sexual purity) was needed and, if the racial stock of Canada were
to be maintained, both men and women had to accept the value
of sexual control.[11]

A final theory to explain Victorian sexual repression has emphasized gender. Historians pointed out that, ultimately, the focus
of repression was female sexuality. They and others have argued
that this reflected men's ambivalence about their own aggressiveness, sexual and otherwise.[12] For example, G.J. Barker-Benfield noted that male attitudes towards female sexuality 'by
definition ... have been linked to man's beliefs about sex and the
position of woman, and his need to separate himself from and
subordinate woman because she was the objective correlative of
his own sexuality.'[13] Peter Gay interprets the denial of female
sexuality as a response to and fear of the woman's movement. In
his words, 'many men ... experienced feminism in all its forms
as nothing less than a threat of castration.'[14] Most of the writers
commenting on the ideology of female sexual repression tended
to view it in a negative way. Women were victims. The ideology
denied them sexual pleasure and it reinforced the aggressiveness
of male sexuality and affirmed a man's right to seek out prostitutes, since no respectable woman could hope to satisfy him.[15]
Yet was the ideology of woman's passivity necessarily a disadvantage to women? Some feminist historians have suggested there
were positive elements to the ideology and, instead of women
being victims, they were participants in the making of an ideology
from which they could benefit. Certainly on the surface sexual
restraint made sense. Restricting access to sexual activity increased its value and, in a society in which it was difficult for
women to 'get ahead,' sex was one of the few assets or 'goods'
with which they had to bargain. Sexual passivity provided a modicum of safety for women endangered by childbirth, since it jus-

tified resisting their husband's sexual importunities. Victorians viewed morality and sexual purity in women as necessary characteristics, given their childbearing role. It was to women's advantage to emphasize this rectitude, for it reminded men of the moral differences between the sexes and the superiority of women over men. Repression (or abstinence) was also one of the only 'reliable prophylaxis against venereal disease' which, as we have seen, doctors believed to be a real danger to women.[16] Moreover, Bacchi has speculated that by denying their sexuality, women prevented their being seen as sex objects and that prudery became a mask hiding women's efforts to achieve freedom of person. Women also down-played their sexuality because it was physical, and any focus on the physical side of the male/female relationship could only emphasize woman's weakness.[17]

The most recent direction in the historiography on sexuality denies repression. In his landmark study *The History of Sexuality*, Michel Foucault challenged the image of sexual repression that had dominated people's thinking about the past and argued that since the seventeenth century, sex had become a focus of attention if not an obsession. He saw the nineteenth century engaged in a constant 'discourse' on the topic and could not envision how a people who talked so much about sex could be repressed. He seemed unwilling to consider that repression is a form of obsession, that they can be two sides of the same coin. What he also ignored was the quality of the discussion. The nature of the discourse on sexuality was not always open and approving.[18] Nevertheless, Foucault's work broke the stereotype of the Victorians as repressive and has stimulated other researchers to re-examine nineteenth-century sexual ideology and reality with new eyes. Carl Degler has done so and, in an analysis of a sex survey given to turn-of-the-century American women, has concluded that the sexual behaviour of women did not correspond to a repressive ideology, although, unlike Foucault, he does not deny the ideology's existence. Peter Gay's opus on sexuality also follows the new direction. According to him, nineteenth-century women revelled in their erotic tendencies.[19]

Foucault's work not only altered the interpretation of Victorian sexuality, but it redirected scholars to the shift in the locale of the discussion on sexuality. Whereas it had traditionally taken place in the confessional, it now occurred in the doctor's office.[20] Both Degler and Gay support this view, although they are not in total agreement with Foucault on the role played by physicians. Degler believes that a sexually repressive ideology did exist but that it was primarily introduced by the medical profession in an effort to help women. Foucault argues that no repression existed and that this can be seen in the discussion within the medical profession. Gay steers a middle course between the two, and views physicians as undecided or ambivalent about the issue of female sexuality.[21] The rest of this chapter will focus on the attitudes of the Canadian medical profession towards female sexuality. Foucault is certainly correct in perceiving a substantive discourse within the profession but he has not appreciated that it is quite different depending on whether physicians are talking about male or female sexuality. The ambivalence of much of the literature tends to support Gay's hypothesis rather than Degler's assessment of medical repressiveness.

Physicians were not antagonistic to sexual activity. They acknowledged its importance but wanted to see it in its proper place – within marriage. Eugene Becklard, in his *Physiological Mysteries*, insisted that marriage was necessary to curb sexual excess and to ensure that sexual intercourse was limited to only one partner. To do otherwise was unwise: 'Promiscuous intercourse enervates the system, oppresses the brain, and blunts the appetite of desire. Variety, in fact, counteracts healthy and vigorous excitements, for its stimulations are but as the passing moments of unnatural strength, during the crisis of fever.'[22] Sexual relations, however, within marriage and with a loved spouse, lay 'at the very foundation of society.'[23] They were a sign of community health and, as such, were significant and of value. According to R. Pierce, love and sex between two individuals became 'a union for life by natural influences which never die out.' So strong were the impressions of a sexual relationship in its rightful setting that he believed if a woman married for the second time she often bore a child who looked like her former spouse.[24]

While sexual relations were important, physicians did agree they had to be moderate and controlled. But control did not mean repression. The concern of the medical profession was indulgence in excess. The sexual instinct was a powerful force that had to be kept in check.[25] If individuals went against the concept of moderation, their health would suffer. Joseph Workman, super-intendent of the Toronto Asylum, discussed the case of an elderly man who, when he was seventy-six, married a woman more than forty years his junior. From this alone Workman questioned the man's sanity and impressed upon his readers that 'of all the old men known to us who have married young wives, how many have not, in a few years, smashed down in both physical and mental competency?'[26] The control of sexuality was important for another reason – it separated humans from animals. William Carpenter made this point explicit: 'A difference exists between the sexual relations of Man and those of the lower animals. In proportion as the Human being makes the temporary gratification of the mere sexual appetite his chief object, and overlooks the happiness aris-ing from spiritual communion, which is not only purer but more permanent, and of which a renewal may be anticipated in another world, – does he degrade himself to a level with the brutes that perish.'[27] Humans were made up of spirit, mind, and body. Sexual desires were natural but civilized people kept them under control of the 'well-developed higher faculties.'[28] Self-control, 'at the root of all virtues,' provided moral freedom to the individual and the ability to be more than an animal.[29] This was not only a medical view but one shared by most in society. Even a fourteen-year-old girl knew that her desire to hug the boy next door was acceptable only 'if ... we had been savages.' But they were not and so she called herself to account, noting that 'he's a boy and one does not hug boys.'[30] Her restraint was not natural, but learned. In his turn-of-the-century sexual exposé *Searchlights on Health*, B.G. Jefferis emphasized the need for parents to talk honestly to their children about sex.[31] If they did not, their children would find out about the facts of life in ways that could lead to their downfall. As an editorial in the *Canada Medical and Surgical Journal* pointed out, newspapers carried obscene ads of all descriptions.[32]

Appealing to male fears about immoderate sexuality, one declared 'Errors of Youth! Sufferers from Nervous Debility! Youthful Indiscretions! Lost Manhood! Be your own Physician.' With such 'advice' readily available, it was important that children be taught properly and, for heir own sake, learn the value of control.[33] Such concerns did not fall on deaf ears. The ladies of the Woman's Christian Temperance Union (WCTU), through their Department of Purity, stressed how important it was for parents to answer all legitimate questions and, in an appeal to a higher authority, reminded its members that 'science has exploded the widely-accepted theory that chastity was incompatible with health.'[34] Canadians believed that control was important in all fields. They established schools to control young people, insane asylums to control the insane, prisons to control criminals. The desire on the part of physicians and others to place limits on sexuality was simply part of this attitude. Control was for the benefit of all. It was not seen as repression but an attempt to moderate, to avoid extremes, and as a way of making living with others bearable.

Although the medical profession agreed that sexuality had to be controlled, not repressed, doctors did perceive and react differently to male and female sexuality. For one, they saw the sexual instinct in man as very strong and consequently believed that restraint for men was going to be difficult. Semen, a concrete manifestation of energy, was proof of this power. It could be secreted, generated, stored up, reabsorbed, or ejaculated at regular intervals.[35] Its loss, however, was not beneficial. Doctors assumed that individuals had only a finite supply of energy and that once energy was lost, as through the ejaculation of semen, it could not be replenished. The body worked as an economic system – spending in one area depleted another. The consequences of wasteful expenditure of energy could be devastating. An American health crusader in the 1840s, Sylvester Graham, believed that one ounce of semen equalled forty ounces of blood.[36] The Reverend W.J. Hunter reminded his large audience of this when he lectured in Montreal at the St James Methodist Church in the 1890s. So debilitating could sexual excess be that William Carpenter warned his student readers that between the ages of eighteen and twenty-eight mortality was higher in men than in women owing to the arousal and gratification of their passions.[38] In addition, their passions did not seem to dissipate very much over time. The *Canada Medical and Surgical Journal* reported in 1877 that a seventy-year-old man who returned to his sixty-year-old wife after an absence of nine years wanted to have intercourse with her. Although his wife objected, he still insisted. She reluctantly agreed but, as a result of the intercourse, she hemorrhaged and had to be taken to the Montreal General Hospital.[39] Doctors also viewed men as more promiscuous than women and, as we have seen, blamed them for infecting their wives with venereal disease. So strong was the sexual urge in men that prohibiting prostitution would only lead to their resorting to seduction and adultery.[40] Young girls especially had to be warned.[41] Physicians saw this as their responsibility but they were not alone in their concern. The Maritime WCTU was disturbed by the vulnerability of young immigrant girls coming to Canada without a protector, 'utterly ignorant of the country and of the evil ways of men.'[42] Man was the seducer, woman his victim.

If men's sexual drives were so harmful to them and threatening to women, why did they exist? Lapthorn Smith, lecturer on gynaecology at Bishop's University in Montreal, believed he knew the answer – perpetuation of the species. In the modern world of the late nineteenth century, men were increasingly caught up in getting ahead. Marriage, from a practical viewpoint, could be perceived to take man away from his work. In addition, marriage and family were expensive propositions. No man would choose to marry except for the fact he was 'compelled to do so by the force of his sexual feelings.' Thus male sexuality drove men to marry. Those who did so had greater sexual drives than those who did not and they passed those drives on to their male children (somehow they were not passed on to their daughters). Survival of the fittest meant the survival of men with the strongest sex drives.[43] Women, too, were more attracted to such men, for sexual vitality in men ensured healthy children, children 'with strong functional vigor.'[44] Male sexual energy could thus overcome the influence of a weak and sickly mother and was needed to ensure the future well-being of the species.

But what of woman's sexual nature? There is no denying that some physicians were quite hostile to the idea of women having strong sexual feelings. William Acton, whose book *The Functions and Disorders of the Reproductive Organs* was continually re-published throughout the century, believed that women had little inclination in that direction. He described one couple who had been married for twelve months and had not yet had sexual intercourse because of the husband's sexual debility. This was a situation the wife was quite willing to have continue, except for her desire to have children.[45] One historian has pointed out that Acton's beliefs, although constantly quoted as proof of the denial of female sexuality, are not dependable. Acton's medical contemporaries were sceptical about his claims[46] and few among them denied the existence of sexual feeling in women as vehemently as he did. Nevertheless, some did not see it as particularly important. Carpenter argued that 'the function of the Female, during the coitus, is essentially passive,' and in 1887 Matthew Mann, in *A System of Gynecology*, echoed those sentiments. While both physicians felt woman's role was passive, they did acknowledge that a woman could experience sexual feeling and that normally she did. It was simply not necessary for her to do so in order to conceive.[47] But in 1890, in a tone reminiscent of Acton, Dr James F.W. Ross, surgeon to the Woman's Hospital, Toronto, could declare that 'fully one-half of the married women are almost devoid of sexual passion.'[48] In the same year Lapthorn Smith hypothesized that, while sexual feelings in women had been strong in the past, they were now decreasing, and concluded that 'women who have no such feelings are perhaps the best off.'[49] Several years later Alexander Skene put forth a similar evolutionary schema. While in primitive races both men and women were polygamous, Skene maintained that in disposition women were monogamous. This tendency had only increased, and women's sexual instinct was no longer as strong as it had been. Unfortunately, men were still polygamous in nature, a trait which for Skene simply highlighted their ethical inferiority to women.[50]

Physicians who denied or down-played the existence of female sexuality believed they could substantiate their view. Some pointed to the smallness of the clitoris compared with the size of the penis.[52] Others appealed to the fact that women needed energy more than men because of the demands of their reproductive system. One way they could preserve their energy was not to exhibit passion to the same degree as men.[52] This was nature's way of protecting women. And there were reasons why physicians may have felt that young women needed protection. The age of puberty was declining and, consequently, women were reaching sexual maturity at an earlier age. The emphasis on controlling or, more rarely, denying female sexuality may have been an effort to offset the earlier development of sexual maturity in women, a way of controlling female youth and imposing standards of behaviour that would protect women from the burden of an illegitimate pregnancy. In addition, strong sexual passion in women would negate the overwhelming belief in the balance between the two sexes. If man was sexually active, then woman had to be less so. Sexual activity in women would suggest aggression and this would contradict the ideology of true womanhood that dominated society during these years. Instead, maternity became passion's substitute.[53]

The concept of balance was more than aesthetic, it was functional. Sexual passivity in women was necessary not just to offset the active sexual drive of men but to protect men from their own urges. Such an idea was particularly strong in the popular medical manuals. In *The Physical Life of Women*, George Napheys argued that women had a sense of shame and modesty that would protect men from their own impulses. Jefferis in *Searchlights* could only agree.[54] Because of the strength of the male sex drive, boys and men were going to have difficulty controlling themselves. C.S. Clark in *Of Toronto the Good* asserted that 'a well developed girl in short dresses' or 'one girl in a bloomer costume ... will create far greater and more widespread corruption among boys than a city full of show bills.'[55] Thus women's control over their own feelings was necessary so they could resist the demands that boys and men would place on them. Henriette Dessaulles at the age of seventeen had already internalized this lesson. When the young man she loved attempted to see her more often, she wrote in her diary: 'Who knows, next he may want to kiss me! But the fact is, I've got my wits about me and keep a tight reign on my feelings so they won't run away with me.' Like Lucy Montgomery, Dessaulles recognized her own desires but felt the need to master them. Even two years later when she railed against 'conventions, etiquette, proprieties' and questioned 'Why can't we live freely and love openly without having to worry about what people might think or say?' she never really challenged those conventions. She continued to resist the entreaties of her lover.[56] The ideology of control not only protected young women, but was also of value to older women. There was a sense among some physicians that whatever sexual feelings women experienced, these passions decreased as they became older. As noted in the last chapter, William Goodell, honorary professor of gynaecology at the University of Pennsylvania, pointed out that this decline during menopause was not serious – since women could no longer conceive there did not seem to be any point to their having sexual desires.[57] Indeed it was necessary that they not have such feelings, for how was a woman to get sexual satisfaction after her husband died? Declining sexuality was nature's way of preparing older women for widowhood.[58] The idea of a sexually mature widow seemed to frighten Goodell. Of course in one respect he was responding to reality – women did outlive men and, perhaps for that reason, doctors stressed the 'necessary' decline of sexual feeling more in older women than they did in older men.

The desire of some physicians to argue against the existence of strong sexual feelings in women stemmed from their inability to reconcile the reality of women as childbearers and childrearers with the concept of women as sexual beings, and their inability to accept the notion of female sexuality existing on its own, separate from male sexuality. What makes this inability and fear striking is that the conclusion drawn went against known physiological phenomenon. As evidenced in the medical concern about female masturbation, doctors recognized that women had sexual urges which were strong and independent of man. Of course, most discussions about the effects of masturbation primarily concerned males. Males had an overwhelming sex drive which, if not satisfied in the accepted way, would seek other outlets. Physicians believed that masturbation was a cause of spermatorrhoea. This was true for Henry McRafferty, who entered the Victoria General Hospital, Halifax, complaining of 'nocturnal emissions.' Twenty-two years of age, he admitted to having masturbated for about three years 'when he was young,' finally giving up the practice before he turned eighteen. Since that time, however, he had experienced the uncontrolled nocturnal emissions.[59] Masturbation could also lead to nervous exhaustion, idiocy, imbecility, and insanity. When asylum statistics are examined, masturbation is listed as a cause of male insanity rather than female.[60] Between 1875 and 1900, thirteen cases of insanity in the Provincial Lunatic Asylum, Saint John, were deemed the result of masturbation. All thirteen were men.[61] And most of the ingenious mechanical devices that were invented to prevent masturbation only made sense if used on men. One such instrument designed to prevent wet dreams consisted of a leather ring with metallic points that was placed over the penis. As the penis became erect the points would cause enough pain to awaken the sleeper in time to prevent ejaculation. Doctors could resort to even more extreme measures. One historian of the American scene reported the use of circumcision and castration, and the placement of a plaster cast over the genital area. To prevent the waste of semen as a result of spermatorrhoea, physicians resorted to leeching, inserted acupuncture needles into the testes and sounds into the bladder, or applied electrical current to the genitals. Less drastic was advice to sit on cane-bottomed chairs and hard benches, rather than soft-cushioned furniture that was liable to stimulate a young boy's erotic imagination. Young men were to avoid reading sentimental novels and sitting for long periods so as to prevent blood from accumulating in the lower trunk of the body, thereby generating enough heat to compel any student to masturbate.[62] Little is known about the treatment resorted to in Canada. One reference does suggest that, while the therapeutics may not have been as extreme, they could be unpleasant. At mid-century the *British American Medical and*

Physical Journal reported the case of a young man suffering from fits. Dr Lawson, a Thomsonian physician, was called in and determined that the young man's fits were 'frequently increased by pumping the seaman [sic] with the hand instead of the uterus or vagina of the female.' Lawson prescribed a 'warm bath ... blistering the stomach ... an injection ... a dose of senna and manna and a decoction of common mullin.'[63] In the case of masturbation, anatomy made males vulnerable to treatment.

Although the discussions of masturbation focused on males, physicians often made passing reference to female masturbation. Becklard, in his early medical manual, maintained that girls masturbated just as much as boys but he did not believe they suffered as much for it. 'It does not drain their system, and hence, cannot cause them so much debility.' This may have been because in male masturbation the ejaculation of semen was a visible sign of loss of energy, whereas in female masturbation the evidence was less apparent. The *Canada Lancet* of 1887 declared it occurred in both sexes, and under similar conditions, leading to equal harm for both, especially in their mental vigour. In his *Sexual Organs: Their Use and Abuse*, John Hett opposed any form of sexual experience and felt that no one was immune from the temptations of masturbation, male or female, for even 'apparently good' children practised it.[64] Physicians generally associated it with the onset of puberty and adolescent sexual awakening. While the tendency was to link masturbation with adolescence, some doctors recognized that adult women masturbated. This was certainly the belief of Henry Garrigues: 'In older female children I do not believe the vice is so common as among boys, but later in life it is probably much more so in women than in men. This cannot be explained merely by the greater facilities offered the male sex for normal satisfaction of the sexual instinct without running the risk of having offspring. There are several reasons for it, one of which is the less degree of orgasm felt by women during normal sexual intercourse.'[65] This is the only reference I have found to the idea that women masturbated because they could not achieve sexual satisfaction through normal intercourse. If it represented the unstated belief or fear of others, it would account for the strong opposition to masturbation in women. It revealed either the failure of men as sexual partners or suggested that sexual feelings in women were so abnormal that only a deviant form of sexuality could satisfy it.

Physicians were convinced that masturbation in women was a cause of disease. According to some, it could occasion vulvitis, leucorrhoea, falling womb, irregular and painful menstruation, painful childbirth, nervous and hysterical affections, deafness, loss of strength and memory, paralysis, imbecility, and insanity.[66] Pierce felt masturbation led to excessive venery or indifference to the opposite sex. In either case the result was to be deplored. If the former, the woman was at the mercy of her body and vulnerable to premarital or extramarital sex; if the latter, her husband would find an indifferent and cold wife. If that was not enough to dissuade women, he warned them that masturbation would make their breasts flaccid.[67] Other physicians also felt that masturbation somehow could accentuate or eliminate woman's normal sexuality. It could lead to 'premature excitement of the sexual desire,' or, owing to the clitoris becoming loose, result in their becoming 'deficient in the sexual orgasm during coitus.'[68] While some warned that the symptoms of masturbation were becoming a bit exaggerated, few denied that ill effects were possible, although Garrigues believed, as did Becklard, that women had more resistance to these ill effects than men did.[69] But whether the repercussions of masturbation were exaggerated or not, and whether women could withstand their effects or not, the medical consensus was disapproval. So concerned did some physicians become about this that they developed painful operations to help women and especially girls stop the habit.[70] Although seldom performed in Canada, doctors elsewhere performed clitoridectomies in an effort to control masturbation.[71]

Belief in masturbation as a cause of disease meant that doctors could account for the ill health of their female patients when no other explanations were available. Mrs S.J. Barrows, a widow, was examined by Dr James Ross on 15 August 1892. She was experiencing fainting fits and her menstruation was clotted and painful. During the physical examination Ross noted, 'All organs normal.

This is evidently a case of onanism. Clitoris erected ... [and] Labia minora very much elongated.'[72] In his text, Garrigues explained to his student readers that female masturbation and its effects were necessary to understand because doctors might find themselves in a situation where 'by knowing the effects of masturbation' their testimony could exonerate an innocent man accused of rape.[73] The medical interest in this topic also provided scope for doctors to give advice. As we saw earlier, many believed they had a right to speak out on a wide variety of topics in an effort to protect the health of their patients. This even extended to bicycle riding. While most concern focused on the physical side-effects of the sport, the few physicians who were against it also raised the spectre of immorality. One author in the *Canadian Practitioner* of 1896 accused the women of Toronto of using cycling as 'a means of gratifying unholy and bestial desire.'[74] An editorial in the journal felt it necessary to refute the slander made against Toronto women, but the next year the *Dominion Medical Monthly* published an article that repeated the accusation that cycling was a new form of evil and argued that it was the duty of the medical profession to sound a warning against it.[75]

The emphasis the medical profession gave to masturbation in women seems excessive from the perspective of the present day. It reflected not just medical views but moral and social views as well. Most doctors saw masturbation as unnatural and it was its unnaturalness that caused disease. It was harmful, not because it was a sexual act, but because it was an anti-social sexual act. The motivation was self-gratification, unlike marital sex which was altruistic because it focused on a loved spouse. Add to this the threat of women's gaining sexual satisfaction without men, and the hostility to female masturbation becomes understandable.[76] Physicians seemed convinced that the body could distinguish between the motivation behind masturbation and the motivation behind sexual intercourse for the purpose of procreation and punish the one and reward the other. But whether punished or not, masturbation was a manifestation of sexual feelings in women and medical concern about it was a recognition of those feelings. It could be argued that this simply substantiates those historians who have viewed sexual passivity in women in the late nineteenth century as a normative value. When Victorians acknowledged sexuality in women, it was deemed abnormal. If masturbation was the only recognition of sexuality in women this would be true. Most physicians, however, discussed female sexuality in a way that revealed their belief in the naturalness of female erotic experience.

The overwhelming tendency of medical literature was to acknowledge the existence of sexuality in women.[77] As early as 1837, in a text that was used for the next few decades in Canada, P. Cazeaux described the physiological changes that women underwent during intercourse: 'During coition, the muscles of the perineum and vulva are excited to involuntary and convulsive contractions, [secretion] ... is expelled in an intermittent manner or by jets, as is the sperm in the ejaculation of the male.'[78] In his *Physiology of Man*, Austin Flint reported on a doctor who deliberately produced an orgasm in one of his woman patients so he could examine the physiological character of it.[79] Physicians recognized that orgasm occurred in women and that it was normal and part of nature.[80] Some physicians even believed that women were particularly susceptible to sexual stimulation. Becklard thought that without the natural release resulting from sexual intercourse, obscene images would come to women's minds.[81] For his part, Pierce worried about women who came into contact with debauched men, especially at dances. Such men could manipulate virtuous women and set 'on fire the courses of nature.'[82] Apparently a certain kind of literature could do the same, especially in unmarried women.[83] What is interesting about the medical acknowledgment of female sexuality was its accuracy. Victorian physicians knew where the centre of sexual pleasure was located in women – the clitoris. This might not appear to have been so extraordinary except for the fact that this information was eventually superseded by the Freudian interpretation of mature female response being centred in the vagina. Not until the modern studies of Masters and Johnson was the clitoris restored to its central place in the physiology of female sexual experience. This recognition on the part of nineteenth-century physicians was not limited to a few. Almost every text written on the subject acknowledged the role played in sexual arousal by the clitoris. As Garrigues made clear, 'The clitoris is the chief seat of sexual excitement in women.'[84] For doctors, it was analogous to the penis in man.

This recognition of female sexuality permeated society. Those running institutions of learning, extended care, and asylums were very careful to assure the public that every effort was made to maintain decorum, by which they most often meant sexual decorum. The Toronto Home for Incurables, in its rules, stipulated that male patients were not allowed in female rooms and vice versa, except in special cases. The bylaws of the Montreal General Hospital did likewise.[85] The sexual inclinations of women were acknowledged in the wider debate over higher education for women. Many critics opposed it because of the dangers co-education presented. Envisioning the consequences of male/female classroom competitiveness, the University of Toronto *Varsity* warned in 1880 that promiscuous intermingling of members of both sexes in the college lecture rooms and corridors would lead to intrigues fatal to those who indulged in them. But male students were not alone in fearing 'the proximity and competition of the "softer sex." '[86] Stalwart figures such as Goldwin Smith saw male/female relations in one context only. Since neither men nor women could avoid their sexual nature, he argued they should avoid needless association to maintain the modesty that decency demanded. Conveniently for men, that modesty meant that women should not enter any sphere in which they would compete with men. Smith feared that if women entered law, male judges, overcome as it were by the feminine appeal of lady lawyers, would be prejudiced in favour of their clients. Since this would happen in any profession women entered, Smith concluded that women should not have careers. And if women were not going to have careers, why give them advanced training alongside men? Considering his strong belief in sexual attraction, Smith could hardly envisage co-education as being conducive to work, unlike those who felt the presence of women would be a prod to male students.[87] Moreover, he and many others feared it would lead to the degeneracy of morals and manners on the part of both sexes, women losing their shy passivity when forced to compete with men and men losing that chivalric deference to the weaker sex when confronted by them as competitors – that is, it would threaten an entire social order.[88] That such contact occurred in the work place and often in a less than desirable environment did not seem to bother these pundits of Victorian morality – they applied the double standard to both sex and class.

Doctors may have recognized that the sex drive was strong in women, but even those who did were not always comfortable with the idea. Many were unable to see it as a drive in the same way as man's sexual nature. Man was active and woman received her satisfaction from him. Sexual feeling in women could exist and still correspond to the Victorian sense of balance if it was seen as less than man's.[89] In this way physicians were able to maintain the views of their society and still be true to the medial facts. Their own fears as men also played a part. This is not as strange as it might appear. Doctors during this period had to be circumspect with respect to their female patients. Canadians were very firm about men not taking sexual advantage of women and about seeing women as victims, not perpetrators, of sexual aggression. Popular wisdom assumed that women could control their sexual feelings; it was men who could not. Doctors, too, subscribed to this ideology except that they, more than most, knew the degree of sexual arousal that women could achieve and, consequently, feared what might happen if patients made advances towards them. Their status was not so secure they could assume they would be given the benefit of the doubt if charges of impropriety were made.

In the medical journal literature there are hints of this fear when cases of seduction brought against physicians are discussed. In 1858 the *Medical Chronicle* described such a case brought against a dentist who had used chloroform on a patient.[90] Although this charge was against a dentist, the medical profession was concerned because of the use of chloroform and the role it apparently played in the case. On 22 September 1858 Mrs Louisa Nichols consulted Dr John Horatio Webster in Montreal about some dental work she wanted done. He administered chloroform to her and, when she became conscious, she found herself not in the dental chair but on a sofa and 'felt the pressure of [Webster's] body' on her. She was aware at that time that he had 'taken criminal liberties' with her. She then sat up and asked that her husband be sent for, but became unconscious again owing to the effects of the chloroform. The next thing she knew was that Webster was sitting beside her with 'his hand in an improper position.' She finally regained enough strength to leave and returned to her home and told her husband what had occurred. After hearing Mrs Nichols's evidence and that of several other witnesses, the jury found Dr Webster guilty of administering a drug with the intent to commit rape and found him guilty of attempted rape. He subsequently spent seven months in jail. The foreman of the Grand Jury and the judge both stressed the need for medical men to be careful about administering chloroform and encouraged them to have witnesses present when they did so. As one historian who has examined the medical reaction to the case pointed out, underlying both the judge and the foreman's statements was a distrust of the profession in its power over patients. The medical press subsequently discussed the problems of using anaesthesia. Some physicians had difficulty accepting that Webster was guilty and felt if he could only prove he had used ether and not chloroform, then an explanation would be possible. They believed that ether tended to excite the mind and body of the patient: 'This had been particularly noticed in the mucous membranes of the generative organs of women.' So reluctant were they to admit the possibility of patients being taken advantage of that they even blamed the victim. Mrs Nichols apparently was menstruating when she consulted Webster and the editor of the *Medical Chronicle* concluded from this that '[she was] in a condition which rendered her peculiarly susceptible to excitement of these [generative] organs on the suspension of the will, and, as a consequence, her dreams or delusion would take their complexion from the excited sexual function.'[91] The attempted rape did not occur, it was in the mind of the patient because of her own body.

In 1883 an editorial in the *Canadian Practitioner* indicated that the charge of seduction against physicians was still a danger.[92] The editor of the *Canada Lancet* agreed and reprinted a paper given by John Gaynor at the New Brunswick Medical Society in 1883 about the effect of chloroform and the vulnerability of physicians because of its effects. Dr Gaynor argued that the anaesthesia made patients, both men and women, emphasize their natural proclivities. In men this was self-preservation and in women preservation of the species. This meant that under anaesthesia men became very combative whereas women's 'thought and sensations usually [ran] in procreative channels.' His moral: 'Never anaesthetize a female excepting in the presence of a third person.'[93] In 1886 seduction was still an issue, for the editor of the *Canada Lancet* felt warranted in reprinting a piece which complimented the profession on how few charges of seduction were made against its members despite the temptations that presented themselves: 'Weak women, who are diffident and shy to all other males, frequently conceive for their physician a passion which it would require but a slight response to convert to a crime. We apprehend there are few of our readers whom professional experience has not convinced of this frailty (which may, after all, be more or less physiological) on the part of the weaker vessel.'[94] When medical practitioners were at risk they saw women's sexuality as something quite aggressive, a trait they seldom recognized in women in any other context.

Although recognizing the physicality of female sexuality, the medical profession was uncomfortable with it. One way to reconcile their medical knowledge with their social beliefs that women were more morally pure than men was for physicians to argue that sexuality in women existed for a higher purpose than individual gratification – the propagation of the species. The idea of woman needing orgasm to conceive went back to the Greek physician Galen and was also taken up and given moral legitimacy in Christian doctrine. Many nineteenth-century physicians simply continued in that presumption, although their adherence to it had lessened.[95] Physicians believed that women were most fertile at or around menstruation, which also was the time when they were more easily aroused.[96] While some doctors recognized that sexual arousal may not have been necessary for conception, they felt it could not hurt and might even help. Orgasm and procreation were different sides of a physiologically normal adult woman.[97] At mid-century one text argued that, although their sexual feelings did not dominate women, the one exception was at the time of childbirth, as a form of compensation for the pain they experienced.[98] As seen in chapter 2, some even suggested that sexual arousal in women was linked to the sex of the child conceived. The *Canadian Practitioner* reprinted an article from the *Medical Recorder* that claimed 'at the generation of male offspring the mother must be in a higher degree of sexual excitement than the father. And, reversely, at the generation of female offspring the father must be in a higher state of such excitement than the mother.'[99] Thus in order to conceive, in order to give birth to male children, sex feelings in women became respectable; maternity endowed sexuality with an important social function and morality.[100] Woman's submission to her sex function was not a recognition of her sexuality but of her reproductivity. Procreation defined the limits of healthy sexual activity in women; refusing to abide by this could lead to ill health.

Ira Warren in *Household Physician* warned women that because their sexual passions, other than for purposes of procreation, and their duty were in conflict with one another, they should not be surprised that stress was visited upon their ovaries and ovaritis could develop.[101] Alvin Chase and Garrigues in their writings both pointed out that masturbation and exciting thoughts as a result of reading novels could lead to disease, although Garrigues also believed that even normal coition could be a problem if engaged in too violently.[102] Napheys believed that too little sexual activity was as harmful as too much.[103] Moderation was clearly the ideal. William Goodell even felt that long engagements were injurious to women owing to the increase in sexual nervous excitement. Unlike men, women were particularly susceptible because they could not work such excitement out of their bodies through engaging in business activities.[104] Of particular concern about sexual intercourse and disease in women was the belief that if coitus occurred during menstruation it placed the women at risk.[105] As seen in chapter 3, the taboo on intercourse during menstruation had a long history behind it.

It is often difficult to know the effect these kinds of beliefs had on physicians' actual treatment of patients. There is some suggestion that, in practice, the profession was not as moralizing as it was in print. For example, a young single woman came to the Halifax Victoria General Hospital in 1900 suffering from syphilis, claiming she had shared a bed the summer before with a girl who had sores over all her body. Although her physician was probably dubious about her story, there was no suggestion of it in the patient record, nor was there any moralizing. She was simply given regular treatment.[106] But what is intriguing about the records is that while doctors did not seem to be judgmental, they did seem to react to sexually transmitted diseases in women differently from in men. In the case records of men who had gonorrhoea there was a tendency to lay the blame on women – that is, a need to write down that the man had had connection with a specific woman. In cases of women with gonorrhoea there was no similar concern to link her disease with sexual intercourse with a man, as if it would not be in good taste to acknowledge that this had actually occurred. For men, women were a specific threat, the carrier of disease; for women the threat was more vague, unrecognized. But if physicians were not particularly judgmental, they could still respond in ways that appear to be excessive. In 1894 the *Canada Lancet* reprinted an article by William Goodell in which he reported two cases of women from whom he removed ovaries because their sexual feelings appeared abnormal. The first was a young woman 'of high intelligence' who had been 'reduced to a pitiable condition of ill-health by menorrhagia and by frequent acts of self-abuse.' The second woman was a middle-aged spinster who he termed 'queer, but not insane enough to be confined.' At her monthly periods she desired sexual intercourse to such an extent that she feared she would eventually give in to that desire. In both cases Goodell operated to reduce the women's sexual urges, and in both cases he claimed success.[107]

But whether or not physicians' attitudes about female sexuality influenced the medical treatment women received, they did determine the advice doctors gave. Because many believed that sexuality in women was for the higher purpose of conception and because unwise experience of sexuality could lead to physical harm, physicians felt obliged to advise their patients and other women about the proper limits of sexual intercourse. Suggestions were made about when the best time was to conceive. Napheys advised the spring, believing that children conceived then had a better chance of surviving.[108] Most physicians, however, suggested what time of the monthly cycle would be most propitious but, as we have already seen, this usually meant giving incorrect advice to women. There was a concern that too frequent intercourse would defeat its procreative purpose. Pierce advised women who were having difficulty conceiving to restrain from intercourse for a while. He also warned them that the nervous excitement resulting from intercourse would be followed by depression and that excess would lead to health problems.[109] In his directions Flint was more specific. He advised women not to engage in intercourse before menstruation, during menstruation, during most of any pregnancy, and only within a legitimate relationship and when both partners were healthy. Ironically, he admitted that few people would follow his advice 'as so few men and women in civilized life are absolutely normal during adult age, and as the sources of unnatural sexual excitement are so numerous.'[110] Nonetheless, doctors continued to impose various restrictions on sexual activity – not after conception, not for three months after the birth of a child, or when the husband was drunk.[111] Only rarely did a physician encourage sexual activity for marital happiness. Jefferis in *Searchlights on Health* seemed particularly sympathetic to women in this regard. He argued that sexuality was important for the marital relationship, but even he counselled intercourse only once a month. What distinguished his advice, however, was the power it gave to women. He exhorted husbands, both new and old, to be much more careful about preparing their wives for intercourse and accused husbands who did not of wife-torturing. He advised husbands that their wives had the right to decide on whether separate beds were necessary. As he phrased it in words that have a very modern ring, 'she has the superior right to control her own person.'[112] But even when sympathetic to women, physicians, like Jefferis, believed they had the obligation to comment on a practice which until then had not been viewed as medical. Physicians had become the counsellors of sex. They were creating a medical sexual norm to which their patients were to adhere. Whereas once the retribution for transgressing sexual norms had been spiritual, now it was physical. Medicine had replaced religion as 'the giver of retribution for immoral behaviour.'[113] And the retribution was not always imagined. Physicians did see the consequences when women apparently strayed from accepted mores. Consider the young unmarried girl who had been engaging in sexual intercourse since she was fourteen. On 25 October 1878, at the age of fifteen, she entered the Burnside Lying-In Hospital in Toronto. Perhaps because of her youth and slight build, she underwent a difficult childbirth and haemorrhaged badly.[114] Or consider Annie Farrady, twenty-eight, single and a domestic servant who entered the Victoria General Hospital on 5 May 1882 suffering from syphilis. After four years of various treatment, doctors believed that surgery was now her only hope.[115] These were not unusual cases and, no matter what physicians morally felt about such women, they, as doctors, more than anyone, other than the women themselves, understood the potential consequences of sexual transgression – whether it was the woman's or her partner's.

In its attitudes towards female sexuality, the medical profession had found one more experience in a woman's life on which to lay claim. As with almost every other experience women had, sexual activity had its medical repercussions. While doctors recognized the existence of strong sexual urges within women, they appeared to be uncomfortable with them. Such desires negated the poplar and widely accepted image of women in society as morally superior to men and contradicted the need for this sexual purity in those whose responsibility it was to bear and nurture children. So strong was the conflict between the two that some doctors seemed to wish for female sexuality to disappear. They were so disturbed by the notion of woman as a sexual being that they denied it or viewed evidence of it as a form of deviance. The majority of physicians, however, could not. The physiological facts were before them, so their challenge was to reconcile reality with normative values. They did not want to repress female sexual activity but to moderate it. Consequently, many continued to link female sexuality with conception. The latter made the former respectable. Take away the possibility of conception and sexual intercourse became unacceptable. It is one reason that the medical profession was opposed to birth control.

Chapter Five

A Modern Issue Emerges:
Birth Control

Just before Henriette Dessaulles's marriage, her future sister-in-law Jos expressed the hope that her brother and Henriette would wait a few years before starting a family. That night, 15 January 1881, Henriette confided to her diary, 'I suppose Jos doesn't know any more about it than I do, but her words "I hope ..." imply that people only have children when they really want to.' She felt this made sense, but the situation of poor families did not suggest to her that it was always possible. She recalled one family she knew in which 'the mother and father were down in the dumps because they are going to have a sixth child, while the other five don't have enough to eat. Surely, when there is no work, that is too many children for their means.' She concluded, 'Isn't it up to them, then, to decide not to have any more?'[1] Dessaulles may have thought the obvious answer to that question was yes, but not all Canadians agreed. Her own education in a convent school had not taught her to control family size and, until her future sister-in-law raised the issue, she had never even considered the possibility of doing so. These two young, French-Catholic women, born and raised in Quebec, were quite typical of women across Canada – Dessaulles, ignorant of birth control and prepared to accept children as they came, and Jos, who clearly was aware that women did not have to bear children they did not want. What method of birth control she had in mind we do not know, but she certainly would have received little information about it from doctors.

Physicians saw most forms of birth control as unnatural and representing women's rejection of motherhood. Ignoring the fact that for some birth control methods to work the co-operation of the male partner was essential, doctors castigated women for limiting the size of their families. And as was the case in other instances when women did not conform to their 'supposed' place in society, doctors argued that birth control would result in physical harm to women. This belief could and did affect their response to their women patients. Birth control was one more issue over which the medical profession laid claim, but their success in doing so was mixed. On the public level they succeeded, for their antagonism to birth control became reflected in stringent laws which made providing contraceptive information and devices illegal. On the private level, however, they failed. Condemnation of birth control simply did not make sense to many women or address the realities of their lives.

Traditionally, historians assumed that people in the past had not practised any form of contraception. Indeed, historians were not aware there were any effective birth control methods available until the advent of the Pill and modern birth control technology made birth control a possibility for most people. But as scholars have probed the history of women and the history of the family, they have discovered quite the opposite – the widespread use of contraception. The general consensus is that middle-class couples adopted some form of family planning first in an attempt to restrict their expenditures and preserve their economic place in society. Only later did working-class families adopt birth control, perhaps because their children remained of economic benefit to them longer than children of the middle classes.[2] While agreeing with this interpretation as far as it goes, Edward Shorter has argued that workers were not simply passive emulators of the middle class but in turn influenced them; the growing autonomy of working-class women, for example, became accepted as an ideal for the daughters of the middle class.[3] But whether from the middle class downward or from the working class upward, increasing numbers of people were restricting the size of their families. How did they do this? Some historians have suggested that the change in sexual ideology was one way of accomplishing this end. Certainly in the English-speaking world the idealization of moderation and sexual control for both sexes, but particularly for women, coincided with the decline in the birth rate and may have partially caused it. In addition, and more surprising from the twentieth-century perspective, active and numerous birth control techniques were available – abstinence, abortion, infanticide, sterilization, pessaries, use of herbal concoctions, vaginal sponges, diaphragms, condoms, coitus interruptus, coitus obstructus, coitus reservatus, douching, prolonged breast feeding, and even an inaccurate version of the rhythm method.[4] The recourse to birth control and the subsequent decline in the birth rate had repercussions for the health of women. Fewer pregnancies reduced a woman's chances of dying in childbirth. And because her body underwent the stresses of pregnancy less often, she was more likely to be healthy when she became pregnant, which in turn lessened the chances of mortality and morbidity for both her and her child.[5]

The evidence is clear that Canadians were using some form of fertility control. The general fertility rate in Canada declined from 189 per thousand in 1871 to 144 in 1871, or by 24 per cent.[6] One factor that accounted for part of this drop was the increase in the average age at which women married. In the 1850s the average age at first marriage for women was 23; in 1871, 25.4, and by 1891 it was 26.7 This delay limited women's childbearing years within marriage and partially bypassed their most fertile years. But why were young women delaying marriage? Certainly they were spending more time in school, consequently prolonging dependency and postponing their entry into the workforce and marriage market. Secondly, material aspirations were increasing at a time when economic prospects in Canada were not keeping pace and for many Canadians, men and women, in both rural and urban areas, it simply made good economic sense to delay getting married until they could afford to set up a separate household. Once married, however, women still restricted family size. In 1871 the legitimate fertility rate was very close to what it had been in the eighteenth century but within the next twenty years it plummeted, especially among older women. For those aged thirty-five the decrease was 35 per cent, and for those aged forty it was 50 per cent. Older women were practising some form of family limitation. As with delayed age of marriage, economic factors appear to have been the reason why this was so.

The decline in family size was particularly noticeable in the urban centres and among the middle classes.[8] Children in urban settings were not as economically useful as children on farms, where cheap labour was needed and willing hands could always be used. In an urban setting, children were an economic liability except for those families who sent their children out to work at a young age. In the early stages of industrialization, children were in demand as workers, but as the century progressed there was less interest in them, especially when employers could hire cheap female or immigrant labour. In addition, by the end of the century, child labour laws began to be passed in several of the provinces and, while they did not apply to all work situations, they did restrict the availability of jobs for young people and signalled a new, disapproving attitude towards the use of child labour. Compulsory school attendance laws in some provinces also added to the difficulty children had in seeking employment. Although neither the child labour laws nor compulsory school attendance provisions were universally implemented, they were applied more frequently and better enforced in urban centres. In the face of such changes, it was difficult for those families aspiring to middle-class status to send their children out to work. Middle-class ideology valued education, and middle-class parents became aware of the need to train their sons in careers if they were to get ahead in life or even maintain their middle-class status. Training for girls was also deemed desirable, either to prepare them for their future role as wives and mothers or to ensure economic security for them if they did not marry or were widowed. Such training resulted in children living at home and being a financial drain on the family longer. The effect of these various changes, pressures, and ideologies was to make supporting a large family costly. While it is understandable why the urban middle class wanted to limit the size of their families, this group cannot account for the general decline of the birth rate. Since most nineteenth-century Canadians lived in rural areas, the birth rate could not decrease significantly unless people on farms began to limit the size of their families as well.

Farm families were experiencing their own pressures to reduce family size.[9] Case studies have revealed that the size of farm families was linked to the stage of development of the farm. In the early years, farm labour was scarce, in part because land was readily available and people did not want to work for someone else when they could work for themselves. Children were, therefore, vital as a labour force. As long as land was available or economic opportunities existed close by, there were few difficulties in providing for all one's children. But when land and opportunities decreased, parents had to be concerned, for a single farm could not provide for all the children when they became adults, married, and had families of their own. Neither could the family farm be divided and still be economically viable. When rural opportunities decreased, more cheap casual labour was available for hire and child labour became less vital than it had been. Farm mechanization further reduced the need for farm labour and limited it to certain seasons. At the same time, farmers increased their debt load by expanding their holdings and/or buying farm machinery.This further reduced the wages that could be paid to farm workers. Farmers' sons could see few prospects for themselves on the land, for as farm labourers they would not earn enough to buy their own farms. Usually only one son inherited the family farm, and this was increasingly coming to him encumbered with debt owing to the father's desire to provide for his other children out of this inheritance. Large families were becoming a liability and the response of farm families was similar to that of families in urban centres – reduce the number of children. This was particularly true in the more settled farm areas in Ontario, where farm land was expensive and little land was available to set up children on farms of their own. Proof of the economic squeeze on farm families was the increasing out-migration by farm sons and daughters during this period. They were unwilling to stay where there was little future for them except as

casual workers. That their parents understood this reaction is reflected in the declining birth rate among farm families and the
resultant demand on the government to allow cheap agricultural
labourers into the country. What was good enough for these immigrant farm workers was not good enough for the children of
Canadian farmers.[10]

Of course Canadians in the late nineteenth century did not make
the above analysis. Those aware of and worried about the declining birth rate blamed the impact of modern life. As we have
already seen, one of the reasons that physicians and many Canadians were concerned about higher education for women was
their not unwarranted fear that it led to women's limiting the size
of their families or rejecting marriage altogether. If this was not
bad enough, physicians also believed that civilization was weakening women's ability to conceive and bear healthy children because it was undermining their health. Men, too, seemed less
inclined to marry and raise a family. According to one author in
the *Canada Lancet* of 1894, 'Thirty or forty years ago young men
used to rush by blind instinct into the toils of matrimony – because
they couldn't help themselves'; but now 'they shilly-shally, they
pick and choose, they discuss, they criticize, they say foolish
things about the club and the flat and the cost of living. They
believe in Malthus. Fancy a young man who believes in Malthus!'[11]
Although realizing that young men feared the economic responsibilities of marriage, the author believed that this had become
a smoke-screen to hide the real reason – that young men simply
were not as capable of reproducing as their fathers. Civilization
by creating an artificial life had weakened them. Even worse, the
effects of civilization were visited more on the 'better' classes
than on others.[12] This did not bode well for the future of Canada.
It also placed physicians in an awkward position, for it was the
'better' classes who were their patients and it was the women
among them who were asking doctors for information on how to
prevent conception.[13] This would not have posed a problem except that most physicians disapproved of birth control – it went
against nature, it challenged women's social role in society, and
many forms of it were illegal.

Of particular concern was abortion. Physicians certainly knew that some of their patients resorted to abortion. The minutes of the 15 December 1863 council meeting of the Nova Scotia Medical Society discussed one doctor who had called on a patient and discovered she had self-aborted by inserting a stick into her vagina. She even bragged to him that she had done so many times before. While she later claimed she had been joking, she did admit she had learned how to bring about an abortion when she was in Boston.[14] In Ontario, Dr Alfred Andrew from Windsor estimated he had at least fifty women a year coming to him seeking termination of their pregnancies.[15] Physicians were also aware of advertisements for abortifacients in the newspapers. Promoted as 'Periodical Pills' to regulate women's monthly cycle – that is, to help menstruation occur – it was clear that such pills could be used to bring about abortion in the warning that accompanied the ads: 'Pregnant women are cautioned against their use.'[16] Such a warning served two purposes. It kept the promotions legal, for the law prohibited advertising abortifacients. It also let the customer know that if the product were used incorrectly, it could end a pregnancy. What the customer did with that information was up to her. Certainly she would have no difficulty purchasing such pills. While an editorial in the 1871 *Canada Lancet* railed against Clarke's Female Pills and Hooper's Female Pills, it acknowledged that many more were available.[17] Dr Holloway's Pills, Ayers's Cathartic Pills, and Dr Rodway's Pills were among those that newspapers frequently advertised.[18] The 4 April 1861 edition of the *Montreal Gazette* had almost one-half of the front page devoted to advertising Dr Holloway's Pills, Dr Rodway's Pills, Spalding's Cephalic Pills, and Moffat's Life Pills. Accessible substances linked to abortion also abounded – pennyroyal, savin, black draught, oil of cedar, tansy tea, oil of savron, ergot of rye, myrrh, hellebore, cantharides, quinine, cotton root, and Christmas Rose. Lyman and Sons in Montreal manufactured 'Ladies Safe Remedies: Apoline.' The Nootka women on the west coast had their own concoctions. They mixed a solution from a three-leaved plant with a white star flower and mashed the roots in water and then drank the solution to effect an abortion. In addition, all types of instruments could be used – soft rubber catheters, male catheters, and female syringes.[19]

With such a variety of pills, medicinal substances, and instruments available, it was no wonder that physicians feared abortion was on the rise. According to the *Canada Health Journal* in 1871, women purchased periodic pills with 'avidity' and, in what was most likely an overstatement, accused the public conscience of becoming so callous that 'the murder of offspring unborn, whether by drugs or mechanical violence, is recognized as the legitimate occupation of many, and the occasional practice of three-fourths of our matrons.'[20] One year later, the *Canada Lancet* in an editorial warned that abortion 'is fearfully on the increase both here and in the United States ...; nor is it confined to that unfortunate class whose only fault is that they have "loved too well," but prevails to an alarming extent even among otherwise respectable married women.' Four years later, Dr Alfred Andrew claimed that the incidence of abortion was so high it was an epidemic worse than typhus or smallpox.[21] In 1892 a British physician writing in the *Canada Medical Record* blamed the use of abortifacients for the rising rate of stillbirth. In such cases the abortifacients had not resulted in an abortion but had caused enough damage to the fetus to prevent a live delivery.[22] By 1900 the perception of some in society was even more catastrophic. A contributor to the *Canadian Churchman* in 1990 warned that the pressures of modern society were such as to embolden 'to put it bluntly, in nine cases out of ten, women to murder their unborn children.[23]

Physicians understood why some women resorted to abortion. The 1870 *Canada Health Journal* acknowledged that poverty often drove women to abort when they discovered they were pregnant with a child they could ill afford. Ill health could also make women reluctant to give birth.[24] Windsor's Dr Andrew believe that those who came to him requesting abortions did so because they were desperate. Many were young, single women who found themselves pregnant. He noted, however, that many married women implored him to abort them as well.[25] In *The Practical Home Physician* published in 1884, Henry Lyman provided a fairly sympathetic account of women who resorted to abortion, seeing them as wives whose husbands forced themselves sexually on them without considering the consequences – pregnancies the women did not want.[26] George Napheys listed several reasons why women might contemplate abortion. He pointed out that bearing too many children was not good for the health of either the mother or the children. Diseases that would prohibit a woman from carrying a child easily sometimes appeared only after marriage and, for such women, pregnancy was 'torture.' He also recognized that some women would die in childbirth. While realizing that women did become pregnant when it was not medically safe, he favoured birth control to prevent the pregnancy rather than abortion after the pregnancy.[27] But whatever the circumstances, Napheys and other doctors agreed that abortion was not the decision of the woman to make but her physician's.[28] They feared that if left on their own, women would resort to abortion for what were essentially selfish reasons.

The *Canada Health Journal* published an article which accused some women of wanting abortions because they viewed pregnancy as decreasing their attractiveness. Certainly economic reasons were not applicable to the middle class.[29] An editorial in the *Canada Lancet* agreed that the dictates of fashion were behind many abortions.[30] One writer to the *Sanitary Journal* of 1876 argued: 'the demands of society in this so-called civilized age are very trying to females. The love of idleness is a most pernicious evil.' As a result, women were forgoing the demands of maternity.[31] Martin Holbrook felt that women perhaps had a sense of shame regarding pregnancy or simply wanted to avoid the cares of maternity.[32] Doctors referred to women seeking abortions as 'unnatural mothers' and to married ones as 'degraded' and 'inhuman' for attempting to avoid maternity, and demanded punishment for those who were perverting 'the highest function of woman's nature, and [turning] blessings into cursings.'[33] Even when a woman aborted naturally, there was sometimes a suggestion it was her fault. One woman, who had given birth to several children and had miscarried others before delivery, was admitted to the University Lying-In Hospital, Montreal, on 19 May 1896 having spontaneously aborted another fetus. The notes on her case remarked that alcoholic excess and frequent coitus were the only known causes that could explain her losing her child.[34] Of more concern, however, was deliberate or criminal abortion. The conscious rejection of maternity appalled physicians, for it called into question what they and others considered to be the natural balance between the sexes and could only result in the collapse of ordered society as they knew it. Despite the rhetoric that abounded at the time about the maternal ideal and how devoted women were to their children, there was a sense that many women rejected maternity relatively easily and would continue to do so unless they were stopped. Physicians felt only they should determine when pregnancies could be terminated, and the indications for this were limited.

Dr Andrew described the case of one woman who he had aborted in 1845. She suffered from a very severe pelvic deformity and, on the three times that she had given birth, a craniotomy or a cutting operation on the child was performed. To avoid this trauma a fourth time, he agreed to abort her but, recalling it thirty years later, wrote that if faced with the same situation he would instead perform a Caesarian section.[35] While this had the virtue of providing some opportunity for the child to survive, the chances of the mother's surviving were not particularly good, maternal mortality rates from Caesarians being very high. Thus he was willing to place the mother's life in jeopardy rather than resort to abortion. For his part, Napheys had no hesitation about where his loyalties lay: 'Better, far better, to bear a child every year for twenty years than to resort to such a wicked and injurious step; better to die; if needs be, in the pangs of child-birth, than to live with such a weight of sin on the conscience.'[36] Such a sentiment was largely rhetoric to persuade women to reject abortion. Most physicians, when faced with the decision to choose between the life of the child or the life of the mother, chose the mother.

Physicians had good reasons to be hostile towards abortion. It was a criminal offense and physicians could be and were prosecuted for performing it. This had not always been the case. Not until 1803 did England pass legislation that prohibited abortion. The penalties, however, were different depending on whether the women had quickened (felt fetal movement) or not. Death was the punishment for performing abortion after quickening, but transportation for fourteen years was the maximum sentence if the abortion occurred before quickening. New Brunswick (1810) and Prince Edward Island (1836) were the first colonies to pass abortion legislation in British North America and each maintained the distinction between an abortion performed before and after quickening. It is difficult to know why this early legislation was passed – there was no public debate on the issue and little evidence that authorities ever enforced the laws. In 1841 when Upper Canada passed its first abortion act it abolished the quickening distinction, as did New Brunswick in 1842. In none of the jurisdictions which had abortion laws was the woman liable to prosecution for attempting to abort herself; the focus was on the abortionist. Amendments to the New Brunswick Act (1849) and the introduction of Nova Scotia's first abortion law (1851), however, removed that protection. The full weight of the criminal law could now be brought to bear against the woman, and this became true across the country when the federal government took over criminal law jurisdiction and in 1869 essentially adopted the New Brunswick legislation. The maximum penalty for abortion was life imprisonment.[37] In 1892 with the consolidation of the Criminal Code, section 179(c) made it clear that in the public realm abortion and birth control were not acceptable. It stipulated a two-year sentence for anyone who 'without lawful excuse or justification, offers to sell, advertises, publishes an advertisement of, or has for sale or disposal any medicine, drug or article intended or represented as a means of preventing conception or causing abortion.'[38] Doctors applauded the restrictive legislation. Many were antagonistic towards the women who sought abortions and believed that the woman should be liable to prosecution as much as the abortionist. Arguing that she 'is the chief criminal, either herself soliciting the performance of the criminal act, or submitting willingly to the influences of the seducer, that it should be performed,' one author in the *Canada Lancet* concurred with the federal government's making life imprisonment the maximum penalty and even suggested that in some cases death might be considered if it would 'prevent a violation of both Divine and human laws.'[39] Abortions debased 'the country both morally and physically.' In 1889 the editors of the *Canada Lancet* even went so far as to urge physicians to report any approach made to them for abortions.[40] Patients who wanted abortions were the enemy. They were women who rejected their natural role and were trying to embroil their physicians in a criminal act.

References to criminal abortion trials in the medical literature reminded physicians of the seriousness of the offence. In 1861 the *British American Journal* detailed the case against an 'unlicensed practitioner' charged with murdering a young woman by administering drugs prescribed to effect an abortion.[41] Seven years later the *Provincial Medical Journal* reported the trial of Robert Notman of Montreal, accused of procuring and counselling abortion. He had made Margaret Galbraith pregnant and subsequently advised her to abort the child. She received ergot of rye from a Dr Patton, but when this failed to work a miscarriage was brought about through use of instruments. Two days later Dr Patton was found dead in his room, the result of poisoning, whether accidental or deliberate was never determined. If not for that, Dr Patton, too, would have been on trial. In his charge to the jury, the judge pointed out that unfair though it might appear, the law did not allow Miss Galbraith to be charged. However, her lover could be. 'The jury would judge if the prisoner would be allowed to sacrifice not only the life of his unborn illegitimate child, but also risk the chance of killing the woman who had given her honor for her guilty love for him.' The jury's verdict was guilty.[42] Any doctor could find himself at risk, vulnerable to the pleadings of his patients, especially when those patients were well-to-do. The 1884 *Canada Medical and Surgical Journal* reported the case of Dr Archibald Lawson of Halifax. Mrs O'Connor, a widow in 'comfortable circumstances,' consulted him and requested an abortion. The doctor agreed and charged her $50, a large sum for those days and perhaps one that made the risk worthwhile to Lawson. Unfortunately, the abortion was followed by puerperal septicaemia and Mrs O'Connor died. Before her death, however, she implicated Lawson. On hearing this, Lawson quickly left the city and so could not be charged. What is significant about this case is that Dr Lawson was not a quack or even a young practitioner in need of patients. He was a prominent member of the Halifax medical profession and a lecturer on the principles and practice of medicine in the School of Medicine.[43] The lessons of such a case were obvious to all – no physician was immune to temptation, but succumbing was not worth the consequences if caught.

The publicity that such inquests, trials, and reports garnered in the popular press did not help the efforts of practitioners to be seen as professionals. They tried hard to curb their own fraternity, but it was not always possible, and when one fell into disrepute he cast his shadow on the rest. Certainly, doctors would have been hesitant to call Dr Thomas Neill Cream one of their own. Under the guise of performing abortions, Cream killed his victims. Suspicion was first cast on him in 1879 when the body of a chambermaid was discovered in a privy near his Dundas Street, London, Ontario, office. Apparently she had come to see him about an abortion. While many suspected that Cream had murdered the woman, no charges were filed. However, with his practice in ruins, Cream left for Chicago where he continued to see Canadian patients. In 1880 American officials arrested him for the murder of another Canadian woman who also had consulted him about an abortion. The evidence against him was not conclusive and the charges had to be dropped. Only in 1891 was he arrested in London, England, for the murder of several young women, found guilty, and executed.[44]

It was not just the illegality of abortion that made practitioners shy away from it. Even if abortion were legal, most physicians did not feel it was moral. A *Canada Health Journal* article argued that it was a crime against God because the fetus was alive as soon as it was conceived.[45] Such an argument was relatively new, for conventional wisdom did not recognize the life of a fetus until the mother felt it move within her at about the fourteenth week of her pregnancy, Quickening had been the basis on which the law had traditionally determined what penalty for abortion should be imposed. Although the law had changed and physicians now recognized the continuous spectrum of life after conception, many in society still made the quickening distinction. Other Canadians were simply not concerned about the issue at all. In 1862-3 a scandal broke out in the Red River settlement when it became known that the Rev. Corbett, an Anglican minister suspected of impregnating his ex-servant Maria Thomas, had attempted an abortion on her. Maria was fifteen at the time and the Rev. Corbett, not being expert in abortion procedures, attempted to effect one five different times. In one instance he used 'a certain instrument or piece of wire, tied with tape to the fore finger of his right hand and with the point of the wire projecting about half an inch or three quarters of an inch beyond the point of his said finger ... he ... insert[ed] it into her *vagina* ... and towards and in the direction of the *os uteri* or mouth of the womb.' What is fascinating about this incident was not just the fact that the abortionist was a minister but that in the trial that ensued, although found guilty, Corbett was sentenced to only six months' incarceration with no loss of property. Even at that, some within the community thought the sentence overly harsh.[46] Doctors were out of step with many Canadians in their attitudes towards abortion.

Those Canadians who supported the doctors' view and disapproved of abortions were often reluctant to raise the issue in a public way because of distaste for discussing sexual issues and from a reluctance to face the reasons behind abortion and the willingness of many women to resort to it. The Dominion WCTU, through its Purity Department, acknowledged in 1891 that abortions did occur, but the hesitancy of that organization to come to grips with it was obvious. After discussing the need for proper health training for young people, the convenor abruptly changed the subject and wrote: 'There is another matter to which I feel reference should be made, and that is, pre-natal infanticide. Immortal souls are thus by the mother's will denied a natural existence. We must remind them of the command, "Thou shalt do no murder."' Having done her duty by recognizing what was obviously an unpleasant reality, she went on to discuss the problems Canadians were facing as a result of newly arrived immigrants.[47] Doctors, then, were the major group in society for whom abortion was a public issue.

The hostility that physicians exhibited towards abortion was directed to non-medical abortions – that is, abortions performed by the woman herself or by doctors and quacks who were operating outside the regular medical fraternity. In the case of the latter, the potential for undermining the economic interests of physicians was great. We have already seen that physicians did not have a monopoly over medical practice until the end of the century. Until then, regular practitioners were concerned about competition from those they believed to be unlicensed and unqualified. They wanted to separate themselves from such individuals in the public mind, and one way to do this was to harp on such irregular practitioners' being the source of abortionists.[48] Abortionists and drug companies offering potential abortifacients competed with physicians. A series of ads by the A.M.C. Medicine Company Ltd of St Paul Street in Montreal promoting its 'all-vegetable' products exhorted women to use the product that 'puts to shame the family doctor.' In an appeal to the reluctance of women to talk over intimate topics with a physician, the promotion told them that at the St Paul Street office 'experienced ladies are in attendance every day ... whose duties are to confer with ladies desiring fuller explanation regarding the action of these great woman's medicines, than can be given in a pamphlet or in a newspaper advertisement.'[49]

Physicians who opposed abortion felt vulnerable when they refused their patients something they obviously wanted. Indeed, in 1889 the editors of the *Canada Lancet* feared that, if doctors refused abortions, their patients would accuse them of performing them anyway, simply to gratify their resentment. Especially at risk were young doctors whose practices were financially precarious. Despite this concern, the editors extolled the profession 'that so few have fallen victim to so alluring a temptation.' But the insecurity remained,[50] and practitioners had every right to feel insecure. Take the case of Emily Howard Stowe. In 1879 a domestic servant, Sarah Ann Lovell, consulted Stowe, wanting medicines 'to bring on her periods.' When Stowe refused, Lovell threatened to drown herself. To calm her, Stowe prescribed tincture of myrrh, tincture of hellebore, and tincture of cantharides, all believed to be abortifacients, though in a harmless dosage. This all came out at a trial to investigate the death of Lovell from congestion of the lungs. After hearing Stowe's testimony, Mr Justice McKenzie directed a not-guilty verdict. Nevertheless, Stowe had gone through an ordeal and her case suggests the vulnerability of doctors to their patients. Even with the not-guilty verdict, Stowe's tribulations were not over, for the *Canada Lancet* described the trial in some detail and the editors could not refrain from commenting on her actions: 'It was a most unfortunate prescription, as Dr Stowe admitted, taking the most charitable view of the case.'[51] For a physician such as Stowe who was already marginalized because of her sex, such pronouncements in the leading medical journal in the country could only serve to increase her vulnerability.

To reinforce their own self-image as health providers and to encourage their patients to reject the idea of abortion because of the awkward and dangerous position in which it placed them, physicians described in vivid detail the health problems that would result to women who underwent abortion.[52] The *Canada Health Journal* of May 1870 was particularly clear on this score. Abortion led to sterility, inability to carry a child to full term, to a general breakdown in health, and, if this was not enough, to loneliness in old age.[53] Others believed it caused leucorrhoea, displacement and falling of the womb, ovarian disorders, inflammation of reproductive organs, fistulae, insanity, and inability to produce any but sickly children.[54] Some of the problems, of course, were a result of the conditions under which abortions had to be performed. Mrs Letitia Smollet, a forty-four-year-old widow, entered the Victoria General Hospital in Halifax on 29 September 1891. Her case history indicated that sixteen years previously, believing herself pregnant, she aborted herself using a knitting needle, another woman telling her how to do it. She hemorrhaged for about a day but, according to her own report, she never felt well afterwards, at times feeling weak after any exertion.[55] But abortion did not have to lead to ill health. After the 1880s abortion was a relatively safe medical procedure. Indeed, in 1881 an article in the *Canada Lancet* detailed how to induce an abortion, concluding, 'it will be very rarely indeed that convalescence will not be prompt and perfect.'[56] But as we have seen, physicians seldom viewed it only as a medical procedure. They feared that women wanted abortion not for health reasons but for social and economic reasons, neither of which were sufficient to end a pregnancy. Doctors viewed the embryo as having the status of personhood. Pregnancy in and of itself was valuable and, as one modern critic has assessed the position, women 'should subordinate other parts of their lives to that central aspect of their social and biological selves.' Refusing abortion to women reinforced woman's maternal role. It limited a woman's ability to control her own body and to make decisions regarding it. It made doctors' control over women more certain. Assuming the responsibility of refusing abortion to women was a way that physicians could increase their own importance to society: 'What the physicians did, in effect, was to simultaneously claim both an *absolute* right to life for the embryo (by claiming that abortion is always murder) and a *conditional* one (by claiming that doctors have a right to declare some abortions "necessary").'[57] Doctors gained from both positions. Windsor's Dr Andrew believed that, in Canada, Protestants practised abortion more often than Roman Catholics because Roman Catholic priests held such sway among their adherents they could prevent a high abortion rate. Because the church did not hold such a powerful position among Protestants, he determined that the medical profession should step into the vacuum. Doctors would become the secular priests of Protestant Canada.[58] They would determine if and when abortion was proper.

The potential control that physicians had over their patients with respect to abortion was impressive. Unfortunately, the hatred of abortion among some physicians was so great that it sometimes distorted the kind of care provided. Recall Dr Andrew's feeling that in 1875 he would have resorted to a Caesarian section when faced by a woman with severe pelvic deformity rather than perform an abortion as he had in the 1840s.[59] Yet not all physicians were as vehement as the public stance of their profession would suggest. When Mrs Farris visited Dr Hugh Mackay of Woodstock in the summer of 1878, she had, as his notes reveal, 'for a long time past much tenderness in the pelvic region. Having so far as I can ascertain undergone operations in London England for ruptured perineum and vesico vaginal fistula.' She was now afraid that she was two months pregnant and terrified that another confinement would be dangerous for her. He examined her and 'found the external vaginal orifice so contracted that a small size speculum could not passed [sic].' He consulted with another physician and both agreed that her safety demanded the premature induction of labour (abortion).[60] Jane Humphries, a patient of Dr Gardner in Montreal, entered the Montreal General Hospital on 29 January 1886. She complained of severe pelvic pains and his examination revealed inflammation and adhesions. The examination also noted that the patient was three months' pregnant. His treatment was to introduce a tent into the vagina. On 30 January a larger tent was inserted and on 31 January the patient aborted. Dr Gardner's records do not indicate that he introduced the tent for the purpose of causing the fetus to abort, but doctors did know at this time that the insertion of such objects could and often did cause abortion. More telling is that his records do not suggest he saw the resultant abortion as unusual, unforseen, or a tragedy.[61] Neither were physicians swift to condemn women in a concrete way, for despite the hostility they expressed towards women importuning them for abortions, they never turned them over to the authorities despite some encouragement to do so. Such entreaties were part of patient-doctor confidentiality and that confidentiality was integral to making the practice of medicine a profession. Breaking confidentiality would alienate patients and, besides, many doctors did understand the desperation of some women who sought abortions. Thus, while the rhetoric on abortion was hostile, when faced with a specific case doctors had difficulty condemning the woman even if they did not feel able to accommodate her.[62]

If the willingness of some women to resort to abortion revealed how desperate they were to avoid having a child, infanticide highlighted that desperation to doctors even more. In a summary of 354 cases between 1843 and 1847 at the University Lying-in Hospital in Montreal, Dr McCulloch told of one case of twins where the physician 'found the patient with symptoms of Labour in her Master's house and very much continued to deny that she was pregnant until she was delivered, and then the presence of a double Placenta, with two cords, disclosed the secret of her having a short time previously given birth to another Infant. Her former residence was immediately searched by the police and the other Twin found concealed in her trunk.'[63] In Toronto alone between 1860 and 1870 there were at least eighteen reported cases of infanticide and, between 1877 and 1894, the coroner investigated fifty-three cases.[64] Despite the sense that infanticide was increasing, doctors seldom discussed infanticide with the same urgency they did abortion. This did not mean they ignored the issue. In the 1840s the *British American Journal of Medical & Physical Science* detailed several cases of suspected child-murder. Of particular concern were instances of precipitate birth where the child born quickly landed on the floor or an equally hard surface, resulting in death. The question for doctors to determine was whether the precipitate birth was deliberate or not. One such case occurred to Hugh Mackay. On the night of 30 March 1876 he was called to the home of Carter McKenzie, where he found McKenzie's step-daughter Merry on the floor with a 'child lying dead beside her.' He noted, 'no marks of violence on the child.' Nevertheless he consulted with Mr Bell the crown attorney 'as to the propriety of holding an investigation as to the circumstances of the case,' but was advised there was no case.[65] Doctors could also become quite graphic in their descriptions of infanticide. In 1873 the Kingston *Canadian Medical Times* provided its readers with instructions on how infanticide could be perpetrated with little evidence. All you needed was to insert a sharp needle in the infant's upper eyelid, thus puncturing the brain. No marks would be left. Only an autopsy could prove that the infant had died from unnatural causes. And perhaps not needing to be said – only physicians had the expertise to perform autopsies.[66]

One way of lessening infanticide was suggested by the *Upper*

Canada Journal of Medical, Surgical and Physical Science in 1852. Registration of births and deaths would prevent concealed births, known only to the mother and midwife. As James Connor has noted, the last is a telling reference. It implicates midwives with infanticide, suggesting they were perhaps not 'wholly trustworthy' in reporting births and might 'tacitly condone' infanticide. Such a view recognized the attempt of practitioners to distance themselves from minority practitioners and to develop a cohesive and unified code of ethics for the practice of medicine.[67] In this case, doctors' loyalty belonged to the state, through the registration of births, and to the fetus. The midwife's loyalty, it seemed to be suggested, was to the birthing mother. But although physicians disapproved of infanticide, they were not up in arms about it; neither were Canadians in general. Constance Backhouse has discovered that when cases of infanticide were brought to trial in which both judge and jury had clear evidence to convict a woman, they refused to do so. There was a sympathy with the usually young, unmarried women who resorted to such desperate acts. Doctors' relative silence on this issue and the courts' leniency suggest there was not a recognition or appreciation of new-born infants as particularly significant beings. That being the case, the hostility doctors showed towards abortion could not have been motivated by concern for the unborn child. Rather, Backhouse has argued that what bothered physicians about abortion was that respectable married women resorted to it and that a medical service was involved. The former threatened the moral purity of the population and the latter the economic interests of physicians.[68] In either case, the result was overwhelming medical hostility towards abortion.

The public antagonism that most physicians exhibited towards abortion and, to a lesser extent, infanticide suggests they might have been more lenient towards other forms of birth control. If successful, birth control would remove the necessity for abortion and infanticide. Unfortunately, the few birth control methods physicians tended to support were not effective and the ones that were effective were those physicians did not support. This had not always been the case. Before mid-century there was some suggestion that physicians were willing to provide birth control advice. Eugene Becklard, in his *Physiological Mysteries*, discussed the ways both to prevent conception and to bring about abortion once conception had occurred. He advised placing a sponge in the vagina before intercourse, or using condoms as a preventive measure. Even eating spicy food was advised. If conception was feared, he suggested that exercise to disturb the embryo within twenty-four hours after conception might be effective. His aim was to limit the number of children being born to the poor and to reduce the childbearing responsibilities of women. He used what would become a very modern birth control argument – the quality or health of the children born was more important than the quantity.[69] Becklard's was one of the few medical manuals that discussed contraception in a positive way and one of the few early manuals that even raised the issue. This may suggest that in the early years family limitation was not a concern, perhaps because, as the birth rate indicated, few were engaging in it, but also because Canadians and others saw birth control as a private rather than a public issue. This did not remain the case and, as the century progressed, discussion on the issue occurred and more often than not assumed a negative tone. Once again, the issue of what was natural seemed to be the factor determining support or opposition.

Self-restraint was one method of birth control that physicians encouraged. Pierce thought that the husband should exhibit this restraint to protect his wife from the trials of childbearing.[70] One article written for the *Queen's Medical Quarterly* of 1898 went even further. The author recommended that, in the case of financial problems or the ill health of the wife, the husband should abstain from sexual intercourse altogether.[71] Both of these physicians acknowledged that pregnancy could be a threat to some women, but instead of recommending an active form of birth control that would allow the married couple to have a normal physical relationship, they instead advised sexual restraint or abstinence on the part of the husband. Perhaps realizing the impracticality in advocating restraint, doctors also advised couples on when conception was most likely to occur. Unfortunately, as we have already noted, their understanding of the female cycle was minimal and, with respect to the fertile period, inaccurate.[72] While believing that male sexual restraint was the best birth control method, Napheys, in *The Physical Life of Woman*, recognized that for many men this led to domestic unhappiness and adultery. Yet control of some sort was necessary as a way of avoiding the more horrendous problem of abortion. Women, he felt, had a right to determine the number of children they bore. His favoured birth control method, however, was not exactly foolproof even if it was nature's way of controlling conception. He recommended that women nurse their children for at least a year and thus inhibit their fertility.[73] In this, he may have been responding to reality, for Reuben Ludlam, in his *Lectures Clinical and Didactic on the Diseases of Women*, noted that while many women refused to nurse their children, others nursed them too long in an attempt to avoid conception.[74] Nursing had a long history as a contraceptive method and knowledge of it was probably widespread. Nursing for a year or more, of course, would simply give women a short respite between pregnancies. It was not a solution for those who did not want or should not have children. Neither did all physicians believe it to be harmless. Goodell in his *Lessons in Gynaecology* explained to practitioners that over-lactation could result in disease.[75]

Abstinence or restraint, intercourse only within prescribed periods, and prolonged nursing were about the only forms of birth control countenanced by physicians. All were non-mechanical and non-interventionist and, consequently, conformed to what seemed natural. Except for abstinence, which was not realistic for the long term, none was very effective. Of those that were, most physicians opposed them, using therapeutic arguments bolstered by appeals to nature. Coitus interruptus had been known for centuries as a contraceptive method. In the 1820s in England, Francis Place advocated it as one form that would be useful in the industrial districts of northern England.[76] Useful it may have been, but physicians disliked it even while they recognized its popularity. Horatio Storer, assistant in obstetrics and medical jurisprudence at Harvard University, argued in the 1867 *Canada Med-*

ical Journal that while some forms of birth control and abortion were harmful to women, withdrawal was harmful to both sexes and could cause 'dyspepsia, functional or organic nervous disease, and at times impotence' in men.[77] In 1883 Edmund King, surgeon to St Michael's Hospital, Toronto, quoted experts who agreed with Storer. In addition to impotence, however, they added insomnia, restlessness, mental depression, and headache.[78] Withdrawal before completed intercourse for women could be equally harmful, leading not only to insomnia, restlessness, mental depression, headaches, and hemorrhage but leucorrhoea, chronic metritis, and fibroids.[79] B.G. Jefferis, too, stressed to his readers the problems that withdrawal caused and recommended nature's way – that is, abstaining for the fertile time of the month. Jefferis's readers were fortunate if they took his advice – he was one of a minority of physicians who approximated the fertile period correctly.[80]

Physicians' opposition to withdrawal went beyond warning their patients about its dangers. They sometimes took a moral stance about individuals who practised it, and the consequences to those individuals could be severe. William Goodell reported a physician who discovered that one of his patients, a woman with uterine troubles, practised coitus interruptus to prevent childbirth. The physician argued that this had weakened her health and he refused to treat her until she and her husband gave up the practice.[81] This they refused to do. Such an episode reveals two things. First, the physician's refusal to help this woman was based on his opposition to her and her husband using a form of birth control that the physician found harmful. While it is understandable that his belief in its dangers would make him frustrated about satisfactorily treating her, his refusal to help her at all seems extreme. Second, the patient refused to take his advice. The reasons for her and her husband not having children were strong enough in her mind that she was not going to be frightened away from a birth control method she found satisfactory.

Using condoms was another method of family limitation. As Angus and Arlene McLaren have discovered, by the 1890s condoms were being mass-produced in both the United States and Britain and were easily available from druggists in large cities in Canada. C.S. Clark in *Of Toronto the Good* reported blatant evidence of this practice: 'I saw a druggist's advertisement a short time ago in a Toronto paper with this significant line: *Rubber Goods of ALL KINDS for Sale.* There is not a boy in Toronto, I dare say, who does not know what that means.' While effective as a birth control device, condoms were resorted to more as protection against venereal disease as a result of premarital or extramarital affairs. In any case, doctors warned about the inflammation they could cause.[82]

Despite doctors' hostility towards any but the most passive forms of birth control, evidence suggests that Canadians were not persuaded. The private papers of some French-Canadian women contain instructions on how to make a diaphragm.[83] At mid-century the *Acadian Recorder* advertised *The Married Woman's Private Medical Companion* in which birth control information was provided.The advertisement asked women: 'How many have difficult if not dangerous deliveries, and whose lives are jeoparded during each time will find in its pages the means of *prevention ...* and *relief?*' What is more, the advertisement advised readers that the book could be purchased either through the mail from New York or at R.G. Fraser's drug store on Granville Street in Halifax.[84] In the late nineteenth century Allen McIntosh, a lay preacher and Ontario appleseed cultivator, worked his way through eastern Ontario selling, along with apple seeds, abortifacients and pessaries which he inventively described as 'Dinosaur Turds.'[85] In 1901 even the Eaton's catalogue notified its readers of 'Every Woman Marvel Whirling Spray.' Whether women used the vaginal spray as a birth control method is unknown, but douching had certainly been a well-known contraceptive practice for centuries.[86] What this evidence suggests is Canadians' willingness to resort to birth control and their resistance to the ideology of procreation that permeated society. It also revealed the determination of women to control their bodies, for all these examples involve women acting in a way that not only challenged the popular and pervasive ideology of motherhood but also forced women to come to terms with their own physicality since such methods involved the handling of the genitalia.[87] For many Canadians, birth control was a private issue and not the public one doctors were trying to make it. While physicians may have felt that birth control attacked the sanctity of the family, many Canadians could view the decision about family size as one each couple had to make for themselves. And, as the declining birth rate indicated, they were doing just that. Ironically, so were physicians, since they were among the groups with the smallest families in Canada.

Physicians' opposition to birth control was strong. When discussing it in general terms rather than referring to specific methods, the theme of its physical and moral dangers becomes even more vehement. For Theodore Thomas, birth control caused disease because it interfered with nature.[88] For Henry Lyman it was 'an evasion of physical ... obligations.'[89] Birth control led to nervous disease, insanity, hemorrhage, leucorrhoea, chronic metritis, and fibroids.[90] In the estimation of John Thorburn, 'there are in fact, no harmless or available means for thwarting nature's plain intention, for if they should not injure the body they assuredly will the mind.'[91] The threat to sanity was an effective one, for Victorians were deservedly frightened of what appeared to be increasing rates of insanity as reflected in overcrowded asylums. Insanity represented total loss of control, loss of humanness – it left the individual at the mercy of her/his physical being. If sanity was important to maintain, so was morality. Both were what distinguished humans from animals. Yet physicians made it clear that birth control was immoral, except for the few methods they agreed did not challenge nature's way. When one advertisement suggested methods to prevent conception, the editors of the *Medical Chronicle* in 1856 exhorted readers to become concerned: 'For the protection of society, and suppression of crime, the authorities should take cognizance of, and vigorously put down, every attempt to give currency to plans for the purpose of effecting the "prevention of offspring."'[92] The emphasis on the moral dangers intensified. The author of *The Practical Home Physician* felt the use of birth control was an evasion of both physical and moral obligation.[93] In his text, William Goodell stressed that physicians were morally obligated to refuse the numerous requests for birth control information they received. In addition, birth control would only dull sexual excitement and consequently lead to unfaithfulness. It cheapened sex.[94] An editorial in the *Queen's Medical Quarterly* of October 1898 expressed the feeling best: 'The men and women of this country must be educated to know and to feel that it is woman's highest functions [sic] to perpetuate the species.' To engage in intercourse when procreation was not the goal was prostitution.[95]

Sexual intercourse was to lead to the procreation of children. Anything that interfered with this process went against nature and would lead to physical, mental, and moral harm. About the only way around this was for individuals to use means that did not contradict nature. Restraint did not. If anything, it revealed mastery over the body by the mind, a condition which Victorians admired. Nursing a child did not, for nursing was a natural phenomenon and part of nature's way of providing food for the child. Any other method was, according to physicians, dangerous, although the evidence for this was slim. Doctors asserted what could go wrong, but seldom could they prove any connection to birth control. Nonetheless, what was unnatural had to be harmful. Yet some physicians recognized the existence of harmless but effective birth control. The *Canada Lancet* of 1893, in a small article, reported that in cases of pelvic contraction, abdominal and uterine tumours, pregnancy could be dangerous. Advising abstention from sexual activity was not very practical since such advice was seldom followed. Mechanical means were not suitable for hygienic and ethical reasons. However, a cocoa butter suppository containing a 10 per cent boracic acid was safe.[96]

If physicians knew of harmless methods, why were they so hostile about their patients' practising birth control? The concern about rejecting nature is an important reason and one that has been a continuing theme throughout this study of doctors' attitudes towards women. The concern about birth control (including abortion) being used by the 'better' classes suggests another reason. Immigration was increasing in the latter decades of the century. There was the fear that the direction that Canada was going could take a turn for the worse if the 'better' people in

society did not propagate as much as the 'lower' orders. Still
another reason was provided by a physician hostile to the public
availability of contraceptive information: 'knowledge is power.'[97]
By controlling access to information, access to birth control of
any type, doctors increased their power and influence. Above all,
the responsibility of women in general but especially women of
the 'higher' orders was to have children. Nature had designed
their bodies for this purpose. The irony of this determinism was
that women and men were rejecting it to some degree, as evidenced by the declining birth rate, and doctors believed that
women's bodies were becoming ill-suited to give birth according
to the dictates of nature. Fortunately for women, doctors were
there to help them perform a natural function that was increasingly becoming less natural for them.

Chapter Six

The Emergence of Medical Obstetrics

August 15 [1832] ... [I awoke] to strange and ominous sensations.

Edward set to work to get the stove up and I lay as quiet as I could on the sofa to wait till they had finished their work.

After dinner I went into Mama's room to get out of their way and from thence I did not very immediately return, for a few minutes made me the mother of another son. The nurse had not arrived, but Mama was so completely taken by surprise that she had no time to be alarmed. With Edward's assistance and Flora's ministration she did all that was requisite for me and the baby.[1]

Tuesday Oct. 14th (1890)
Awoke about two feeling very miserable & continued ill until half past three when our little daughter was born the last few hours I suffered very much Mrs Crosby and Martha Ryan were with me we got all settled down & I felt quite comfortable. Slept well.[2]

Although almost sixty years separated the childbirth descriptions of Mary O'Brien in rural Ontario and Nellie Bailey Bolton in Port Simpson, BC, the similarities between them suggest that little had changed. And for women in rural and outpost areas this was true. Many women were on their own with no one to help them except relatives, friends, and perhaps a midwife. Elsewhere in Canada, however, much had altered and, while the focus of this chapter is on some of those changes, we must always keep in mind the continuity of experience that was the reality for women such as Mary O'Brien and Nellie Bolton.

As noted elsewhere, in the latter half of the nineteenth century the image of woman as mother was a powerful one. Although the number of children in the average family fell, the emphasis placed on the children who were born intensified. Increasingly, the raising of children became a significant task and one which was the primary responsibility of the mother. Motherhood as a social role had emerged. As one woman declared, 'Whether we shall be a strong, pure, intellectual people depends most of all upon our women, and their just apprehension of all the possibilities attaching to the holy office of motherhood.'[3] But maternity not only dominated popular imagery of women, it determined how physicians viewed women's bodies. Indeed, historians have suggested that in the nineteenth century, physicians and others no longer saw women's bodies as a lesser reflection of men's but as quite different, with that difference being centred on 'woman's automatic reproductive cycle.'[4] Young bodies were preparing themselves for motherhood, mature bodies were potentially capable of bearing children, and older women's bodies were paying the price of that childbearing. Whereas 'paternity rests on *knowledge* rather than experience,'[5] maternity is experienced and it was the physical act of that experience – childbearing – that held centre stage in the medical treatment of women. Medical assistance during childbirth remained limited for many women, although the number who received some medical support increased as doctors extended their sway over childbirth and assumed the position that traditionally had been held by women. That this was happening at the same time that the domestic image of women was strengthening and the fertility rate declining is ironic. The ideology of domesticity deemed the domestic sphere the only respectable one for women and the one in which women would be protected from the influences of the outside world. The reality was that even the most intimate occurrence of the private world – childbirth – was becoming more open to scrutiny, either by having a male physician in attendance or, more rarely, by taking place in a hospital. In gaining ascendancy, male practitioners had greatly enlarged their professional influence not only in the advice proffered to women but in the medical treatment provided to them. Obstetrics became a major field of medical specialization in this period and *the* medical specialty with respect to women. Certainly there was a great deal of attention given to obstetrics in the Canadian medical journals of the time and obstetric texts were among the most frequently listed in medical college curricula. Childbirth was one of the most common cases that practitioners of medicine would face and indications are that it was becoming more so. Obstetrics became the field in which medicine and women as patients most often came together. As William Tyler Smith in his text *Parturition and the Principles and Practice of Obstetrics* clearly appreciated, 'obstetricy ... may fairly be considered as an expression of our social condition – of our humanity towards women and children.'[6]

When assessing practitioners' attitudes towards and treatment of women in childbirth, it is necessary to remember that the general information available to physicians about fertility was limited. Until 1832 when the human ovum was discovered, doctors could only speculate on the association between menstruation and the reproductive process.[7] Until the fusion of sperm and egg was seen in 1854,[8] few understood that both women and men contributed to the creation of a child and that the mother was not simply the host for the active seminal matter. These two discoveries alone would go a long way to help explain the strength of the maternal image of woman. Not only did the image have cultural support, it had a scientific foundation. While information we consider basic was relatively new for Victorian medicine, some of the technical knowledge was impressive. For example, in the *Canada Lancet* for October 1870 an article reprinted from the *Lancet and Observer* entitled 'On Artificial Fecundation' went into explicit detail on how artificially to inseminate a woman.[9] Despite the technical advances and the strides medical science made in understanding some aspects of conception and fertility, those practising it were not able to divorce themselves completely from the social biases of the time. An excellent example of how the understanding of science and the social perception of gender role could come together was revealed in Pierce's *The People's Common Sense Medical Adviser*. In it, he describes the process of conception in which male and female involvement corresponded to what Victorians considered appropriate gender characteristics for each in society:

Generation requires the concurrence of *stimuli* and *susceptibility*, and to perfect the process, two conditions are also necessary. The first is the sperm, which communicates the principle of action; the other is the germ, which receives the latent life and provides the conditions necessary to organic evolution. The vivifying function belongs to the male, that of nourishing and cherishing is possessed by the female, and these conditions are sexual distinctions. The former represents *will* and *understanding*; the latter, *vitality* and *emotion*. The father directs and controls, the mother fosters and encourages; the former counsels and admonishes, the latter persuades and caresses.[10]

Medicine confirmed conventional gender roles in society by providing 'scientific' justification for them, even though the interpretation of that justification was clearly influenced by the Victorian rhetoric surrounding those roles.

The medical view of fertility could and did have consequences for women. As we have already seen, since scientists did not accurately understand the changes behind women's monthly cycle, most physicians gave incorrect advice to their women patients about when they were most likely to conceive.[11] Only in rare cases did doctors acknowledge that the mid-part of the menstrual cycle was the fertile period and, when they did so, some suggested this was an abnormal situation due to sexual stimulation caused by coition, immoral excesses, or drinking.[12] Because of the lack of accurate information on the menstrual cycle and reproduction in general, doctors' pronouncements on fertility problems often reflected their own prejudices. George Napheys tended to link inability to conceive to the fault of the woman rather than the man. As long as men were not impotent, he concluded they could impregnate a woman. If they could not, there was something wrong with the woman. Napheys referred to wives who never became mothers as sterile or barren, assuming, first, that it was their fault they had not conceived and, second, that all women wanted children and that only sterility or barrenness could account for childless married women. To correct the problem, he advised stimulating the breasts, which in turn would act on the womb, resting on the bed after sexual intercourse, and horseback riding to the point of fatigue.[13]

One of the more curious exercises of those specializing in obstetrics was to discuss what determined the sex of the child. The interest in this issue stemmed from the desire of parents to determine and thus possibly control the sex of the child conceived. Underlying this interest was the belief that boy children were more valuable than girl children, hence the greater emphasis on the condition needed to conceive a male. As mentioned in chapter 4, some physicians comforted themselves that women were capable of sexual arousal in order to conceive 'male offspring.'[14] But this was not the only theory of sex determination that had adherents. P. Cazeaux, in his early nineteenth-century text, believed, not surprisingly, that the stronger the husband was, the more likely his wife would bear a male child.[15] William Carpenter felt that several different factors favoured the birth of a boy: the time when conception occurred relative to the menstrual cycle – towards the end a boy would be conceived owing to, as he put it, the advanced stage of maturation of the ovum; living in mountainous countries; having a food scarcity; and when the father was older.[16] Two decades later, doctors were still engaging in similar speculation. Austin Flint noted that two theories to account for the sex of a child were popular in medical circles: one focused on the nutrition received before conception and the second on the time when sexual intercourse occurred. Flint, himself, favoured the latter view. He also theorized that when just enough of the 'male element unites with the ovum to secure fecundation,' a girl child results, but when a 'greater number of spermatozoids unite,' a boy child is created.[17] Both B.G. Jefferis and Henry Lyman in their health manuals supported the time of conception within the menstrual cycle as being the main determinant. Jefferis even harkened back to Carpenter when he explained to his readers that female babies resulted if conception occurred within four days of the close of menses 'because the ovum is yet immature.'[18] In his *Common Sense Medical Adviser*, Pierce offered a different explanation, which had its origins in Greek medicine. The right ovary furnished the egg for boys and the left for girls, and the right testicle provided sperm for males and the left for females. He did not explain why this was the case; he merely presented it as one of the common beliefs of sex determination.[19]

Because the woman carried the child, physicians understandably believed in the very close association between the two. This bond was one reason that Canadians in general and physicians in particular were so concerned about the morality of women. It was inconceivable that those who bore children and nurtured them could be immoral, not because it was impossible but because of the consequences of this for the child – the morality of the mother could not help but be visited on her child. Maternal influence went beyond the psychological bonding that modern theorists discuss; many physicians and Canadians believed that maternal impressions were absorbed by the child in vitro. Canadian temperance women were convinced that Frances Willard, founder of the American WCTU, a woman they idolized and idealized, had been profoundly influenced by her mother's desire, while pregnant with Frances, that her child work for the temperance cause.[20] The *Medical Chronicle* of 1856 explained in one article that a mother's thoughts could influence the foetus physically, morally, and mentally.[21] In the *Canada Health Journal* of February 1870 Professor J.C. Sanders agreed, although he maintained that the physical, moral, and mental characteristics of the child could be influenced by both parents. His concern was to ensure that only the 'right' people had children and warned those who were 'contaminated' in any way to avoid marriage. If they did not, their actions would be a crime against the children of that marriage, a crime against the race, and a crime against God.[22] So strong was the belief in moral characteristics being transmitted either through the maternal or, to a lesser extent, paternal line that some physicians advocated castration of male and female criminals so they would be unable to pass on their criminal tendencies to their children.[23] This concern reflected the perceived increase in crime during the latter part of the century and a preliminary understanding of the laws of heredity which doctors and others applied to all characteristics. John Hett in his sex manual even suggested that the influence of parents, especially mothers, was increasing simply because the minds of people were becoming more powerful than they had been in the past owing to the modern need for brain power.[24] Such a notion reinforced physicians' concerns about who had children. Flint admitted it was sometimes difficult to predict what the mental and physical characteristics of the child were going to be, not only because there were two parents involved but because, if the woman had had a previous husband, the child of the second husband often looked like the offspring of the first. At a time when remarriage was quite common, such a superstition could have raised all sorts of anxieties for families.[25] Napheys, in contrast, was quite explicit about the influence of father and mother on the child. According to him, 'The father transmits to the daughters the form of the head, the framework of the chest and of the superior extremities, while the conformation of the lower portion of the body and the inferior extremities are transmitted by the mother. With the sons this is reversed.' Thus smart men had smart daughters and smart women had smart sons.[26]

Although many physicians believed that both parents influenced their children, most believed that maternal impressions were more significant. Despite the often accepted belief that the male was the active participant in conception, the actual carrying of the child by the woman made up for her so-called passiveness in the initial creation. To convince his student readers of the power of maternal impression, Flint related the case of a janitor at the College of Physicians and Surgeons of New York whose child had a deformity of the ear identical to the deformity of a man about whom his wife had dreamed. Hugh Mackay on 9 February 1878 performed a craniotomy on a child with a hydrocephalic head and noted in his record that the mother had been so 'affected when three mos. advanced in gestation with one of her children having taken a convulsion on her lap that she was apprehensive that her child would be wrong.'[27] When a young woman at the Burnside Lying-In Hospital gave birth on 4 May 1881 to a deformed child, many of the medical students who came to see it thought it had the features of a rabbit. When questioned, 'the mother state[d] that early in her pregnancy a boy frightened her with a dead rabbit.'[28] Henry Lyman, author of *The Practical Home Physician*, was not willing to believe such stories but, while denying that the thoughts and emotions of the mother could influence the physical nature of the child, he granted they could influence the child's emotional nature.[29] What is striking about all these views on maternal impression is the power they attributed to women, power over which doctors had little control.

While doctor may have been concerned about the power of maternal impressions, the women giving birth had their own worries. At mid-century the average number of children a woman would give birth to was approximately seven, so that five and a quarter years of her life were spent being pregnant. When the recuperative period, the nursing period, and the pregnancies ending in spontaneous miscarriages and abortion are added to this total, the centrality of childbirth to many women is undeniable.[30] For some women this reality started at an incredibly early age. In the 1860 to 1889 general practice of Fredericton's Dr Theodore Clowes Brown, the youngest obstetrical patient was fourteen years of age. While obviously not typical, it reveals that for some women childbearing could begin almost as soon as they were biologically capable of it.[31] In Hugh Mackay's Woodstock practice from 1873 to 1888, his youngest patient was also fourteen and his oldest forty-seven. Although most of his patients were in their twenties, approximately 22 per cent were in their thirties and over 10 per cent were forty years of age or older. And while 28 per cent of his patients had come to him for their first labour, over 35 per cent were having him assist with their fourth or more childbirth.[32] Similarly, in the Toronto practice of James Ross in the latter half of the century, over 50 per cent of his patients were having their fourth or more child.[33] For women, childbirth was not only an ideological reality but a physical one as well.

Although they believed it was necessary for women to give birth, physicians were also convinced women were having difficulty doing so – primarily because of the effects of civilization.

Ira Warren described to his mid-century readers what he saw as the major dilemma. Brain power was needed in a modern society and natural selection was accommodating this need through the birth of children with larger heads than had occurred formerly. But larger-headed babies creating birthing problems since the pelves of women had not increased proportionately.[34] Another problem reported by the *Canadian Practitioner* was the excess of females over males owing to the increased death of boys in infancy, the proportionally increased number of boys among still-borns, and the lower conception of boys compared with girls. In order to have male children, parents, particularly the mothers, needed to be healthy. But civilized life had resulted in the gradual decline in the physical strength of women and, consequently, more girl babies were being born.[35] The question for physicians was what could be done about it? How could they control the situation so that more male children would be born? Lapthorn Smith of Montreal, in a popular Darwinian stance, advocated the survival of the fittest. He argued that civilization was allowing women with small pelves to survive labour and breed more daughters with equally small or smaller pelves. Such breeding had to stop and he was willing to advocate the removal of the uterus of such women to prevent it. Harkening back to Warren, he also argued that, at the same time that the pelves of women were becoming smaller, the heads of *male* children were becoming larger owing to the need for brain power in the modern society of the nineteenth century: 'While nature, if left to herself, would exterminate at their birth these big-headed men who are able to amass so much wealth, civilization comes to their rescue and saves them.'[36] Of course the rescuer was the medical practitioner as he increasingly became involved in the process of managing childbirth. The irony of Smith's analysis was that, while believing in natural selection, he was not willing to accept the consequences of it – small pelvic women unable to give birth to large-brained males. In this scenario, nature did not know what was best and intervention on the part of the physicians was required. Of course, not all women had difficulty giving birth to healthy children of both sexes. There was a general belief that poorer women, immigrant women, and women living in less rarified settings than modern cities had little trouble. It was modern woman who could not fulfill her destiny.[37] As we have seen earlier, physicians tended to extol the primitive woman and her ability to work and be healthy. Napheys did point out the fallacy of such a view when he acknowledged that many so-called primitive women were not fertile, died in childbirth, and had a short life expectancy. Admitting that, however, did not change the fact that the modern woman, because she was finer, more delicate, nervous, and frail, could not be expected to bear as many children as her primitive sister.[38]

How accurate were these perceptions of physicians is difficult to assess. Often they were responding to the social reality around them and seeking medical explanations for it. Women *were* having fewer children. When coupled with the belief that women should naturally want children, the explanation had to be that women were having more difficulty than previously in bearing them. Physicians were also consulted more by women who had had complications in previous pregnancies than by those who had not, which may have reinforced the perception of women's experiencing birthing difficulties. In Dr. Langis's late nineteenth-century Vancouver practice, 70 per cent of his obstetric patients engaged him before delivery and those who did had a much higher rate of complications than those who did not, which suggested they had come to him because they anticipated difficulty. That most of those who engaged Langis beforehand had already had a pregnancy supports this view.[39] The clientele of physicians was definitely among those women whom observers would deem 'civilized,' not primitive. This allowed physicians to maintain a utopian vision of the way primitive or poor women gave birth. In examining doctors in England, Judith Lewis has noted that they, too, believed that aristocratic women had more difficulty and pain in labour and more trouble reproducing than poorer women, despite all indications to the contrary. To explain this contradiction, she argues that 'doctors may have been too pushy or too indifferent to pay attention to the cries of their lower-class patients. It was an easy step from there to the belief that lower-class women suffered less than did upper-class women.'[40] Doctors had a vested interest in viewing their patients in more need of assistance than women who could not afford to pay them. Women themselves may have helped to promote the idea that childbirth was difficult for them. Two American historians have partially traced the ideology of female frailty to women who were trying to avoid numerous pregnancies. In an effort to convince their husbands of the need for sexual restraint, they appealed to a medical imperative – they physically could not undergo a multitude of pregnancies.[41] In this situation, women used medicine for their own needs.

If doctors had a vested interest in viewing their patients as in need of assistance, they also had one in determining who was qualified to provide that assistance. Traditionally this had been the responsibility of other women – friends, family, midwives – but trained physicians increasingly argued they were best suited for that role. The importance of their success cannot be underestimated. When women believed that physicians were required or preferable in childbirth, birth became a medical as opposed to a natural phenomenon. Why midwifery declined, particularly in the United States, has been a major subject of historiographical debate. Ann Oakley has argued that midwifery and regular medicine pitted two systems of therapeutics against one another. The first saw reproduction as a normal process. Understanding it was just a matter of empiricism – that is, experiencing it – rather than professional training. The second system viewed reproduction as a medical condition fraught with all sorts of dangers that could be avoided only by the intervention of professional medicine.[42] What has particularly aggravated the hostility of many feminists about the victory of the second system is that 'the group that is not at any risk from reproduction (male) control[s] the group that is at risk.'[43] But it is more than simply power that modern critics of obstetrics object to – they feel that the way midwifery was practised was safer and more humane than the delivery of babies by trained physicians.[44] Those supportive of the midwives have argued, for example, that midwives were less interventionist than physicians and that this was of benefit to both mother and child.[45]

Not that all historians have agreed. In particular, Edward Shorter is much more supportive of the medical profession and more critical of midwives, unless they were formally trained, than feminist scholars until quite recently have been.[46]

Although there is disagreement over the quality of care provided by midwives, there is no disagreement about the fact they declined in importance. Jane Donegan has linked this to William Smellie (1697-1763), a Scottish physician, who opened up training in childbirth to men by teaching them to make precise measurements of the female pelvis 'and thus revolutionized obstetrics by coming to understand the true nature of the mechanics of parturition.' Donegan argues that by 1800 midwives in the United States had been partially replaced by general practitioners simply because midwives could not compete with the anatomical knowledge of physicians. If they had, the cultural mores of feminine modesty would have favoured the continuance of female control of childbirth.[47] While interesting as a theory, it does not explain why midwives continued to flourish in Britain.[48] Other historians have argued that formal anatomical knowledge was no substitute for the experience that midwives brought to their patients and so other reasons must also have existed. The fact that physicians were men and midwives were women did not always work in midwives' favour. First, there was a belief, particularly in the nineteenth century, that women were not as intellectually inclined as men, which suggested to many women about to give birth that male physicians with their formal training would be able to provide safer childbirth. Second, midwives, unlike physicians, did not have their own organization to lobby for them. Like women in other areas of economic endeavour they were isolated. Third, the increasing prestige of science during this period aided physicians. Because physicians were able to align medicine with science in the popular mind, they argued that they could provide better care than midwives, especially midwives who were untrained. In addition, free outpatient obstetrical care through hospitals undermined the clientele that midwives had largely depended on – those who could not afford the services of a doctor.[49]

Very little research has been done to explain the decline of midwifery in Canada. James Connor, in his study of the relationship between midwives and doctors in nineteenth-century Ontario, has suggested that no one factor accounts for the decline of midwifery but rather a congruence of social, economic, and political factors. Midwives in Canada were not organized and, unlike in Britain, where they received the support of the medical elite, they were without powerful advocates. Compared to the situation in Britain or in Europe, the mobility and transiency of people in late nineteenth-century society accentuated the midwives' isolation by restricting feminine networks. Medical technology, for whatever reason, was associated with physicians rather than midwives and, as medical advances occurred, particularly the introduction of anaesthesia, women could see physicians as scientific practitioners. This latter point is important for it emphasizes the active participation of women in choosing whom they preferred to deliver them. The declining birth rate resulted in women giving birth to fewer children and, as Connor has suggested, it may be that women determined to get the best possible care they felt was available for those fewer births. Less important for him in explaining the decline of midwives was the opposition or ambivalence of some physicians to them. Whatever the reason for the eclipse of midwifery in Canada, few deny that early in the century midwives and other women dominated childbirth. The isolated nature of much settlement ensured that many British North Americans had little access to physicians and that there was little opposition to midwifery practice. This did not mean that male practitioners were totally excluded. In the 1820s in York (Toronto), the Society for the Relief of Women attempted to aid women in childbirth by providing a midwife or 'if required' a physician.[50] 'If required' meant in cases of complication when the midwife could no longer help the woman.

Dr John Dickson, a Kingston doctor, reported a case he attended on 29 July 1850. On arrival at the patient's home the midwife, who had been supervising the case, informed him that it was the patient's first child and that 'the *vagina was completely closed*.' Not wanting to make a visual exploration (perhaps to save the dignity of the patient) he requested Mrs S, the midwife, to do so and discern whether there was any kind of aperture. Meanwhile he returned home to get his scalpel. On his return, Mrs S told him she could find no opening and, after confirming this himself, he cut into the imperforate hymen to facilitate the birth of the baby.[51] In this situation midwife and physician co-operated. At times, however, the actions of the midwife left no room for co-operation. Such was a case attended by Dr Verity from Hemmingford. On arrival at his patient's home he was appalled to find the right arm of the child was 'protruding through the vulva,' wrapped in a piece of cloth 'for fear of cold,' as the midwife said, and carefully tied to the patient's thighs 'for fear it should go back again.'[52] In 1872 a doctor from Fingal, Ont., reported a case he had had several years before that had been attended by a midwife before he had been called in. He arrived to find the dead child missing each of its arms because, as the midwife confessed, she had 'by means of a noose, above the elbow of the child, connected to a towel around her shoulders ... succeeded in extracting, first one arm without much trouble, and then the other after a great deal of trouble.'[53] While Dr Verity and his colleague from Fingal were distressed by the care provided by the midwives, their experience and that of Dr Dickson underlines the fact that very early on midwives themselves or the families of the women concerned perceived that in difficult childbirths a trained physician did have a particular kind of expertise to offer.

The importance of midwives was recognized by the legislation surrounding medical practice in the early years. The first law regulating medicine in Upper Canada apparently prohibited midwifery by declaring that 'no person ... shall be permitted to ... practise physic, surgery or midwifery within the Province, for profit, until such person or persons shall be duly approved of by a board of surgeons.' While this did not prevent women from acting as midwives on a charitable basis, it did stop them from doing so as a way of making a living. Subsequent legislation revised this 1795 law and in 1815 midwives were exempt from control. This remained the situation until 1865 when the Medical Act removed that exemption. But did this mean that midwifery was illegal? It would appear that the aim of the 1865 act was not to prohibit midwifery but to prevent individuals from passing themselves as licensed and registered physicians. Since midwives seldom claimed to be licensed, they were not the focus of the legislation. Nevertheless they were in an awkward situation – the legislation had not made midwifery illegal, neither had it made it specifically legal. Consequently from 1865 onwards, at least in the province of Ontario, midwives could practise with impunity but not with the assurance of legal protection.[54] Elsewhere the situation was different. In 1872 the legislature of Nova Scotia formally recognized midwifery when it insisted that females might practise in Halifax once they had satisfied the Medical Board as to their competency.[55] Yet in 1889, only eleven midwives, all married, were practising midwifery in that city.[56] Outside of Halifax, control was more lax, and little was done to impede midwives' work in Nova Scotia before the First World War.[57]

It is almost impossible to know who the midwives were or how wisespread midwifery was in the nineteenth century. There certainly was a disparity of skills among them. Some were formally trained while others had apprenticed with a practising midwife, just as aspiring doctors apprenticed themselves to a licensed practitioner. Still others were women who may have acted as midwives but did so only occasionally when their services were needed and no one else was available. Such women would not have considered themselves midwives and certainly would not have identified themselves as such for the census enumerators. Since many physicians were hostile to midwives and since the law in some jurisdictions was vague about the legality of their practice, women who were midwives may have been reluctant to identify themselves as such. As a result, the census figures are guaranteed to underestimate considerably the number of midwives. Nevertheless they do give some sense of the use of midwives at mid-century. In 1850–1 Upper Canada had seventeen practising midwives whereas Lower Canada had only eight. This compared to 382 and 410 physicians and surgeons, respectively. By 1860–1 the number of midwives had increased by one in Canada West and had doubled to sixteen in Canada East. The 1871 census reported the number to have increased to twenty-one for Ontario and up to forty-five for the province of Quebec. In New Brunswick there were eight reported and for Nova Scotia there were fifteen.[58] After this point it is almost impossible to trace midwives through the census since they were categorized along with nurses. However, we do know that in Ontario 16 per cent of births in 1899 were unattended by physicians and 3 per cent of births were attended by women who considered themselves and were considered by others to be midwives.[59] Although midwives did seem to be increasing in absolute numbers, what the above figures suggest is that by no means did this expansion keep pace with the growth of the population. More significantly, by the end of the century physician-attended births were becoming the norm.

The rise in physician-assisted childbirth and the relative decline in midwife care can also be seen in the history of obstetric treatment in hospitals and refuges for women. In the early decades of the century women had no alternative but to give birth at home since few institutions existed to provide care for birthing women. Not until June 1848 in Canada West was the Toronto General Dispensary and Lying-In Hospital established to provide help for destitute women and to train midwives.[60] Such an occurrence suggested two things. First, until mid-century, at least, there had been little interest on the part of Ontarians about the problems of childbearing women who, through lack of means or circumstances, could not have their children at home. Second, the willingness of the dispensary to train midwives indicated an acceptance of these women and a recognition of their importance. The skill that some midwives brought to their task was also recognized by the University Lying-in Hospital in Montreal between 1844 and 1886, when eight midwives served as matrons. All were British and two had diplomas from the University of Edinburgh.[61] The by-laws of the hospital insisted that the midwife could not attend labours outside the hospital and that within the hospital she had to be present at every birth and 'never trust the patient to the medical knowledge of any Student.'[62] In 1886, however, when the residing midwife retired, her non-medical duties were given to a matron and a resident physician assumed her medical duties. The break had occurred. No longer was the management of the hospital willing to accept midwives, even trained ones, as suitable childbirth practitioners.[63] Similarly in Ontario, 'An Act to Regulate Maternity Boarding-Houses and for the Protection of Infant Children' passed in 1897 stipulated that only a 'legally qualified medical practitioner' could attend births in hospitals or maternity homes.[64] Among Catholic orders who provided shelter for unwed mothers and their babies, the decline in midwife care was more complex. The Sisters of the Miséricorde in Montreal had often acted as midwives until 1860, 'when Rome decreed that midwifery was incompatible with the vow of chastity.' After that, the sisters had to hire either a physician or a lay midwife to provide assistance to those in their care.[65]

Although the historiography on midwifery suggests hostility on the part of doctors towards midwives, the reality was not as clear cut. No doubt midwives did provide a certain amount of economic competition for physicians, many of whom believed there already was an oversupply of medical practitioners. It is difficult to know whether this was true, but the ratio of doctors to population was increasing and many physicians did have difficulty making ends meet. To try to offset competition among themselves, the Medical Society of Nova Scotia adopted a scale of fees in May 1861. A major operation could run from £10 to £20, a minor one from £1 to £5. Midwifery cases were charged from £2 to £5 and those which necessitated an instrumental delivery anywhere from a minimum of £2 to £10 to a maximum of £7 to £10.[66] Such a fee schedule reveals that the members of the Nova Scotia Medical Society believed that childbirth was equivalent in cost to a minor operation and, if necessitating instrumental intervention, could cost almost the same as a major operation. Such fees were well beyond the means of most people. Midwives charged much less and, since they were often willing to stay throughout the whole labour and help with the household chores, their services would certainly seem to be cost efficient. It is no wonder that many families looked to midwives for help – most had no other choice. This undercutting of physicians' fees, however, meant that doctors were unable to break into this kind of practice without drastically

reducing what they charged. This they may have been unwilling
or unable to do. Midwifery was a way for women to make money
to help in the raising of their families, but seldom was it a full-
time occupation.[67] For physicians, however, medical practice was
the main source of their livelihood. One physician, who wrote
to the *Canada Lancet* and signed himself 'A Correspondent,' ar-
ticulated the problems a practitioner might have to face. Describing his competition as being two women acting as midwives and
one quack, he admitted they had 'been pretty successful in their
attendance on [midwifery] cases. They charge $2 (while I have
$5) for their attendance, and they get about 60 cases a year, which
would amount in my hands to a very decent living for my small
family.'[68] Between 1827 and 1867 Dr Harmannus Smith of Ancaster
did not raise his fee of $4 in obstetric cases, and for many patients
the charge was much less depending at what stage in the delivery
he arrived.[69] In 1881 the ledger of Dr Samuel Burns of Shelburne
and South River, NS, indicated that he charged approximately $8
for a birth, although in some circumstances it could be less. The
same charge was also true of Dr J.R. Collie of River John, NS, from
1875 to 1894.[70] Although the price had remained stable, it was still
beyond the means of most working-class and agricultural families.
The result was that, if given a choice, people would prefer to use
a midwife if they used anyone at all or, if they called in a physician, would be unwilling to pay the full fee.[71] Certainly James
Langstaff's practice in the 1850s reveals the plight of physicians.
Only one-half of all his patients paid him at the time of his visit
and the situation only became worse – in the 1870s only 1 per cent
did. In this case, Langstaff supplemented his income by running
a sawmill.[72] Eliminating the midwife option would not necessarily
have secured full payment for physicians but it would have increased the number of labour cases they attended, for which they
might receive partial payment.

Attendance at childbirth was important not only for the fee it
generated but also for the future business it could bring. One of
the problems many young physicians had to face when they set
up their own practice was attracting clients. Childbirth cases
tended not to be isolated events. If the physician were able to

bring about a quick and safe delivery, the woman, more than likely, would consult him during her next pregnancy. Even more, the family would be inclined to call him in for any medical problems they experienced. Mary O'Brien referred to the lack of work for doctors early in the century. On 15 November 1837, recalling her assistance to a neighbour in childbirth, she noted that the child was born before the doctor arrived and that it was 'the second time I have cheated the doctor within four weeks ... Doctors have no chance at such work here. We make so light of it.'[73] As doctors began to involve themselves more with midwifery cases, the importance of such cases became clearer. Obstetrical patients were only 6.8 per cent of the rural Ontario practice of James Langstaff in the 1850s, but 12.4 per cent in the 1870s.[74] Theodore Clowes Brown did not have a large obstetric practice but his Fredericton records for the 1860s through the 1880s indicate he averaged twenty-five to forty-three cases a year. If each woman represented her family, it indicates the significance of gaining access to such cases for general practitioners. Equally important was the fact that almost 50 per cent of the women he attended, he had cared for in a previous pregnancy.[75] Obstetrical practice was an entrée into family practice, which was the financial mainstay for most general physicians.[76]

Non-economic reasons motivated some physicians against midwives. As in the case of female physicians, the fact that their competition was female, in and of itself, threatened the prestige of male practitioners. In an early edition of his popular manual, William Buchan challenged women's involvement in midwifery. He even went so far as to claim that most problems in pregnancy and labour 'might be prevented by allowing no women to practise midwifery but such as are properly qualified.' Such an argument would be in keeping with the profession's focus on formal training and might seem to be a reasonable request. Buchan, however, reveals his true feelings when he asks the question, 'Was any female ever duly qualified?' and answers, 'I believe not.'[77] Buchan's views were extreme and few physicians were as intransigent as he. But what seemed to bother physicians most about many midwives was their lack of formal training, training which physicians had undergone. Perhaps one of the reasons for the difference in attitude between Dr Dickson and Dr Verity, both of whom had been called in to take over cases from midwives, was that the midwife involved with the former was educated and had not allowed the patient's condition to deteriorate before relinquishing her to a physician. Such was not the experience of Dr Verity. Neither was it the experience of Dr Charles Rolls from Wardsville, Canada West, who reported in 1851 a case he had attended some time previously. Mrs McK was a 'stout, healthy person, aged about thirty' and had borne several children with little difficulty. When he arrived, she had already been in labour for two full days and the two midwives attending her did not seem to know what to do since the action of the uterus had stopped and the birth was not advancing. In summarizing the case he castigated the midwives' actions:

There cannot be the least doubt, had this patient been left without further assistance than she had for the first forty-eight hours, in the course of a short time she must have been a corpse – her husband a widower – and her children motherless. She had been attended by two professed midwives (one of whom is esteemed by the public quite a village oracle): and yet the poor creature had been allowed to remain in strong labour two days and nights, unassisted, in a case in which every medical man knows, the instant he examines, that assistance is necessary, no attempt had been made in the right direction by these midwives, but the labour had been encouraged to proceed, and the woman tortured and worn out, by their fruitless efforts to deliver in the preternatural condition in which I found it; they actually expecting to effect the accouchment by tugging at the arm, and wondering *what in creation* prevented the child from being born. Can there be a doubt in the mind of any unprejudiced person that such practice should not [sic] longer be tolerated?[78]

Yet even Dr Rolls did not condemn all midwives. He concluded his report by calling for properly qualified midwives, women who were trained and examined in the field. Certainly the *Medical Chronicle* in 1855 agreed that training was essential and that men were gradually taking over midwifery because of their superior knowledge and skill.[79] Even Tyler Smith, practising in England where midwives were accepted and often formally trained, believed their day had gone owing to the fact that 'the great mass of our obstetric practice is a ministration of education and experience, such as no endeavours could impart to a body of females.' Women had not added any useful discovery in childbirth. Progress had only come when medical practitioners entered the field.[80] The *Canada Lancet* of 1874 published an article that reiterated the points made by Tyler Smith. Obstetrics had become a modern science when men took it over. It was men who invented the instruments of the obstetric armory, not women. If only women understood this they would feel a 'debt of gratitude' to physicians that would overcome any 'lingering repugnance there may be to the employment of the accoucheur.'[81] Such was the feeling of one practitioner writing to the *Globe* in 1875 when he claimed that he had 'never ... met [a midwife] who had any knowledge of anatomy, who could act whenever the slightest complication occurred.'[82] Clearly it lowered the esteem of doctors to have uneducated women doing the same job as they. It may even have bothered some to have any woman, trained or not, doing the same job.[83] While the arrogance of some doctors' statements is extreme, the situation that physicians found themselves in, vis-à-vis midwives, helps explain why they made them. The only time a physician in private practice would come into contact with a midwife was when he was called in to take over a case she could not handle. No wonder some were antagonistic and saw midwife care as less than advantageous to the patient.

There is a certain irony in physicians insisting on proper training for midwives considering their own training in this field, especially at mid-century when most of the expressed hostility to midwives emerged. In the 1840s students received lectures on obstetrics at the Rolph School of Medicine and at King's College Faculty of Medicine. A Bachelor of Medicine degree required an apprenticeship of six months' attendance at a lying-in hospital,[84] although what that entailed is difficult to know. Despite such training, the *British American Journal of Medical & Physical*

Science still supported students learning to assist in childbirth through the touch method – that is, not through visually examining the woman in labour but by estimating the situation through feel.[85] We have already noted Dr Dickson's reluctance to examine a woman visually, preferring the midwife to do so. At mid-century the University Lying-in Hospital and the Montreal Lying-In Hospital were among the few in North America that allowed their students to view an actual birth. Certainly McGill University did not before the 1870s. Only after completing their McGill courses did students apprentice at the University Lying-in Hospital for six months and attend at least six births, which seemed to be the number required by most medical schools at the end of the century.[86] Until 1890 the Burnside Lying-In Hospital was the only institution in Toronto where students could gain real clinical obstetrical experience.[87] At the Halifax Medical College in 1900 the courses in obstetrics revolved around an artificial pelvis and mannequin, although for practical midwifery students did attend the lying-in ward of the City Alms House.[88] Even as late as the 1920s medical students received more surgical training than they did obstetrical, despite the fact that obstetrical cases would be more numerous in their practice than surgical.[89]

The point of describing the training that physicians received in obstetrics is not to belittle them but to place their objections to midwifery in perspective. Most physicians apprenticed with a physician or graduated from medical schools with little experience in childbirth. They had theoretical knowledge and some had viewed though not assisted in childbirth, although by the end of the century this was no longer the case. Yet they maintained they were trained better than midwives. Their assurance came from their belief in book learning, that theory was more important than experience. Yet it was experience that many midwives had. Most midwives in Canada were probably not trained in any formal sense but they did have certain advantages over physicians. As the Halifax situation points out and as other studies have suggested, they were usually older, married women. These were women who more likely than not had borne children. They knew from their own experience what childbirth was like. Because they were women, their patients may also have been less inhibited in talking to them about their symptoms and certainly less inhibited about having their bodies examined. Tradition has it that midwives often apprenticed with another midwife. If this is true in the Canadian context, it would mean they had probably seen and assisted in many more births than had new medical graduates.

Despite their criticism of the lack of training for midwives, doctors were not particularly supportive of their being trained. When the National Council of Women (NCW) wanted to celebrate Queen Victoria's Jubilee in 1897, it decided to create a nursing body, the Victorian Order of Nurses (VON), that would assist women in isolated areas of the country where physicians were few. The most obvious need both urban and rural women had was help when they went into labour. Keeping this in mind, the NCW envisioned that Victorian Order nurses would be educated in midwifery. The Canadian medical profession was so aghast at the idea that they opposed the concept of the VON altogether. Only when the NCW agreed that the nurses would not take over midwifery cases, and assured doctors that the nurses would only be assistants to them and not substitutes, was the approval of the physicians gained and the VON formed.[90] The entrenched hostility against even trained midwives reflected the changed position of regular practitioners from mid-century. Earlier their status had been tenuous and they felt pressured by competition on all sides, particularly from those who called themselves physicians. To raise their own position, to eliminate others in the field, and to protect patients from the unskilled, doctors emphasized the formal nature of their training. Gradually their definition of training held sway and, by the end of the century, they had few professional competitors. Their main competition was from other colleagues. In the decades in which this medical monopoly was occurring, midwives were a minor annoyance compared to those physicians following Thomsonianism and homeopathy. Indeed, there never was a concerted movement to eliminate midwifery, only isolated voices complaining.

Generally speaking, doctors left midwives alone. Indeed, over time, their interest in midwives seemed to decline, for the most vociferous attacks came at mid-century. Such attacks, however, were without bite since physicians themselves had no organized power. In subsequent decades even these outbursts declined as doctors' increasing domination of midwifery practice took place. James Connor has suggested that the first generation of midwives, the pioneer generation, was unable to recruit younger women to take over from them, and the abating concern of physicians about midwives seems to support this conclusion.[91] A rejuvenated midwife threat, however, endorsed by the foremost women's organization in the country, was a possibility physicians would rather do without. Doctors now dominated childbirth and preferred to keep it that way. They could argue that women had come to choose them over midwives because they had something to offer them. Developments had occurred in medicine that had changed the experience of labour. Three major ones were the introduction of anaesthesia and its possible use in childbirth, the acceptance of antiseptics and the popular belief that this guaranteed safer delivery, and the rise in the number of hospital births. All were linked to physician-attended births.

Before the advent of anaesthesia doctors could only offer their patients alcohol, opiates, or in some cases resort to mesmerism as a palliative to the pain of surgery. Seldom did physicians attempt to alleviate the pain of women in childbirth. On 4 November 1847, however, Sir James Simpson at Edinburgh University used chloroform in a childbirth case and, shortly after, on 25 January 1848, Dr A.F. Holmes, professor of theory and practice of Medicine at McGill, followed suit and administered chloroform to a woman in labour.[92] On 8 March 1848 Dr James Johnston of Sherbrooke, Canada East, reported three similar cases in childbirth and related that he had also used chloroform to reduce morning sickness. With other Canadian physicians quickly following,[93] it would appear that a new day had dawned in obstetric care. Not all physicians were convinced of the efficacy of using anaesthesia in childbirth. What concerned opponents was the question of morality. Was it right to remove the pain of childbearing? Dr Charles Meigs, one of the leading gynaecologists in the United States, considered the pain of childbirth to be 'a desirable, salutary, and conservative manifestation of life force.'[94] Tyler Smith, just two years after Simpson's use of anaesthesia, argued against its use on the grounds that it took away the pain of a natural process and that sexual orgasm would become its substitute.[95] Without the pain of childbirth, women would simply bear children like animals. The debate over the use of anaesthesia in labour was such that the *British American Journal of Medical & Physical Science* asked Abraham De Sola, a McGill lecturer on the Hebrew language, to write an article on its use with respect to the Bible's admonition laid out in Genesis 3:16: 'Unto the woman he said, I will greatly multiply thy sorrow and thy conception; in sorrow thou shalt bring forth children; and thy desire shall be to thy husband, and he shall rule over thee.' If anaesthesia took away the pain, it took away the sorrow. How could God-fearing doctors reconcile medical therapeutics with God's direction? The concern here was not the medical repercussions of anaesthesia in childbirth but the moral. In the ensuing article De Sola asserted that there was no prohibition against using anaesthesia unless it harmed either the mother or the child. With this article and the example of Queen Victoria demanding chloroform in childbirth, the morality of its use was answered. After this, discussion centred on when it should be used.[96]

Dr Hanmet Hill of Ottawa believed that physicians should avoid chloroform in all instrument births. Only if the birth was normal or not necessitating instruments could chloroform be safely utilized. Not all agreed. At the University Lying-in Hospital in Montreal between 1843 and 1860, chloroform was seldom used. Dr Archibald Hall, physician accoucheur to the hospital, claimed it was prohibited in 'all ordinary labours' but used 'whenever anything untoward occurs which demands an artificial assistance.' It was used 'in all cases of version [6/1949 cases], and in forceps cases [19/1949], after the blades of the instrument have been introduced and locked. Such are the cases to which its employment has been as yet restricted, because no others have as yet occurred to require it.'[97] Of course, the Lying-in Hospital was designed for unwed and/or destitute mothers and such women may not have been the major recipients of chloroform. Considering some physicians' beliefs that poorer women did not experience birth pains to the same degree as middle-class women, doctors may not have felt anaesthesia was indicated for such women. And unlike their middle-class sisters, they would not have been in a position to demand anaesthesia. In addition, since most of the patients would have been unwed mothers, doctors may not have seen their pain as deserving of sympathy. The mid-century rural practice of James Langstaff, however, suggests that the difference between hospital and private practice may not have been great, for in his practice he used chloroform only once in every 600 cases, and a contemporary did so only once in every 900 cases.[98] After mid-century, most discussion of anaesthesia assumed its use. One reviewer of an American text compared the pain of childbirth to that of a tooth-ache.[99] While such an analogy suggested that childbirth was a pathological occurrence, it also highlighted the willingness to see labour pains as no longer having moral overtones. Even Tyler Smith changed his view on the subject.[100] President of the Medico-Chirurgical Society of Montreal, T.A. Rodger made it clear that the only real debate was not whether anaesthesia should be used but what kind should be given – that is, chloroform or ether.[101] Napheys agreed. In his manual he argued that labour should be without severe pain and felt that physicians could use either chloroform or ether if it were needed. In 'Parturition without Pain,' Dr Holbrook clearly felt there should be no pain in childbirth if the birthing woman was healthy and, like many other physicians, he appealed to the example of savage women as his proof. Granting, however, that not all women were savage, and that for many women there was pain in childbirth, he believed that doctors should alleviate it.[102] Despite this seeming consensus, some physicians remained unsure about when to use anaesthesia. W.S. Muir of Truro, NS, did not think it warranted in every case of instrumental labour, whereas R.S. Black of Halifax did.[103]

As suggested by Drs Muir and Black, the use of anaesthesia depended very much on the physician. At the Burnside Lying-In Hospital, doctors used anaesthesia in only 3.6 per cent of the cases.[104] In his Woodstock, Ont., obstetric practice Dr Hugh MacKay used it in only thirty-five out of 816 cases. Among the reasons for Mackay's disinclination to use chloroform were some of the problems associated with it. On 17 May 1876 he noted that he had given chloroform to Mrs John Malton and that afterwards he observed 'patient pale, pupils dilated and pulse weak ... Suspended the chloroform and gave brandy and water pretty freely which had the effect of steadying the pulse.'[105] Mackay's form of anaesthetic conservatism was urged in an editorial in the 1885 *Canada Lancet*, which sounded the alarm at how 'fashionable' the administration of ether and chloroform had become and warned its Canadian readers that women had more difficulty overcoming the effects of anaesthesia than the pain of labour.[106] Not all Canadian doctors were convinced. Dr Alexander McPhedron's casebook for 1884–7 indicates little hesitation about using chloroform in his Toronto practice.[107] Even the Montreal Maternity Hospital was providing anaesthesia in 50 per cent of its maternity cases by the turn of the century.[108] Whether this was a result of more paying patients being cared for, the fact that physicians and not midwives were in charge of even normal births, or a change in attitude about the use of anaesthesia is difficult to determine. While the Fredericton years of Theodore Clowes Brown indicated a 15 per cent use of chloroform,[109] in 1896 G.E. Coulthard, president of the New Brunswick Medical Society, analysed 1000 of his own obstetrical cases and found he used chloroform in all but 211 of them. In those, the women either refused it or he arrived too late through the delivery to administer it.[110] This indicates not only the greater use that was being made of anaesthesia but also that women had a certain degree of autonomy in determining what kind of treatment they would receive. It would have been very difficult for doctors to reject anaesthesia altogether, for their patients quickly heard about its wonderful pain-killing properties and demanded its use. Dr Johnston's patient in February 1848 'begged' him to give her chloroform to ease the pain – this within six months of its first being used in midwifery practice.[112] In 1868 William Canniff reported the same experience. He carried chloroform with him on all midwifery cases 'to be given *if desired by the patient*,' and noted that more and more women were demanding it.[112] Understandably when faced with patients' demands, physicians would prefer to acquiesce if they possibly could. Doctors did not enjoy seeing patients in pain and the pain of childbirth, coming as it did from a natural function, may have made them question how much they deserved the thanks of women. By being able to offer women a way of avoiding pain, physicians could feel they had done something worthwhile.

The initial hostility to the use of anaesthesia in childbirth on the part of a few physicians such as Tyler Smith and its eventual endorsement represented two ways of approaching the female body. These differing approaches also raise the ever-present theme of nature versus nurture or, in this case, culture. As one historian has concluded: 'For obstetricians who oppose anesthesia, woman's body belongs to the realm of nature, which requires a man's monitoring; only Tyler Smith, for example, can recognize in her cries sexuality subdued through pain. For obstetricians who advocate chloroform, this same body must be stilled; only then can it be delivered from nature into the culture where, once so mastered, it properly belongs.'[113] Whether midwives saw a birthing woman as part of the 'realm of nature' is unknown but, if so, it may help explain their apparent non-use of anaesthesia. There was no legal prohibition against their using it, and James Connor has point out that anaesthetic agents could readily be purchased at drugstores and easily utilised.[114] Practical and financial considerations, however, may have militated against their use. Most midwives lived in isolated areas and would have had little access to drugstores. Also, the cost of such drugs was likely prohibitive, considering how little midwives charged their patients. And although there may have been no legal prohibition against the use of anaesthesia by midwives, there may have been general disapproval. Commenting on the death of a Port Hope woman in 1864 after she was chloroformed by a dentist, the inquest jury made clear 'their disapprobation to the giving of chloroform by unqualified persons. The jury consider that no person ought to be allowed to administer chloroform, except a physician.'[115] By not using anaesthesia, midwives may have assisted in their own decline. Anaesthesia was something tangible which physicians could offer women, and the indications are that women were willing to accept it and even demand it.

Of less obvious value than anaesthesia from the patient's perspective but of more significance was the introduction of antiseptic medicine, particularly with the increase in medically managed childbirth. Traditional medical historiography has viewed pantiseptic techniques as a revolutionary breakthrough and argued it was one reason that medicine was able to earn the prestige it did. Antiseptic procedures made treatment safer. While such an interpretation is not incorrect, it does not tell the whole story. Not all physicians embraced antisepsis and it took a great deal longer to be implemented than previously thought. Dr Adam Wright of the Burnside Lying-In Hospital in Toronto indicated that when stringent rules concerning asepsis were introduced, they were not popular. In fact, 'the resident assistants sometimes ignored them, or obeyed the directions in a half-hearted way.'[116] In her study of the Montreal Maternity Hospital, Rhona Kenneally points out that not until 1925 did authorities at the Montreal Maternity acknowledge that the wearing of a mask in the delivery room was important.[117] And while medical mythology credits antisepsis for declining mortality rates from surgery in the nineteenth century, David Hamilton has argued that such rates altered as a result of better nutrition and the decline in infectious disease.[118] Nevertheless, doctors believed it to be the result of their adoption of antiseptic techniques, and this encouraged them to intervene in the human body in ways they had never dared to do before.

How important was antisepsis in childbirth? Certainly the connection between germs that could be carried on a physician's clothing or on his person and infection in patients was crucial in making physicians more aware of the need for cleanliness. This would lessen the chance of doctors unknowingly carrying disease from one patient to another, a possible cause of much of the puerperal fever of the period. Dr Adam Wright maintained that mortality from septicaemia had declined at Burnside between 1888 and 1897 because of the introduction of aseptic procedures and he gave much of the credit to Miss MacKellar, the head nurse.

Adopting such antiseptic procedures put physicians on a par with the best of midwives who, because they only cared for women in childbirth and seldom travelled from one patient to another, were not the source of infection that doctors potentially were. The medical press was positive about the notion of cleanliness in practice, although there was some reluctance to acknowledge the existence of germs and the need to carry out what appeared to be extraordinary measures to ensure antiseptic cleanliness. In any event, interventionist antisepsis – the use of carbolic sprays which sometimes made pools in hospital surgical rooms – were of little use in midwifery practice given that most women gave birth at home. Antiseptic douches were a possibility, however. Dr Adam Wright did not resort to vaginal douches in his own practice, but when he became physician to the Burnside Lying-In Hospital in Toronto he found that douching was used quite frequently.[119] The author of 'Meddlesome Midwifery' in the 1885 *Canada Lancet* worried that perhaps too many physicians were resorting to them. While such intervention might be necessary in the case of an instrument birth and 'exposure to contagion,' in ordinary cases it was uncalled for. Antiseptic douches, he felt, were just another fad that had come and would go, 'but that obstetrician who has most faith in Nature, and who makes patience, discrimination, cleanliness and moderate conservatism his guiding star, will be able to show a record second to none.'[120] The minutes of the British Medical Association in Nova Scotia in 1892 suggest his was not a lone voice. The association's members discussed the use of antisepsis in midwifery cases and at least one expressed dismay at the 'general indiscriminate use of antiseptic injections' and deemed them 'harmful.'[121] There was a reluctance on the part of some physicians to changes occurring in medicine, as if change was acknowledgment of previous error. George Armstrong, a Montreal physician responding rather defensively and perhaps belligerently to the publicity surrounding Joseph Lister and antiseptics, pointed out that women still gave birth to healthy children even when antiseptic procedures were not followed. And to illustrate the absurdity of those procedures, he envisioned what the future held in store unless more reasonable heads prevailed:

I think we might recognize a momentum in antiseptic theories – a momentum that seems to be carrying us into irrational and absurd practices, that after a time we shall be compelled to give up, but not without the loss of prestige and influence with the public. According to the present rate of progression we shall soon, when called upon to attend a case of midwifery be compelled to retire to our bath-rooms, wash and scrub in disinfectant solutions, don a fresh suit of disinfectant clothes, and, like the Romish priests, when called to administer the communion at a person's residence, we shall go forth, preceded by couriers to clear the way and open doors, etc., etc., not daring to touch even a door bell knob, less, possibly, an unclean mendicant has first handled and defiled it.[122]

More reasonable heads did not prevail, for a more perfect description of obstetrics in our day could not be imagined! But before this became the reality rather than an absurd vision, childbirth would have to leave the home and enter the hospital. This it would not do to any major extent until the twentieth century.

As long as births continued to occur at home, physicians were restricted in the kind of antiseptic care they could provide, which pleased those who saw childbirth as a natural physiological event. But home births also limited a physician's power, for in a home birth the physician is an interloper and must fit his needs with those of the household. He is visibly and directly accountable to the patient's family, a member of which always seems to be around when he calls. In a hospital, in contrast, the physician is on familiar ground. It is an environment in which he has power, not the patient or the patient's family. They have to play by the hospital's rules, and these are rules that favour the physician. In recent years there has been a great deal of criticism about hospital births. Barbara Rothman has pointed out that giving birth in a hospital makes a natural process into a medical event: 'You do not put someone in a hospital gown, place her on a hospital table under hospital lights, and affix little bracelets to her arm so that you can always tell whose baby is whose, and not create the image of "patient." A woman cannot view herself as healthy while all the external cues proclaim illness.'[123] Especially if accompanied by interventionist midwifery, birth in a hospital creates fear in the pregnant woman, leading to tension and difficulty in birth. Nonetheless, for many women advantages exist to giving birth in a hospital. For poor and overworked women, a hospital stay, no matter how limited, provides a much needed rest away from the stresses and demands of family. For others, it represents convenience and, above all, safety in the constant professional care received.[124]

Very little of this is applicable to nineteenth-century Canada, for the real shift to hospital birth did not come until the twentieth century. As late as 1939 more births occurred at home than in hospitals in the province of Ontario. For most of the nineteenth century few women would give birth in a hospital unless they absolutely had to. Hospitals were not particularly attractive places, and many refused to accept midwifery cases except in cases of emergency. Nevertheless, hospital authorities did make some attempts to help poor and needy childbearing women. At mid-century the Halifax Visiting Dispensary was established. One of the by-laws allowed annual subscribers of twenty shillings or more the right to recommend one midwifery case which a medical student would attend under supervision of the resident or visiting physician. However, midwifery cases were not many. In 1868 there were only nine cases, although twenty-nine cases of diseases of pregnancy were treated. In 1875 midwifery cases had only increased to ten.[125] The pregnant women attending the University Dispensary of the Montreal General Hospital in the early 1880s were usually suffering from extreme symptoms of pain. Thus medical assistance in a hospital setting seemed to be for a very small minority of women who were having difficulty with their pregnancies or had nowhere else to go. Margaret Coady turned to the University Dispensary for help when she found herself, at the age of twenty-eight, unmarried but pregnant. She first came on 18 March 1882 complaining she had not menstruated since 23 December 1881 and had been suffering from headaches, nausea, and vomiting after meals, constipation, and leucorrhoea. Found to be four to five months pregnant, the physicians gave her medication to help alleviate the constipation. Further medication was prescribed on 23 March. On 11 April she again came to the dispensary suffering from vertigo and on 20 May of pains in her back and side.[126] She was clearly seeking physical relief, but she may also have been searching for some kind of support in facing a society generally antagonistic to unwed mothers. At the dispensary she received care with a minimum of moralizing. This also seemed to be the situation of Digby resident Lilias Harmon, aged twenty and unmarried, who came to the Victoria General Hospital, Halifax, on 5 November 1894 and was admitted for two days. She complained of the absence of menstruation for the last seven months and, on examination, was found to be seven months pregnant. The hospital arranged for the Salvation Army to come in and assist her.[127] Lilias Harmon's case could reveal one of two things – that she was so unaware of what was happening to her own body and ignorant of the basic knowledge of reproduction that she was not conscious of her pregnancy or, more likely, that her approach to the hospital was one last desperate attempt to stop the pregnancy and, failing that, to get some kind of assistance.

In addition to dispensaries and general hospitals willing to take in emergencies, maternity homes existed for normal cases of pregnancy for the poor and especially for unmarried women. As early as the 1820s both Montreal and York (Toronto) each had organizations for the care of pregnant women, the former founded by Catholic lay societies to provide for unmarried women and the latter to supply food, clothing, and medical care for women who had homes of their own. Homeless women in York had no alternative but to go to the General Hospital, which was certainly not set up for maternity cases. In 1841 Dr MacNider of the Montreal School of Medicine opened a Lying-In Hospital in that city as a teaching aid for his students, but it lasted only five years. In the 1840s as well the University Lying-in Hospital (Montreal) was established and the Hôpital de St Pélagie (Montreal) run by the Sisters of St Pélagie and the Maternity Home of Mercy (Quebec City) were founded.[128] The wives of the medical professors from the Montreal General Hospital had set up the Lying-in Hospital to aid working-class women, and a board of management of ladies oversaw the domestic running of the institution and appointed a visiting committee. The purpose of the hospital was two-fold; first, to provide care for destitute women when 'sickness is impending' at no fee, to take in paying patients, and to provide for out-patients, such as wives of labourers or mechanics, who, because of the needs of their families, could not enter a hospital; second, to instruct medical students from McGill University and at mid-century any women 'desirous of acquiring an acquaintance with the duties and practice of Obstetrics.' Staffed by the medical faculty of McGill University, it was a voluntary hospital – that is, it was supported by donations and administered privately. As in the case of the Halifax Visiting Dispensary, each annual subscriber could recommend a pauper patient for admission within two weeks of her delivery, although the midwife or physician accoucheur had to approve the admission. Otherwise a patient had to provide letters of recommendation and present them to the visiting committee. No woman who presented herself in actual labour, however, would be refused admission. The matron could admit any woman, if recently widowed or married, into the hospital earlier than two weeks before delivery in cases of distress or destitution as long as the woman could provide proof of destitution. In special circumstances, the monthly visitors could even give 'refuge for some young female' if a parent, priest, minister, or guardian requested it. This latter case was a response to the dearth of shelters for the casual poor or lonely woman.[129]

Elsewhere in the country similar institutions were being founded. In Toronto a five-bed General Dispensary and Lying-In Hospital opened in 1848, and two other homes for the care of pregnant women in 1856. In 1869 all three amalgamated to form the Burnside Lying-In Hospital which, in 1877, became part of the Toronto General Hospital. In 1888 the Salvation Army opened its first Rescue Home in Toronto, which soon became a maternity hospital for unwed mothers.[130] Unlike many hospitals, the Kingston General Hospital provided a lying-in ward.[131] In Ottawa the Sisters of Mercy opened the Misericordia Lying-In Hospital offering medical assistance and long-term residence in 1879. In the same year local women founded the Ottawa Home for Friendless Women, a Protestant-supported institution to give refuge to 'friendless women, discharged female prisoners, and those desiring to forsake a life of sin.'[132] Under the auspices of the British Columbia wCTU, a Cottage Hospital in New Westminster opened that was for women patients, there being little accommodation for women in the general hospitals of that province.[133] The establishment of so many charitable institutions for pregnant women responded to a need in society. Although it is difficult to know the rate of illegitimacy in Canada, it has been estimated at somewhere between 2 and 4 per cent. Between 1875 and 1900 alone this constituted at least 16,000 births.[134] Many of these women were friendless with nowhere to turn. Poor married women, too, needed assistance, since the circumstances of many prevented them from being able to afford a physician or a midwife.

The charitable aspect of these institutions is reflected in the women who entered them. Of the 1301 patients whose ages were known at the University Lying-in Hospital, Montreal, between 1843 and 1859, 822 were under the age of twenty-five. This is not surprising given that most of these women were unwed. Indeed, between 1843 and 1886, three-fifths of the 7000 women delivered there were single.[135] The majority of women entering the Kingston General Hospital Maternity Ward in the 1860s and 1870s were also unmarried. At the Burnside Hospital between 1878 and 1882, just over half the women were aged twenty-one or younger, with fewer than 9 per cent over the age of thirty. And 80 per cent of the patients were unmarried.[136] This is quite different from private practice where the vast majority of patients were married. The length of stay in these institutions accentuates their charitable purpose.[137] Almost one-third of patients attending the University Lying-in Hospital entered two weeks before their delivery, and the women who gave birth in the Kingston hospital stayed on average twelve weeks. Unwed women would have limited resources to fall back on as they neared their time of delivery, and the social hostility towards them would ensure they had few people to care for them. Consequently, early entry into the hospital was a charitable act, not a medical necessity. Until they gave birth, these women were expected to help with the housework of the hospital. Over 20 per cent of the University Lying-in Hospital patients stayed longer than two weeks after delivery despite the regulation of the hospital not to keep a patient more than ten days after childbirth. Those who stayed longer were those who had entered well before their delivery and, because length of stay was not linked to any birth complications, it seems safe to assume it was because of socio-economic needs. Burnside's records, too, reveal early entry with approximately 35 per cent of the women coming to the hospital more than fourteen days before delivering; thus Burnside was acting as more than a hospital, especially when just over 60 per cent stayed in the hospital two weeks or more after delivery. Early entry was not linked to the mother's health before entry or to the age of the woman, although women thirty or over were slightly overrepresented among those admitted early, the number of deliveries she had previously undergone or, surprisingly, her marital status.[138] Unfortunately, the records are not detailed enough to know the class or familial background of the women, but since early entry was not linked to medical needs, it was probably the result of financial and personal needs of the patients. The University Lying-in Hospital responded to the economic needs of their patients even more explicitly. Hospital authorities would arrange for their patients to be sent out to wet nurse. At mid-century employers had to pay a fee of ten shillings and the woman herself had to pay £1 to the hospital.[139] Wetnursing was a form of employment that allowed these young women an opportunity to support themselves.[140]

Despite the obvious concern about providing childbirth assistance to these women, little sympathy was expended on them. The inspector of prisons and public charities for Ontario reported in 1879 that maternity cases stayed for an average of eighty-three days at the Kingston General Hospital and noted that '[pregnant] women sent to the hospital are chiefly prostitutes ... apt to look upon [it] as a convenient bedding place.'[141] Since so many of the patients were unwed, there was an air of rehabilitation about their care and women who did not exhibit signs of rehabilitation were not considered deserving. For this reason the University Lying-in Hospital, among others, insisted that an unwed woman could only be admitted once. Repeat offenders need not apply.[142] Once admitted, rules were stringent – no visitors were allowed on the wards, no extra eating or drinking, a patient had to obtain the permission of the matron before she could leave the ward to visit friends in the hall, and such visitors could not stay more than one-half hour and needed permission either from the matron, midwife, or physician to visit. When well, the matron could also require patients 'to make themselves useful.'[143] If the women did not adhere to the rules, they could be discharged.

The medical care provided in these early facilities varied. At Burnside the need to call in physicians in emergencies could cause delay in treatment. One young woman who entered on 4 February 1881 and delivered on 28 February ruptured her perineum to the rectum and had to wait for four hours before the doctor arrived to sew it up.[144] Assessing the situation in the 1890s, Dr Adam Wright believed that the weakness in protecting the health of patients in Burnside was the fact that the 'resident assistants have charge of all normal deliveries.'[145] At the Montreal Maternity Hospital, a midwife delivered the normal cases. There was no resident doctor and only the chief obstetrician (McGill's professor of obstetrics) could use forceps, provide medication, and perform emergency intervention. According to one historian, he did not appear at the hospital with any regularity. By the 1880s, however, the situation had changed. As we have already seen, the last mid-wife retired in 1886 to be replaced by a physician. Doctors became more visible – they took over routine births, the training of medical students at the hospital, brought in consulting specialists, and became more involved in administration. The number of patients increased and they were staying a shorter period of time.[146] The University Lying-in Hospital did remain a training hospital, which meant those who entered free often had less privacy than paying patients. Usually two students attended each birth, but in the case of one woman admitted 11 June 1894 ten students witnessed her delivery, with the use of low forceps as part of their exam.[147]

As can be seen, the lying-in hospitals served numerous functions. In her excellent study of the Ottawa Maternity Home, Kathleen Pickard pointed out they were rescue homes, childcare institutions, rehabilitation centres, employment training facilities, and teaching hospitals.[148] The refuge aspects of institutional maternity care, however, did start to decline by the end of the century. In the 1890s the percentage of patients at the Montreal Maternity Hospital who were married increased. In 1893 one-third of the patients were married and only two years later, one-half. This increase did not solve the financial needs of the hospital because many of these women could not afford to pay. At its annual meeting in 1894, Dr Craik alluded to the hospital's financial problems and the difficulty the lady managers had raising money owing to 'delicacy of feeling' in talking about their work in a public forum. If money were to be raised, the male supporters of the hospital would have to do it.[149] Certainly depending on paying patients was not going to suffice. Between 1884 and 1905 no more than twenty were admitted in any given year.[150]

Elsewhere this was not the case. Facilities for paying patients were increasing. In 1893 the Doran Wing of the Kingston General Hospital was built and designed for non-charity gynaecological and obstetric cases.[151] In 1896 the directors of the Royal Jubilee Hospital in Victoria remarked they were considering building and maintaining a maternity ward as a separate institution to meet the needs of women.[152] A year earlier, the Ottawa Maternity Home opened with the intention of serving the needs of married women and, if possible, paying patients. The women behind its establishment 'focused on the physical risks of childbirth, not the social consequences of unwed motherhood.' This did not mean they were no longer interested in providing charity – they were. Part of their mandate was to care for unwed mothers and nurse women who delivered at home. But the hospital would not provide a refuge for patients. Although charitable cases never comprised more than 17 per cent of the patients, the Ottawa Maternity had little difficulty in filling its beds. By 1903 11 per cent of the births in Ottawa took place in the Ottawa Maternity Hospital, and most of the married women admitted chose semi-private or private accommodation despite the $10 per week charge for private patients.[153]

Why was the shift towards hospital births beginning to be supported? Some historians have suggested that women went to hospitals assuming it would decrease their chances of dying in childbirth because of their belief that the hospital was the major repository of medical science.[154] This was an idea that many physicians wanted to encourage. They disliked having to deliver in women's homes where their expertise would be under the scrutiny of other women who came to keep the pregnant woman company. William Buchan, in giving instructions to his readers on the proper care of a parturient woman, noted 'that ridiculous custom ... of collecting a number of women together on such occasions. These, instead of being useful, serve only to crowd the house, and obstruct the necessary attendants. Besides, they hurt the patient with their noise; and often, by their untimely and impertinent advice, do much mischief.'[155] Dr Rolls of Wardsville, Canada West, agreed. He had gone to a patient and in an exasperated tone described how he had found 'the house ... filled with women, all eagerly on the *qui-vive*, to know whether the patient was to die or live.'[156] Despite physician hostility to these women, recent research has indicated that the presence of a supportive woman during labour shortens its duration and may even decrease childbirth complications.[157] Hospitals were the domain of the physician, not of the patients or their friends, and from the doctor's perspective had much to recommend them. However, we should not exaggerate the shift to hospital births among those women who could choose where they gave birth. The vast majority of women still gave birth in their own homes.

But if the locale of birth had not changed to any great extent, who delivered the child had. In the latter half of the nineteenth century physicians came to manage childbirth. They did not do this through any overt efforts to prohibit midwives (except at the end) but rather through offering women an alternative portrayed as safe and scientific. We have already noted the strength of that kind of appeal. What they offered may not have been as accurate as they believed, for physicians had not escaped all age-old superstitions surrounding birth. Nonetheless, they were able to couch their superstition in scientific rhetoric. What doctors offered their patients was a willingness to try to understand, in a way that appeared rational rather than mystical, *how* women's bodies worked. The perception of many physicians was that women's bodies were not working well, that women were no longer giving birth as easily as they once had. Modern society had separated women from a natural life and it was doctors' responsibility to assist women, not to return to that life, but to cope with the problems of childbirth that were now facing women. The real test of a physician after all is in the care of his patient.

Chapter Seven

Changing Obstetric Care

Rose MacDonaugh entered the Victoria General Hospital in Halifax on 24 March 1893. According to her records, she had begun to menstruate at fifteen and was regular in doing so until her marriage in 1887. Her first child was a forceps delivery and since that birth she had suffered from lower back pain and a leucorrhoeal discharge. Despite her weakened condition, she gave birth to her second child just thirteen months after the birth of her first. Now, several years later, and diagnosed as having a lacerated cervix and perineum, on 30 March doctors at the Victoria General stitched the perineum. On July 11 they discovered that the stitches had never been removed and that the procedure had been unsuccessful in mending the tear. Consequently on 15 July the perineum and the cervix were again stitched, this time with the stitches being subsequently removed.[1] Lucille Bouvier entered the hospital three months after MacDonaugh and revealed that in nine years she had given birth to six children, only four of whom were living. She had miscarried two months previous to entering the hospital and afterwards had remained in bed for one month but on getting up felt pains 'of a dull aching character' in her pelvis and lumbar region. She informed the attending physician she had not menstruated for two months. On examination she was found to be pregnant.[2]

How typical the experiences of MacDonaugh and Bouvier were is impossible to know. Judith Leavitt has pointed out that the nature of nineteenth-century childbirth depended on the wealth of the woman concerned, what medical providers were available, and which one the woman preferred. Nonetheless Leavitt categorized women in childbirth into four groups. The first were the 'institutionals,' those women so poor they had to go to a general or a lying-in hospital. Women of the urban working class and rural women were 'traditionalists' in that they had midwives to provide assistance. The urban middle class were women who could afford a physician and Leavitt refers to them as 'integrationists.' 'Privileged' women had access to the obstetric specialist.[3] While such categories are not exclusive – a wealthy woman might choose to have a midwife and a working-class woman might be willing to pay a physician – they do reveal that care must be taken when generalizing about childbirth. While this study will not examine the support provided by midwives, it will touch upon the other three. Records of lying-in hospitals provide insight into the treatment of the poor; records of private general practitioners document the treatment of rural inhabitants, the middle class, and some among the skilled working class; and the instructions of textbooks and some of the medical periodical literature outline the treatment which the most privileged in society might have received. But regardless of the wealth of the patient, physicians provided little pre-natal or post-partum care. The focus of their energies was the actual birth process. They recognized its naturalness but at the same time felt the need to intervene, to be a participant. The irony was that many physicians were increasingly concerned and vocal about the intervention occurring in childbirth or, at least, the type of intervention that was taking place. Only rarely in the debate over intervention were the demands of women heard, but when they were it was clear that intervention was not always imposed on women against their will or with their being unaware of its repercussions. At times, women insisted on relief from pain, from prolonged labour, or from birth complications, and instructed doctors on how to provide it.

In the present day, doctors carefully monitor women throughout their pregnancy. So standard has this become that some critics have accused doctors of treating pregnancy as a disease. A physician looks for *symptoms* of pregnancy, then *diagnoses* a woman as pregnant, and then compares her to her *normal* or her non-pregnant state.[4] This concentration on the pre-natal phase of a pregnancy is relatively recent. In the nineteenth century the medical literature makes little reference to the care of pregnant women before they went into labour. When it did, it centred on the difficulties in diagnosing pregnancy and the problems this created for male physicians, especially early on in the century. The notes of one medical student clearly reflected his lecturer's discomfort about performing an internal examination to determine pregnancy: 'As this is a disagreeable operation to modest Ladies we ought to be particularly cautious and avoid giving offence by the manner in which we touch and endeavour to render it as agreeable as possible by advising it to be done at their own houses, where they may have their own servants about them, and people they are used to, a strict attention to this Part of your business will be of greater consequence to you in your practice.'[5] The description of the surroundings and the expressed consideration for the sensibilities of the woman assume that the student's future patients will be respectable and relatively affluent. It suggests the care that male physicians had to take when examining their women patients and that an internal examination by a man, even if a doctor, was still not a normal occurrence. The willingness of the physician to allow the woman to have people around her protected the doctor from charges of impropriety and indicates that physicians were relatively open about the wants of their women patients and prepared to accommodate themselves to them.

The diagnosis of pregnancy was not straightforward in the nineteenth century. There was no ultimate test for pregnancy before quickening and physicians depended on other symptoms, ones that could just as easily apply to other conditions. In his 1837 textbook, P. Cazeaux stated that a strong indication of pregnancy was whether the woman experienced a 'voluptuous sensation' during intercourse, a belief which reflected the popular notion that vigorous sexuality in women was advantageous for conception. A more dependable symptom was 'ceasing-to-be-unwell' – that is, no longer menstruating.[6] This was what brought Anne Palmer, aged thirty, to the University Dispensary of the Montreal

General Hospital early in 1883. Although unmarried, she admitted to having had sexual intercourse once, on Christmas Day 1882. On diagnosing her as pregnant, her physician noted that along with cessation of her menses other symptoms of pregnancy were present, namely nausea and uneasy sensations in the breasts.[7] The records of Hugh Mackay's practice also revealed the guesswork involved in diagnosing pregnancy. Called to a patient who was not normally his, she informed him her physician had determined that her 'uterine hemorrhage was due to some disease associated with the "change of life."' He had treated her by passing something up her womb, and had daily placed medicated lint on the os. When Mackay saw her, she was experiencing pains similar to labour pains, which she claimed was impossible given what her own doctor had told her and from the fact that she had been menstruating for the past month. Mackay examined her, found the os dilated, and a five-and-a-half-month-old foetus presenting itself. As he laconically wrote, 'I then told her that something more than clots would have to come away before she was better.'[8]

Most women would not consult a doctor for a diagnosis of pregnancy and most did not receive pre-natal care. Exceptions to this were those patients who had had previous complications in childbirth[9] and those who entered the charity maternity homes before they went into labour. But the latter did so for socio-economic, not medical reasons. Nevertheless, because such hospitals were often teaching establishments, when monitoring procedures became available these women were among the first to receive them. The 1898 report of the Montreal Maternity revealed it now had a testing room for urinanalysis designed for use on a daily basis by waiting and convalescent patients. The next year the physician accoucheur to the hospital, Dr Cameron, stressed how important 'careful systematic observation of pregnant women during the last two months of gestation' was in detecting potentially complicating conditions.[10] The majority of women, however, only saw a physician (if they did at all) when they went into labour. Throughout the century, most Canadian women lived in rural regions where there was a strong tradition of self-reliance, where access to physicians was limited, and where hard currency with which to pay a physician was scarce. The records of several private practices confirms the pattern – attendance at birth only. James Langstaff, in his Richmond Hill, Ont., practice from 1847 to 1875 seldom saw a woman before birth and at the birth attended for only an hour. He would remain for another hour afterwards, but only medical complications dictated any more extensive post-partum visits.[11] One of the reasons for this limited supervision was the cost of multiple visits to the patient and her family and the time it took from a practitioner's other patients. For example, Langstaff visited seven to nine patients a day or over 3000 a year. He simply would not have the time to visit expectant mothers (or post-partum ones) on a regular basis. Most pregnant women, then, relied on the advice of their neighbours and their own experiences in previous pregnancies.

The actual labour was the arena for physician participation. Critics of modern-day medical texts have accused the authors of not describing what it feels like to be in labour – that is, they do not take into account the participation of the woman.[12] Some nineteenth-century texts were little better in their descriptions of the actual birth phenomenon. They tried to generalize labour for their student readers and in so doing ignored the trauma of the patient. Kenneth Fenwick, in his 1889 *Manual of Obstetrics*, summarized labour in a statistical way. For a primipara (a woman who had never had a child before) he estimated the average duration of labour at seventeen hours, for a multipara twelve hours. The first stage of labour lasted approximately ten hours, the second two hours, and the third ten to fifteen minutes.[13] While Fenwick may have lost sight of the parturient woman in his attempt to quantify, not all of his colleagues did so. In Gunning Bedford's 1861 *Principles of Obstetrics*, the author describes a doctor's first visit to a patient in labour (note the assumption that the doctor has not seen the patient before). He advises the physician to act like a gentleman and to talk generalities with the woman in order to calm her fears.[14] Later in the century, Montreal's Dr D.C. MacCallum also counselled treating the pregnant patient gently and being sensitive to her sense of decorum. And in a manner that harkened back to the early decades of the century, he suggested that when a doctor wanted to perform a vaginal examination he should acquaint the patient of this through a third party, either a nurse or an elderly friend. MacCallum went on to state that 'the better the patient's rank in life is, the more docile will she prove at these times, and the more resolute to undergo whatever she is told it is necessary to submit to.'[15] While clearly seeing the patient as relatively passive, MacCallum accepted the need for restraint on the part of a physician, especially when the woman was wealthy and being delivered in her own home where the physician was the outsider and dependent on her to see that his needs were met. He acknowledged the presence of other individuals either in the birthing room or close by and was indeed willing to take advantage of their presence.

The latter fact is important, for much has been made in recent years about the reluctance of physicians to have outsiders in the birth chamber. However, as is suggested by the MacCallum example, this was not always the case. And MacCallum was not alone in appreciating the support that others could give to the expectant mother. Earlier in the century Cazeaux insisted that the physician should be responsive to those the patient wanted in the room with her. Some patients wanted their husbands, others did not.[16] William Playfair in his 1880 text agreed – it was up to the patient whether she wanted her husband with her.[17] As we have seen, not all physicians were so open and dissenting voices were heard, especially if the woman wanted the presence of an untrained midwife or several neighbours or friends. Pye Henry Chavasse was even hostile to the husband's being present.[18] What seemed to be occurring was a switch from birth being a community event where the woman's friends and neighbours would be present to a privatized experience where only the husband or one close woman friend or relative provided support. Physicians disliked the former, perhaps because they had less influence in such a situation, but, with some exceptions, seemed willing to countenance the latter. Whether they would have preferred removing everyone, leaving only the patient and themselves, is not known, but the chances of doing so were unlikely as long as birth took place in the home.

Some doctors' openness to the wants of their pregnant patients was exhibited in another way – the position of the woman during labour. There are references in the literature to allowing a woman to move about as much as was comfortable for her, at least until the hard pains began.[19] And unlike the mid-decades of the twentieth century when the lithotomy position (this has a woman on her back with her legs in the stirrups) became standard, there were several alternatives from which the doctor, or in rarer cases the patient, could choose. In 1874 one article in the *Canada Lancet* pointed out that the English tradition was to have a woman giving birth lying on her left side whereas in France, Germany, and the United States the normal position was on her back. The author of the article, however, supported the lithotomy position, not because of its advantages to the patient but because of its convenience to the physician and in case instrumental or operative interference was necessary.[20] At the end of the century MacCallum still advocated the British position, for 'the patient lies more comfortably to her own feelings; her face is turned from the practitioner who sits behind her, and who, from this posture, is able to examine or to perform any other necessary manipulations without her feelings being annoyed by seeing what is going forward.'[21] While such a position removed women from full participation in the birth process, there is little suggestion that this was the purpose behind it, although it is clear that this position made the doctor feel more comfortable. While some physicians preferred certain positions, for others it was not an issue. One practitioner in rural Quebec advised letting the woman take whatever position she wanted. He had found that his French-speaking patients preferred a half-sitting position on the floor, whereas his English-speaking patients preferred to be on a bed or lounge lying either on their back or on their side.[22] In his practice the woman, not the physician, decided what birthing position to take.

There was also some acknowledgment that the physician was not always needed. In discussing the third stage of labour, George A. Tye, a Chatham, Ont., physician noted that it, like the preceding stages, was a 'strictly physiological process' requiring little, if any, assistance from an attendant. Only when conditions

were pathological was interference by a practitioner justified.[23]
In a back-handed way Dr MacCallum, too, recognized that in normal cases the efforts of physicians were not really essential and
warned students, after the os uteri had dilated to the size of a half
dollar, not to absent themselves from the birth chamber for very
long. This was not because they were going to be needed but
because delivery could occur at any time; if the physician was
not there at the actual birth of the baby (even if he did nothing),
he could well lose his reputation.[24] It would also lessen his own
sense of professionalism.

In most cases a physician's involvement in the childbirth process ended with the birth of the child. Little advice was provided
about after-care. Some physicians expressed the hope that women
would nurse their children, seeing it as good for the children and
helpful in preventing flooding and milk fever.[25] So important was
breast feeding considered that the 1859 by-laws of the University
Lying-in Hospital insisted that patients must 'suckle' their children unless the physician approved otherwise.[26] Such a regulation
made sense at a time when there was no satisfactory substitute
for breast milk. It also made care of the children easier, and
authorities may have hoped that breast feeding would forge a
bond between mother and child so that on discharge the unwed
mother would accept responsibility for her child. In a non-insti-
tutional setting such enforcement was impossible and doctors
were sorry to report that not all women wanted to breast feed.
Some texts claimed that the dictates of fashion were enough to
persuade women against it, particularly those of the 'better class.'[27]
While most doctors supported breast feeding, they did argue that
not all women could or even should nurse. Among the latter were
women who were 'hysterical and nervous, subject to violent per-
turbations of the mind.'[28] Maternal influence was so strong that
practitioners believed mental disorders could be transmitted to
her child through a mother's milk. In such a case or when the
woman was physically unable to breast feed, wet-nursing was an
alternative. George Napheys's *Physical Life of Woman* even described what kind of woman the wet-nurse should be – moral,
clean, and cheerful, under thirty, having had children of her own,

the youngest of whom was under six months.[29] Whether Canadians believed that unwed mothers sent out from the University Lying-in Hospital met such standards is doubtful, but those in need of wet nurses were probably not in a position to be overly particular.

The issue of breast feeding was related more to the health of the child than to the health of the mother. In general there was a dearth of instructions on maternal post-partum care. One of the earliest was published in the *Upper Canada Journal of Medical, Surgical and Physical Science* in October 1852. The physician, in the straightforward manner characteristic of mid-century medical advice, ridiculed giving tea and cold water to a new mother as others advocated. He believed that the woman had earned a better portion than this and advised giving her whiskey or brandy.[30] Not all physicians had a similar sense of the occasion or the ability of the woman to appreciate it. In fact, many tended to treat new mothers as if they were invalids. *The Practical Home Physician* advised women to stay in bed for at least two weeks after delivery.[31] An article in the 1881 *Canada Medical Record* favoured one to four weeks, noting that modern women could not resist disease as well as their predecessors and thus had to take precautions.[32] In his textbook Paul Mundé complained that women left their bed too soon after childbearing and, while he acknowledged that 'a very valid objection may be made to this view that in the lower walks of life women rise after labor and attend to their duties with impunity on about the ninth day, and yet enjoy a marked immunity from uterine affections,' middle- and upper-class women could not. Their weaker system would break down. Others suggested lying in bed from ten days to only a few days. If women did not follow doctors' advice (which varied from physician to physician), they would have to pay the price in poor health.[33]

While the advice on post-partum care revealed concern on the part of doctors, few women giving birth at home were able to stay in bed long afterwards because of the needs and demands of their families. Only the wealthy and in some cases the very poor received post-partum care. Wealthy women giving birth at home could afford servants to take care of their families while they were recuperating and even nurses to care for themselves. When the Ottawa Maternity Hospital opened, largely for paying patients, the average stay was sixteen days. Women who could afford this attention had the resources to hire help to care for their families in their absence. Ironically, women whose poverty enabled them to receive aid from such institutions also received extended care. The founders of the Ottawa Maternity even had the naïve belief that a two-week stay for such women could offset years of deprivation.[34] For women giving birth in the charity institutions their stays could be quite lengthy. As noted in chapter 6, approximately 20 per cent of all patients at the University Lying-in Hospital remained for more than two weeks after delivery between 1850 and 1900 and the percentage who did so increased over time: whereas in the 1850s only one in seven women stayed more than two weeks, by the 1890s more than one in three did. While such stays were not linked to the health of either mother or child, the fact the woman remained so long meant that she may have had an easier recuperative period than did women who gave birth in their own homes.[35] Certainly the 3 per cent of women at Burnside who received specific medical treatment after delivery might very well not have received it if they had had a home delivery because of the prohibitive cost.[36] Out-patient departments also provided follow-up care for poorer women in their own homes. For instance, in 1896 the Montreal Maternity Hospital (formerly the University Lying-in Hospital) provided daily attendance by both nurse and physician for a period of ten days to 'seventeen poor and deserving married women' in their own homes.[37] Such care would have been beyond the means of most Canadians. Beyond rest and medical care when needed, there was little to distinguish post-partum care in these institutions. At mid-century, the University Lying-in Hospital placed its patients on an invalid diet for the first three days after birth. This consisted of:

Breakfast   1 pt tea; 2 oz, bread or 1/2 pt porridge and 1/2 pt milk
Dinner   1 pt water gruel; 4 oz bread
Supper   1 pt tea; 2 oz bread or 1/2 pt porridge, and 1/2 pt of milk.

After this time patients went on a half diet for three more days and finally a full diet.[38] While such a repast may suggest punishment more than benevolence, lying-in hospitals could offer more nourishing fare if needed. After the birth of her child on 7 July 1879 at the Burnside Lying-In Hospital, one woman complained of pain for several days afterwards. She was examined and nothing found amiss, but as the notes on her case indicate the next day she was eating better – brandy, an egg and milk mixture, and ice milk with lime water.[39]

Despite the fact that most physicians recognized the naturalness of childbirth, the medical literature of the late nineteenth century abounded with references to excessive interference or what was known as 'meddlesome' midwifery.[40] This had not always been true. William Tyler Smith in his 1858 textbook, *The Modern Practice of Midwifery*, criticized physicians who did little in childbirth cases because of what he called their 'timidity' in interfering with nature. The result was real harm to the patient.[41] An article in the *Canada Medical Record* almost twenty years later confirmed that at mid-century physicians had been so opposed to interference that many women were left in labour for hours without assistance. Physician to the University Lying-in Hospital, Archibald Hall, described the case of Mattie Gould, an unmarried woman, aged thirty, who had been admitted on 22 January 1855 and went into labour on 18 March. The medical student, whose case it was, was sent for and, confident he could handle it, refused to consult with the matron. Complications set in and, because of his delay in seeking assistance, the child was stillborn and Mattie died.[42] Times changed, however, and the concern by the mid-1870s was that there was too much interference.[43] Certainly for the rest of the century there was a constant emphasis on the importance of conservative treatment in a normal labour and criticism of meddlesome midwifery.[44] Lapthorn Smith of Bishop's Medical College advocated a form of natural childbirth, even letting the baby feed before being washed so the child could become accustomed to her/his new surroundings.[45] Smith and physicians like him saw childbirth as a physiological process as opposed to a pathological one. Only when something went wrong during birth were physicians to assist, otherwise they were to attend.[46]

Although there seemed to be strong support for rejecting meddlesome midwifery, its continuing presence is suggested by the fact that physicians writing in the literature continued to rail against it.[47] There was a sense that too many physicians were not following conservative principles. The very nature of the profession may partially account for this criticism. An editorial in the 1874 *Canada Lancet* pointed out that obstetrics had become a major specialty in recent years and 'will be held to worthily distinguish the present epoch in medical history.'[48] Status in the profession came with specialization but also with the degree of intricacy of that specialization. Status would accrue with difficulty to those whose job it was to attend a birth. Medical teachers taught their students to acknowledge the reality of normal birth but they also had to prepare them for what could go wrong. While the need for this is understandable, the tendency was to emphasize the abnormal aspects more than the normal. When faced with his first obstetrics case, the conscientious doctor understandably looked for any sign that the birth was going to be difficult and, being human, could well have found what he was looking for. The periodic literature was even worse in stressing the difficult case. The articles published were to interest the reader and to introduce him to 'new' ways of practising medicine. A description of normal childbirth was not going to accomplish either. Descriptions of complicated births, and the ways in which the attendant physician coped with them, would. Consequently, at the same time that the profession acknowledged the need to intervene only when necessary, its own literature was prompting the opposite. When coupled with the tendency on the part of physicians to compare a pregnant woman with a non-pregnant woman instead of a healthy pregnant one, the predisposition to intervene in childbirth would be difficult to resist.[49] Even when physicians compared pregnant women to each other, it did not necessarily reduce intervention. At the University Lying-in Hospital, detailed records were kept on the length of labour, the length of each child born, her/his weight, the amount of amniotic fluid, the weight of the placenta, and the length of the umbilical cord. When enough data was compiled, physicians would be in a position to describe a 'typical' birth. While interesting as an intellectual exercise, what such data collecting did was to create a norm by which practitioners could judge their patients. It revealed the increasing medicalization of birth, with physicians looking to clinical details rather than the patient for information on how the birth was progressing and its results. If a patient's experience did not conform to the norm, then a doctor might deem intervention warranted. In addition, what was the point of having a doctor in attendance and having to pay for that attendance if he did not 'do' anything or was not seen to 'do' anything? Intervention made the physician an active rather than a passive participant.[50] At times doctors did not have the choice of remaining passive, for the patient and her family insisted on intervention. Hugh Mackay related the case of Mrs Wilbur Woods, who he first saw at 2 PM on 6 June 1875. Returning at 11 PM he stayed until 3 AM. During the protracted labour, Mackay considered using forceps but decided against it, feeling it 'is much better not to interfere.' Mrs Woods's family was not so inclined and Mackay in an exasperated tone wrote in his records, 'My patience was tried by the *im*patience of pats. mother and motherinlaw *who thought something ought to be done.*'[51] It was not easy for physicians to resist such importunities.

The intervention in childbirth that many physicians criticized took several forms and varied from one era to another.[52] From the eighteenth century to the middle decades of the nineteenth century, bleeding pregnant women was an accepted medical procedure. Behind it was the assumption that pregnant women had an overabundance of blood and the view that bleeding could offset the dangers of eclampsia (convulsions and coma).[53] But women bled throughout their pregnancy entered labour in a weakened condition. As well, considering the high rate of anaemia or iron deficiency in women during this period, bleeding only accentuated an already existing problem. William Buchan advocated bleeding when the labour was exceptionally long.[54] The register of the University Lying-in Hospital for 1843 to 1847 indicated that venesection was used, although only in two cases, once before delivery and once after.[55] The *Upper Canada Journal of Medical, Surgical and Physical Science* of 1851 published an article in which Dr John George Bethune supported bleeding to bring a woman out of puerperal convulsions. He reported how in April he had been called to see the wife of a young farmer in the district and had found her stretched out on the floor 'in strong epileptic convulsions.' She had just given birth to a living child and the birth itself had been easy. Dr Bethune at once extracted thirty ounces of blood from her right arm in a 'full stream.' In addition, 'her hair having been removed from the upper and posterior parts of the head, cloths steeped in cold water were applied to the bared scalp, and constantly renewed; her feet placed in a warm bath, the body having been previously elevated into a semi-recumbent posture. Mustard frictions were applied to the calves of the legs and inner surface of the thighs, and warm cloths to the abdomen.' Eventually the convulsions subsided and he left her comfortable. Seven hours later finding her undergoing convulsions again, he reopened the vein in her arm and 'relieved her of twenty additional ounces of blood.' Fortunately, these convulsions, too, lessened and the patient made a good recovery.[56] Bleeding in this case may have caused a severe enough shock to the system to succeed in stopping the convulsions.

Another use for bleeding in obstetrics was to weaken an hour-glass contraction of the uterus which would not allow the child to be born. In one case in Canada West the patient was bled to the point of fainting.[57] In 1856 doctors at the University Lying-in Hospital bled Mrs Eliza Feeny because of her protracted labour and the rigidity of her uterine opening. Looking back four years later, Dr Hall, physician accoucheur to the hospital, advised using tartar emetic in such cases rather than bleeding.[58] Certainly after mid-century doctors were recognizing that pregnant women really did not have an abundance of blood. The result was a significant decline in bloodletting, especially for hemorrhages in childbirth. Its replacement was the use of ergot post partum, the placement of ice in the uterine cavity, or the pouring of cold water on the abdomen.[59] Even for puerperal convulsions its popularity had waned. At the University Lying-in Hospital between 1867 and 1875 in seven cases of convulsions, venesection was used only twice, in one instance on a girl of nineteen from whom twenty-five ounces of blood was removed. According to D.C. MacCallum, professor of midwifery at McGill, the rarity of bleeding was due not to doctors' lack of faith in its efficacy in cases of puerperal convulsions but 'to the fact that the class of patients admitted into the hospital will not ... bear depletion; and the same ... may be said generally of women living in cities.'[60] Thus for him the weakened condition of women's bodies necessitated a change in medical therapeutics. Burnside's Dr Adam Wright also noted the decline in venesection but questioned whether 'we neglect it too much in these modern days?'[61]

Hand intervention was another technique that nineteenth-century physicians resorted to. At times doctors needed to change the position of the child in utero when it was not going to present properly. Podalic version, which turned the child from a more unfavourable presentation to a footling one, was such an example. Archibald Hall noted that it had been used only six times in over 1200 cases at the University Lying-in Hospital but still he was not satisfied. Because it necessitated internal manipulation, he preferred a form of external turning. Unfortunately external version was seldom done, being a procedure 'scarcely taught in the schools, and rarely alluded to even in obstetrical works.'[62] Doctors would have preferred to avoid any hand manipulation, external or otherwise, but it was not always possible. In Theodore Brown's Fredericton practice, fewer than 1 per cent of his cases had a non-head presentation.[63] Both Dr James Ross in Toronto and Dr Mackay in Woodstock had a 4 to 5 per cent non-head presentation rate,[64] which was the approximate figure for the Burnside Lying-In Hospital. What such figures meant was that, sooner or later, physicians would face the decision of whether to turn the child to a more favourable position or to deliver in whatever position the child presented and cope with the complications that might ensue. Unfavourable presentation was not the only situation in which a physician might intervene manually. In 1884 George Tye of Chatham criticized the Credé method of using external pressure to encourage the expulsion of the placenta in the third stage of labour. He recalled that for ten years he had used it and, as a consequence, a large number of his patients hemorrhaged. He further admitted that when he had arrived too late to follow the procedure, flooding had not occurred, nor had it, or hardly so, in women attended by midwives. As a result he abandoned the procedure and for the last seven years the results to his patients had been more than satisfactory. For him the Credé method was unwarranted and he did not hesitate to criticize Henry Garrigues, a leading American physician, for advocating it in all cases.[65] A year later the *Canada Lancet* took up the subject of hand interference and, associating it with meddlesome midwifery, castigated the physician who constantly inserted his hand during labour and after 'to fix' things.[66] On 9 April 1891 the British Medical Association of Nova Scotia met and recorded the following entry: 'Dr — opened a discussion upon the management of the third stage of labour. He laid stress upon keeping the hand over the uterus as a guide to its condition. After waiting a few minutes after the child is born, he aids in the expulsion of the placenta by exercising some pressure during pains.'[67] This was a description of the Credé method that Dr Tye had earlier rejected. What is noteworthy about the above description is that the doctor is describing what appears to be a normal birth. There are no indicators that his assistance was needed to expel the placenta and he relates the assistance given in a way to suggest it was routine. In the past, he may have found the procedure of use in cases where the placenta remained adhered and subsequently introduced it as a preventive measure in all his cases. In such a way, childbirth could easily change from being a phenomenon that nature managed to one that doctors managed. How typical such physicians were is difficult to know, for hand intervention varied from one doctor to another. The records of the lying-in hospitals in Montreal and Toronto reveal minimal interference – certainly under 2 per cent. But the records of James Ross's and Hugh Mackay's practices indicate approximately 5 per cent and 9 per cent manual interference, ranging in Mackay's case from turning the child, removing the placenta, or inserting fingers into the vagina.

Mackay seemed to have been somewhat of an obstetric specialist and often consulted by his colleagues in difficult cases, a situation which may have raised his rate of intervention. Nevertheless, before the acceptance of antiseptic medicine and aseptic procedures, such intervention could have increased the chance of puerperal infection.

Another procedure that came under criticism and entered the rubric of meddlesome midwifery was the overuse of ergot. Ergot of rye became part of midwifery early in the nineteenth century. It was a poisonous drug, but its value was that it caused severe abdominal contractions which could be beneficial in protracted labour. It was also used to stop hemorrhaging after birth and in case of eclampsia.[68] In Canada there seemed to be a strong respect for its strength and physicians used it sparingly. Doctors at the University Lying-in Hospital between 1843 and 1847 used ergot only twice[69] and at the Burnside Lying-In Hospital in only four out of 517 cases between 1878 and 1882.[70] This reticence may have been one reason why Dr Verity was incensed that a midwife had dared to use it on a patient and indeed boasted that she always used it in cases of protracted labour. Verity's temper was, as he confessed, 'ruffled' and he proceeded to chastise 'her soundly, for her presumption and rashness in administering such a powerful remedy without a knowledge of its properties, and the circumstances under which it was proper to give it.'[71] The reluctance to use ergot may also have stemmed from the fact that ergot was an excellent abortifacient.[72] Considering the profession's opposition to abortion and public hostility to it, doctors may have been reluctant to be seen using a substance that clearly had its darker side. Whether for this or its powerful nature, some physicians were interested in finding a reliable substitute. Dr Parker advocated Tartarized Antimony to the Halifax Medical Society in 1861, arguing that unlike ergot it did not result in continuous uterine contraction and that it stimulated the mucous membrane in the vagina to overcome dryness.[73] Others suggested injecting vinegar or cold water or placing ice into the uterus to stop post-partum hemorrhage.[74] Electro-galvanism was also a possibility. Doctors would place one pole of the galvanic current in the uterus and the other over the abdomen and hope that the powerful contraction that resulted would stop the hemorrhage.[75] Not all physicians were agreed, however, on the limited use of ergot. At the same 1 October meeting of the Halifax Medical Society where Dr Parker was expressing caution, Dr West maintained that ergot could be used safely at every stage of labour.[76] In Hugh Mackay's practice, he used ergot in just over 2 per cent of the cases, and, while not often, his use was certainly more frequent than in the two lying-in hospitals. Dr James Ross was even more adventuresome. A study of his practice between 1853 and 1891 (over 1400 cases) determined that he used ergot on 16 per cent of his patients.[77] In the first five years of his Richmond Hill practice, James Langstaff only employed ergot five times, but by the 1870s he was doing so nine times a year or in almost 9 per cent of all his obstetric cases.[78]

What the discussion and reality of ergot's use and other forms of intervention reveal is that there was no accepted way of treating women in childbirth and that obstetrics was as much of an art as it was a science. As each work of art is slightly different, so was treatment in each childbirth case. Medicinal intervention was particularly varied. While Hugh Mackay was not especially dependent on ergot, he relied on some medicinal aid ranging from anaesthesia to brandy to morphine in approximately 17 per cent of his cases, although the combination varied from case to case. This was also true for James Ross. In addition, medicinal intervention in his late nineteenth-century practice increased significantly. From 1853 to 1891 the overall rate of such intervention was 23 per cent, but in 1881 it was 44 per cent, in 1886, 51 per cent, and by 1891, 70 per cent. The art of medicine was in working with nature, the science in deciding when nature needed assistance and how to provide it. But doctors at times seemed to be redefining what was natural. When one women gave birth at the Burnside Lying-In Hospital in 1881 and, as a result, ruptured her perineum, the physician advised leaving the wound to nature to heal. In this case, leaving it to nature necessitated that the patient 'be on her left side with her knees tied together and to be syringed out with warm water twice daily.'[79] Underlying such redefinitions and all forms of intervention was the sense that leaving it to nature was no longer enough. What concerned critics of meddlesome midwifery was that too many doctors were becoming nature's substitute.

The form of intervention that generated most debate was the use of forceps. An instrument with a long and somewhat clouded history, forceps had been invented in the seventeenth century by Peter Chamberlen, who shared the secret of them only with his family. While ridiculed by physicians and midwives alike, there was no denying that he and his descendants had something that allowed them to bring even difficult childbirth cases to a successful conclusion. Only in the 1720s did the 'secret' become public and by 1833 their design was available for all to copy and use[80] – all physicians, that is, for in England forceps were legally classified as surgical instruments and since only physicians could practise surgery, midwives were effectively prohibited from using them.[81] It would appear that this interdiction became customary elsewhere, for seldom is reference made to midwives using these instruments or being prohibited from using them, although it may be that their use would be interpreted as the 'practise of medicine' and thus illegal for anyone but a licensed practitioner.

Properly employed, forceps were a blessing. Physicians could shorten prolonged labour, for which many women must have been thankful. The records of the Burnside Lying-In Hospital (1878–82), the University Lying-in Hospital (1851–1900), Dr Hugh Mackay's Woodstock practice (1873–88), and Dr James Ross's Toronto practice (1853–91) reveal that approximately 6, 10, 12, and 16 per cent of their patients, respectively, were in labour for twenty-four hours or more. In the case of Ross, his use of forceps was directly linked to protracted labours. Of those women experiencing drawn-out childbirth, 22 per cent eventually had an instrumental birth, whereas only 7 per cent of all his patients did.[82] Forceps were also an aid in turning the child who was positioned unfavourably. One historian has graphically described what childbirth was like for many women before forceps were used: 'Until then the arrival of a surgeon or man-midwife to assist a woman in labour was only too often a death sentence for the child and the beginning of a long period of incapacity for the mother. Many a woman prayed for release by death, rather than be split apart by levers or lacerated by hooks which were man-midwife's stock and trade. Forceps overcame this but had to be used delicately.'[83] Forceps became part of meddlesome midwifery when physicians did not use them delicately and/or used them in a routine way.

As with most medical technology, the use of forceps had its own ebb and flow. Lecture notes taken by a Canadian medical student overseas revealed that resorting to them was rare in the late eighteenth and early nineteenth century. The lecturer recommended stealth when introducing them 'without the knowledge of the Patient or her Friends.' For example, the physician could carry the forceps in his pocket and then place them under the bed clothes. Inserting them into the patient was admittedly more of a problem but students were advised that 'you ought before to have used your fingers firstly freely otherwise the deception will be found out.'[84] Such advice given to medical students suggests, first, the amount of interference by hand that this lecturer was acknowledging and, to a certain extent, advocating; and, second, the subterfuge to which a physician should go in order to bring about a successful birth. In Canada, too, the frequency of forceps use was limited. Between 1843 and 1847 the University Lying-in Hospital employed forceps in only one out of 354 obstetric cases, although by 1859 it had increased to one in sixty-four and by 1883 to over one in fifty.[85] But was this typical? Judith Lewis, in her work on maternal care in England, has pointed out that in the early nineteenth century upper-class women were more likely to have experienced an instrumental birth than lower-class women.[86] Forceps were still exotica, and kept for those women who could pay for their use. The charity patients of the University Lying-in Hospital could not. Not that this was necessarily a problem. Until the acceptance of germ theory in the late 1870s and the adoption of antiseptic or aseptic procedures, the use of forceps, while alleviating the problems of a difficult birth, could introduce a death-causing infection. Because not all physicians knew how to use the forceps properly or because the results were not as splendid as their reputation had led physicians to believe, there remained hesitation about their use – so much so that Tyler Smith, in his 1858 work *The Modern Practice of Midwifery*, felt safe in encouraging students to take advantage of them, assuming that the bias against them was such that they would not be overused.[87]

Not all were as sanguine as Tyler Smith. Just a few years later Gunning Bedford explicitly warned his student readers against the dangers of forceps and estimated that doctors were using them in almost 10 per cent of all midwifery cases, a tendency which he clearly believed was extreme.[88] He certainly would not have approved of Dr R.S. Black from Nova Scotia, who estimated that in 1454 midwifery cases occurring between 1838 and 1877 he had employed the forceps 191 times, or on approximately 13 per cent of his patients.[89] Yet it is difficult to know how typical Dr Black was of other Canadian practitioners. The obstetric practice of Dr James Ross indicated a less than 4 per cent use of forceps between 1852 and 1877.[90] The complications that many of these forceps' cases presented was reflected in the fact that in 20 per cent of them the child was born dead. Use of forceps depended on the nature of a physician's practice, whether his patients were healthy or malnourished, and whether, as Ross's practice revealed, they experienced birth complications or not. Until the mid-1870s the use of forceps did not seem to be a major issue in Canada. Lecture notes taken by Alexander MacLaren at the Trinity Medical College in 1870 indicate that students were cautioned about applying forceps, that in cases 'where head of child is making very slow but sure progress ... leave it to nature.' In cases of forceps use, the mother had a one in thirteen chance of dying, whereas without interference she had a one in thirty chance.[91] In 1873 the *Canadian Medical Times* published a piece lamenting that doctors were still reluctant to use forceps, preferring to keep their patients in long, painful labours while nature took its course.[92] This did not seem to be a situation that was going to last. One indicator that forceps were becoming more popular was their introduction into the Woman's Hospital in Montreal. The annual report for 1878 claimed a 10 per cent rate in the use of forceps.[93] This was in stark contrast to the minimal use at the University Lying-in Hospital.

In the last two decades of the century physicians expressed more concern about the use of forceps. At the 1882 meeting of the Canada Medical Association, Chatham's Dr Tye 'said he really thought they were passing through the iron age in the matter of obstetrics. After seeing all the forceps and scoops and other iron instruments, he really congratulated himself that he was not a woman.' In his practice he preferred to rely on nature. To this another physician responded that 'while he disapproved of undue multiplicity and complication of instruments, yet the valuable assistance rendered by them could not be overlooked.' No one denied the value of forceps when properly used, but underlying the criticisms was the suspicion this was not always the case. Dr Stewart of Brucefield pointed out at the meeting in reference to one patient that 'from certain *post mortem* examinations made the vagina had been found ruptured by the forceps and death had been the result.'[94] Patient records provide reasons to support Dr Stewart's perceptions. In December 1886 Rose Millard entered the Victoria General Hospital suffering from a prolapsed uterus. Ten years earlier she had given birth to her last child during which 'she had an injury to the organs of generation,' the result of forceps. The same was true for Mrs MacDougall, who entered the hospital on 11 July 1893 suffering from a burning, dragging sensation, the cause of which she was sure was the instrumental birth of her first child twenty years before.[95] Faced with the results of what they interpreted as poor forceps use, critics believed better training was needed. The authorities of the Burnside Hospital must have agreed. Its regulations prohibited the use of forceps by any resident assistant except with 'the permission of the medical superintendent or a member of the visiting staff.'[96] Unfortunately, even when supervision occurred, women still paid the price of medical students' learning their craft. The records of a patient admitted in 1881 reveal that whoever used forceps on her did so for the first time, 'but by patience and perseverance in applying and delivering safely, the only mishap was a slight laceration of the perineum due to the hand having come down with the head.'[97] But such cases were the exception, since Burnside was able to keep forceps cases to under 2 per cent.

The concern that many physicians expressed about forceps was not unwarranted. Their use had increased. In 1891 the doctors at the Montreal Maternity used them in 8 per cent of the cases, and at the Ottawa Maternity forceps were used in one-quarter of all deliveries well into the twentieth century.[98] The significant increase at the Montreal institution may reflect the changeover that had occurred from midwife-delivered births to physician-delivered births.[99] Certainly, forceps were prominent in the list of instruments in stock there on 1 April 1889.[100] The difference between the Montreal and Ottawa facilities was that the paying patients at the Ottawa were under the care of their own physicians who may have been more willing to resort to forceps use because of the demands of their patients and because of their patients being able to pay for their use. Charity patients at the Montreal institution could not, but, more significantly, it was a teaching hospital and physicians in the university medical schools were among the most vocal about the need to teach conservative management of birth. Those in private practice seemed more inclined to interfere. In his Richmond Hill practice in the 1850s Dr Langstaff used forceps in approximately 2 per cent of the cases; by the 1870s, in 40 per cent.[101] Dr Walter Burritt delivered over 1800 babies between 1835 and 1886 and used forceps only 104 times, but whereas at the beginning of his practice he used them only once in every sixty deliveries, by the end he resorted to forceps in 10 per cent of his cases.[102] Dr Brown's Fredericton practice closely resembled Langstaff's. Whereas in the 1860s he employed forceps in just over 5 per cent of his cases, by the 1870s he used them in 19 per cent and in the 1880s in over 40 per cent. In most cases, the use of forceps and chloroform went hand in hand. Not all practitioners were so quick to use instruments. Hugh Mackay's practice from 1873 to 1888 revealed only a 4 per cent rate.[103] In 1882 Mackay had two patients who illustrated the problems of forceps application and the dilemma of the physician in using them. In the first, the patient, Mrs Willard Milkener, provoked the use of forceps by becoming 'much excited and intolerant of her pains.' In the second case Mrs Mallory went into labour, during which Mackay used forceps which resulted in 'an abras on forehead of child and back of neck & rupt perineum on mother to sphincter.' Forceps could speed delivery, but their use could harm both mother and child.[104] The physician had to weigh one against the other.

If forceps could cause problems, why did some practitioners persist, as critics claimed they did, in using them to the point of abuse? Dr Clark from Hastings, Ont., could not have been more blunt when he wrote in the *Canada Lancet* of 1885 that 'the forceps are sometimes used to save time, sometimes to gain a little notoriety, sometimes for the double fee, and sometimes from ignorance.'[105] In a review of obstetrics and gynaecology published in the *Canada Medical Record* of 1898, Dr W. Japp Sinclair of Owen's College, Manchester, blamed the increase in forceps use to the overconfidence that the era of antiseptic medicine had given to many practitioners.[106] In earlier decades the use of forceps could lead to infection and puerperal fever. If stringent antiseptic and aseptic measures were taken, doctors believed that the chances of infection decreased, allowing them more flexibility in what they could do.[107] For their own part, critics of forceps use may have been responding to the rise in gynaecology as a medical specialty. As will be seen in chapter 9, many of the physicians who specialized in this field were overwhelmed by the number of their patients whose difficulties seemed to originate in birth complications, many of them the repercussions of poor forceps use. At the same time, by belittling the expertise of others they boosted their own prestige.

Intervention by hand and by forceps appears minor when compared with some of the surgical interventions that took place in the past. Today we take for granted the birth of a live child and the survival of the mother in childbirth. But this was not always the case. In the nineteenth century the birth of a live child was problematic. Many women suffered from rickets, caused by a Vitamin D deficiency and, while men did as well, it did not pose the same kind of problems for them. Rickets often resulted in small or deformed pelves, which created complications in childbirth. In some cases it made it impossible for a woman to give birth naturally. In such situations physicians faced an agonizing choice. They could perform a Caesarian section in an effort to save the child. However, there was no guarantee the child would survive and it was almost certain the woman would die. The alternative was to save the mother through the dismemberment of the child. Mutilating operations on the child were performed to reduce its size 'or divide it in pieces' so that delivery could occur. When the operation focused on the head of the child it was a craniotomy and when focused on the body it was known as an embryotomy.[108] Although performed in order to save the mother, one historian of midwifery has estimated that 18 per cent of mothers died when craniotomies were performed.[109] The number of cutting operations performed will never be known but they occurred throughout the century. A case involving a midwife took place in 1865 when a doctor called in to take over from her found the unborn child with missing limbs. On his confronting the midwife, she 'produced the *two arms of the child, with the clavicle and scapula attached to one, and the clavicle to the other.*' The doctor proceeded to anaesthetize the patient and deliver the remainder of the child.[110] James Ross, in his mid-century Toronto practice, encountered four cases necessitating craniotomy[111] as did Theodore Brown in Fredericton.[112] On 18 January 1877 Hugh Mackay faced a classic case in Amelia O'Brennan. She was deformed, with her 'spine curved laterally as well as antero posterior so that the uterus stood forward over pubes almost at right angles to spine.' The child was already dead and Mackay proceeded with a craniotomy.[113] In 1879 at the Burnside Lying-In Hospital a craniotomy was performed.[114] In 1889 the gynaecology casebook of Dr Gardner of the Montreal General Hospital refers to a young woman, aged twenty-two, who had had a craniotomy performed on her unborn baby,[115] and in 1900 a craniotomy occurred at the University Lying-in Hospital.[116] Doctors were horrified at having to intervene in such a way and looked forward to the day when abdominal surgery became safe enough to ensure the survival of both mother and child.[117] Until that day arrived, however, doctors had little choice – 'the value of the mother's life must be allowed the preëminence.'[118]

The reality of craniotomies must be kept in mind when assessing the cutting operations that were performed on women in childbirth. King's *Manual of Obstetrics* in 1884 pointed out that at least two were available; symphysiotomy and Caesarian section.[119] The symphysiotomy was an operation where the union between the two pubic bones was divided and the bones pushed forcibly outward so as to increase the capacity of the contracted pelvis. It was used when the pelvis was needed to be made larger, usually in the case of deformity. However, because symphysiotomy often impaired the movement of the mother afterwards, it was seldom employed in the late nineteenth century.[120] In 1893 only three cases had ever been performed in Canada,[121] although in 1895 G.P. Sylvester of Toronto referred approvingly to its increase, and in 1897–8 two cases occurred at the Montreal Maternity and yet another in 1904.[122]

While one reason for the rarity of symphysiotomy was clearly its unacceptable consequences for the woman, another was the emergence of a safer alternative – Caesarian section. Until late in the century its mortality rate was prohibitively high. Those performed in Britain up to 1860 resulted in a 70 per cent mortality rate for the women and only a 56 per cent survival rate for their children.[123] Statistics for the United States for the period 1876 to 1886 were even worse. Out of the thirty-seven operations performed, only eight women survived.[124] The reason for the high mortality rate was that until 1882 only the abdominal wall and not the uterus was sutured and thus infection from the wound seeped into the peritoneum. Also before antisepsis was rigidly enforced, infection in any abdominal surgery was difficult to avoid. Other factors, too, played a part, 'previous exhaustion (both of woman and womb) from protracted labor; previous injury from unsuccessful attempts to deliver by version, forceps, etc.; bungling from lack of skill during the operation; and injudicious after-treatment.'[125] This does not mean that Caesarian sections were never performed. The papers of William Canniff indicate that in the early 1830s the father of Dr Thomas Sterling of Halifax had performed such a procedure.[126] But such cases were rare. Even after the introduction of antiseptic surgery, King's *Manual of Obstet-*

rics cautioned practitioners that Caesarian sections should only be done in one of four situations: in cases of extreme deformity of the pelvis in which a craniotomy would be more dangerous than abdominal surgery for the mother; in other cases of deformity in which a Caesarian section had been agreed upon in order to save the life of the child; in cases where the pelvis was obstructed by tumours; and in cases when the woman was dying.[127] To reduce post-operative infection, a variation on a Caesarian section was developed which was known as Porro's operation – the removal of the womb and ovaries during the operative procedure.[128] It is unlikely that Porro's operation was performed very often in Canada, but Canadian physicians did know about it. In the *Canada Medical and Surgical Journal* for 1884 Dr Gardner, at McGill, pointed out its advantages and disadvantages. On the one hand the removal of the womb and ovaries unsexed a woman, but on the other if a woman could not give birth to a child in the normal way it was safer for her not to have children.[129] As we have seen, many physicians believed that sexual desire in a woman was linked to her ability to have children. Thus without the ability to have children, these physicians would not see the absence of sexuality as significant.

Throughout the nineteenth century the overwhelming issue surrounding Caesarian section remained safety. The chief obstetrician of the Montreal Maternity Hospital in 1888 was very cautious in teaching his students about the procedure, fearing they would resort to it too often. He impressed upon them the sanctity of the mother's life: 'The life of an adult woman who has already contracted relations with society is of incomparably greater value, as judging by human standards, than the problematical existence of an unborn babe. Moreover, the expectancy of life in such children is less than those of normal birth.'[130] With the social relations that a woman had already built up over the years of her life and the incredibly poor survival rate for children in nineteenth-century Canada, the doctor's choice was clear.[131] Abdominal surgery of any kind was risky and most physicians appreciated that fact. When Mrs Mary Savon entered the Victoria General on 17 November 1893 she was diagnosed as having an extra uterine pregnancy of about two to three months. The next day doctors applied hot poultices and douches three times a day. By 4 December the poultices were omitted but the hot douches continued until on 23 January 1894 she was discharged. In Mrs Savon's case, conservative treatment was deemed superior and safer to any surgical intervention.[132] When in 1897 a woman died as a result of a Caesarian section performed at the Montreal Maternity Hospital, ten years elapsed before another was attempted.[133]

The image that emerges from the examination of nineteenth-century physicians and their care of patients in childbirth is a mixed one. There does seem to be evidence to suggest an increase in intervention. However, there did not seem to be any consistency in practice. Charity institutions intervened least despite their responsibility for teaching students. When all types of interference are considered from craniotomy to forceps, the interference rate for the University Lying-in Hospital was 2.5 per cent in the latter half of the century, although by the 1890s it had risen to 6.5 per cent. Especially noteworthy was that interference was linked to protracted labour.[134] Burnside was not significantly different, with a manual, medicinal, and instrumental interference rate of 5.2 per cent linked to non-head presentations and birth complications.[135] Private practitioners were more willing to intervene, whether because their patients demanded it, because they did not have the time to spend with their patients, or because they felt the need to be seen to be earning their fee. James Ross's intervention rate (manual, medicinal, and instrumental) was 27 per cent between 1853 and 1891. However, it increased considerably in the 1880s and early 1890s. In 1881 it was 48 per cent, in 1886, 53 per cent, and in 1891, 72 per cent. Although Hugh Mackay did not resort to forceps often, his rate of interference, when combined with his hand interventions, was just over 18 per cent. If medicinal intervention is added, then it rose to almost 30 per cent and was linked primarily to primipara women and to women in protracted labour.[136] While such connections reflect accepted medical reasons for intervening, the medical press was still uneasy. There was a fear that intervention was occurring too often and that physicians were losing respect for the dangers that accompanied intervention. It was the constant reminder of those dangers that the medical literature kept to the forefront. It may account for why, although intervention increased, it nowhere approached that which would occur in the twentieth century.[137]

Most physicians writing for the medical press emphasized that intervention, whether by hand or instrument, should occur only in problem births. The difficulty in assessing whether or not physicians intervened too much or not is in estimating how often problem births occurred. As we have already seen, both a non-head presentation and protracted labour could pose difficulties. The health of the mother was also certainly significant; 5 per cent of the women admitted to the Burnside facility were in poor health to begin with, whether from general weakness or more specific ailments such as syphilis. Neither should the wear and tear of previous pregnancies on a woman's health be discounted. In Theodore Brown's practice, 50 per cent of the women had given birth within twenty-six months of bearing their last child and almost one-quarter within nineteen months.[138] As the practices of both Mackay and Brown revealed, first labours could present more problems necessitating interference and, while the charity institutions obviously did not view this as a reason for expecting difficulties, the medical literature of the time did.

A suggestion of what physicians had to face in their practice comes from a study of the obstetric patient records for Dr Langis of Vancouver for the years 1888, 1891, 1893, and 1894. During these years miscarriages and stillbirths accounted for 11, 10, 6, and 15 per cent, respectively, of his obstetric cases. Difficult deliveries were 23 per cent in 1893 and 30 per cent in 1894.[139] However, these latter figures only refer to those women who engaged Dr Langis before their labour, women who had already preselected themselves and were not representative of the population or even Dr Langis's practice as a whole. Yet Langis's practice does not appear atypical when compared to others. Complications in childbirth (real and perceived) were quite high. At Burnside, almost 10 per cent of the women did not leave hospital with a living child (this includes miscarriages). Non-head presentation and other complications in delivery were the predominant causes of this loss.[140]

If other infant complications, including low weight (under 6 lbs) are added, almost 37 per cent of the cases experienced problems, although some were minor, such as having the umbilical cord wrapped around the child's neck. At least 5 per cent of the women experienced health problems (including death) after delivery and, if combined with those in poor health to begin with, just under 10 per cent were unhealthy. The University Lying-in Hospital experienced an infant death rate of 6 per cent (including stillborns and miscarriages), with the total of infants experiencing any kind of difficulty at almost 18 per cent. Mothers experiencing problems in delivery or afterwards (ranging from premature delivery to dying) reached 7 per cent, and if coupled with protracted labour, interference in labour, and non-head presentation they accounted for almost 16 per cent of all cases. Approximately 28 per cent of labours had some complication to either mother or child. This does not mean that only 70 per cent of the births in these institutions were normal, but what it does suggest is that complications in birth did occur and that doctors in these institutions were very exact in detailing the least occurrence they felt was out of the ordinary. No wonder they perceived women in childbirth as in need of assistance. Theodore Brown's practice did not seem to pose so many challenges. He had a just over 4 per cent death rate for children, and complications in delivery were less than 8 per cent. But his records were not very detailed except for the use of chloroform and forceps, and if the use of forceps is indicative of Brown's perception of birth complications, then their frequency was quite high. Certainly Ross's and Mackay's records detail problems or abnormalities with consistency. In Ross's practice complications in birth ranging from placenta praevia, eclampsia, to post-partum hemorrhage were generally linked to women enduring long labours.[141] Those whose infants experienced difficulty represented 6 per cent. When combined with women with health problems before or after labour, 35 per cent of Ross's cases experienced some kind of complication. In Mackay's practice over 11 per cent of his patients did not have a living child, and in many cases this was a result of a non-head presentation and protracted labour.[142] When Mackay's listings of any form of complication to the child are tallied, almost 24 per cent of births had problems. Birth complications to the mother in delivery occurred in almost 19 per cent of all cases and, if the mother's experience before and after delivery are included, 24 per cent of all births were problematic for the mother. Especially at risk were primipara women. Farm wives seemed underrepresented among those experiencing difficulties, which lends some support to doctors' perceptions of rural women being much stronger and healthier than urban women.[143]

If it is difficult to know the rate of problems in childbirth, what we do know is that the medical profession was extremely sensitive to complications accruing from childbirth and particularly to poor management of it. Hugh Mackay took pride in delivering a patient safely and well and, when in the week of 18 January 1886 he had two cases in which extensive ruptures of the perineum occurred, he resolved 'to make the most determined effort to avoid a recurrence.'[144] But doctors were not always able to protect their patients from harm. Time and time again women and their physicians date medical problems from previous childbirth trauma. Several examples bear this out. Mrs McMaster, aged forty-nine, entered the Victoria General Hospital in Halifax on 14 June 1882. In her file her physician wrote that 'her present trouble dates from 20 years ago. After her first confinement she travelled by coach from Liverpool N.S. to Halifax before she was strong enough.' His examination of her revealed a prolapse of the vagina and uterus. Mrs Calley, a patient admitted a month later, had developed puerperal fever after the birth of her first children – twins – when she was thirty-six. After their birth she had had one more child and then miscarried another. Since then she had not been in good health.[145] At the Montreal General Hospital in the same year Mrs Margaret Lange, aged twenty-nine, had come to the dispensary on 17 August. At that point she had had four children, each delivered by forceps, and in the last four years she had experienced seven miscarriages. Doctors diagnosed her as suffering from subinvolution and chronic endometritis. Another patient at the dispensary, Mrs Hilda Cookson, aged thirty-eight, had gone through even more. She had brought twelve pregnancies to full term but, during her third, had been torn in the process. Fourteen months after her fourth child was born she was finally operated on for a lacerated perineum. After the fifth she was as bad as ever.[146] Mrs Oalringer, aged twenty-six, noticed after the birth of her last child that her womb was protruding through her vagina. Five years later in 1900 she entered the Victoria General Hospital for treatment.[147] Dr McPhedran's private casebook indicated that one of his patients, a Mrs Dougan, aged twenty-six, had gone blind for a short period owing to the medication he had given her during her confinement.[148]

Several themes emerge from these cases. One is the trauma that childbirth could cause women. The fact that so many had undergone numerous pregnancies suggests the possibility that their health was being undermined simply by the wear and tear placed on their bodies. Second, is that many women and their physicians dated their ill health to one of their pregnancies and blamed the attending physician (assuming there had been one). Third, and very important, is that while many of these women experienced ill health for years, they continued their lives and continued to bear children. The health complications they presented to their physicians goes a long way to explain why so many practitioners perceived women as sickly and why they connected this ill health to the nature of the female body itself. But what the actual patient records also underline is the strength of these 'sickly' women who had lived for years in weakened health and had somehow managed to carry on. Physicians understandably focused more on the ill health of women resulting from childbirth than on the strength of women who endured that ill health for years on end. Some comforted themselves by maintaining this was not a physician-induced problem but resulted from the nature of the experience. There was a general sense throughout the latter half of the century that childbirth, even if not interfered with, could result in the ill health of women.[149] Indeed Henry Lyman in his *Practical Home Physician* told women that gynaecological problems stemming from childbirth were really latent – that is, the problem had always been there and it was only when the reproductive system was taxed with the stresses of pregnancy that the problem became manifest.[150] The unspoken corollary to this was that women should not blame their attending physicians but rather fate that had given them a woman's body. Not all physicians were so sanguine. By the late nineteenth century increasing numbers of voices were being heard which pointed the finger at poor obstetrical care given to women as the cause of their ill health.[151] Not surprisingly, many of these voices belonged to gynaecologists, those men who saw the results of bad technique in the patients who came to them for help. As one leading gynaecologist put it, 'the accoucheurs are the providers of material for the gynaecologists.'[152] Not willing to accept such pronouncements, Dr James Russell, superintendent of the Asylum for the Insane in Hamilton, fought back, asserting that although many women experienced abnormalities in the pelvic area owing to childbirth, many of these problems were minor and would never have given trouble except that 'meddlesome gynecologists' got hold of these patients and persuaded them that an operation was needed.[153] Gynaecologists had to beware – they were not beyond criticism themselves.

Complications arising from childbirth fade into relative insignificance when placed next to the possibility of death. Particularly dangerous was puerperal fever. Puerperal fever results from infection originating in the birth canal, which can spread throughout the body causing septicaemia and eventual death. In a pre-aseptic era, doctors often introduced the infection by attending a birthing woman without taking adequate precautions, specifically without changing their clothing or washing themselves and their instruments after attending other patients. In 1847 Viennese physician Ignaz Semmelweiss put forward the proposition that puerperal fever was transmitted by the contaminated hands of doctors. This was difficult for physicians to accept – that they who were to save lives were the cause of so many losing them. It also did not make it easier to acknowledge that those women cared for by midwives in European hospitals experienced much lower rates of puerperal fever.[154] Looking back, the reasons for the difference are clear. Midwives were only concerned with one type of patient – expectant mothers. Doctors treated a variety of patients and so transmitted the germs from their infectious ones to those not infected. Only with the acceptance of the germ theory of disease propagation did physicians finally recognize Semmelweiss's indictment of medical practices and begin to follow antiseptic and aseptic medicine. Unfortunately, this took time.[155] The fear that puerperal fever incited in physicians was reflected in an 1850 text entitled *Essays on Puerperal Fever*. The author of the text, Fleetwood Churchill, expressed his frustration about 'the inutility of all precautions to guard against its attacks, and, in the majority of cases, the utter failure of all attempts to arrest its progress or to prevent its fatal termination.'[156] Hospitals, in particular, had difficulty preventing its spread. At the University Lying-in Hospital there were two cases in 1847, three in 1852, two in 1857, three in 1871, and four in 1872. In each, it had begun as a single episode in a patient and then spread to other women. The vulnerability of hospitals was a result of patients being in close proximity to one another and doctors going from one patient to another. The chief obstetrician of the hospital believed there was another cause. In commenting on six puerperal fever deaths between 1879 and 1882 he blamed the 'more frequent manipulations and greater interference with the patient which ... instruction demanded.'[157] Even antiseptic conditions could not eliminate totally the heightened threat such interference raised.[158]

Puerperal fever raised the spectre of death in childbirth and some historians have linked women's lower life expectancy compared with men's in past centuries to the dangers of childbirth. While this may appear to be straightforward before the nineteenth century, the equation becomes more problematic afterwards. In the nineteenth century women's life expectancy began to exceed men's, yet this did not correspond to a decline in maternal mortality. One study of English mortality rates has pointed out that the mortality advantage of women over men in the middle years (aged twenty-five to forty-four) increased *before* the decline in birth rates, not after.[159] In actual fact, tuberculosis was the prime killer of women in their middle years and its decline accounted for women's increased life expectancy. But if childbirth was not *the* major killer of women, it still remained a significant one and one to which men were not exposed.[160] Physicians recognized this distinction. In 1869 William Carpenter claimed that 'from about the age of 18 to 28, the mortality is much greater in Males, being at its maximum at 25, when the viability is only half what it is at puberty. The fact is a very striking one; and shows most forcibly that the indulgence of the passions not only weakens the health, but in a great number of instances is the cause of a very premature death. From the age of 28 to that of 50, the mortality is greater and the viability less on the side of the Female; this is what would be anticipated from the increased risk to which she is liable during the parturient period.'[161] Thus men's active sexuality placed them at risk during their younger years, whereas women who followed the natural role set out for them, the maternal role, were at risk in their middle years. Even in cause of death, the social norms were adhered to: men were active and women were passive.

Some births placed women in more danger than others. We have already seen that those with rickets often had to undergo horrendous procedures in order to survive. If the child did not present normally, either manual or forceps interference could be needed and the mortality rate for both mother and child would rise because of the increase likelihood of infection.[162] Napheys pointed out that women undergoing their first labour experienced more complications than women undergoing subsequent births. Maternal mortality figures for first births were higher and the incidence of childbed fever among primipara patients was twice that for multipara women. Such was not a comforting thought for a young woman facing the birth of her first child. While modern statistics bear Napheys out in this respect, some of his other pronouncements seem more closely aligned to superstition than clinical reality; for example, he rather offhandedly mentioned that mortality for women increased if the child they bore was male.[163] A study of infant weights in late nineteenth-century Montreal has posited another reason for childbirth mortality. Peter and Patricia Ward have suggested that infant birth weights depended on the health of the mother, the history of the pregnancy, and the genetic or constitutional character of both the mother and her unborn child. What they discerned for the period 1850 to 1905 was that

infant weights actually decreased and they linked this to the malnourished condition of the mothers.[164] Burnside's statistics are
particularly disturbing in that regard: approximately 23 per cent
of its patients gave birth to live children under 6 pounds. While
the Wards were concerned with how the state of the mother's
health affected that of her baby, it is clear their conclusions would
have a bearing on maternal mortality rates. Malnourished women,
compared to nourished ones, would have a higher rate of morbidity and mortality, although good obstetrical care could lessen
this significantly.[165]

Estimating the actual maternal mortality rate for nineteenth-
century Canada is fraught with danger. To begin with the statistics
are simply not reliable. Doctors were not obligated to report deaths
and, even when some encouragement was given for reporting,
the accuracy was questionable. Thus census figures can only provide a very rough estimate. They can be supplemented, however,
by examining the records of maternity hospitals and private medical practices. Some suggestion of what the mortality rate was in
an early nineteenth-century maternity institution is contained in
the register of the University Lying-in Hospital for the years 1843
to 1847. According to its data, only two women died as a result
of childbirth. The first died of uterine inflammation after a long,
hard delivery; the second, as a result of falls she had taken before
she was admitted to the hospital. After a relatively easy delivery
she slipped into a comatose state and died.[166] These two deaths
suggest that just over 5 deaths per 1000 deliveries occurred. This
rate was roughly what it was in mid-century Britain. While it was
not as high as for the pre-1800 period when, in Europe, 10 per
cent of mothers died in childbirth, it still represented a sorrowful
toll in lives.[167] Some practitioners at mid-century had even higher
rates. One eastern Upper Canadian practice had a rate of 21 deaths
per 1000 deliveries.[168] Langstaff's maternal death rate was 12.5 per
1000 deliveries in the 1850s, the major cause being puerperal fever.[169] Statistics for the general population appeared to be much
lower, at 4 to 5 deaths per 1000 births.[170] Rates did not significantly
change for the rest of the century. Census figures indicate a maternal mortality rate of roughly 4 to 4.5 per 1000 births in 1870-1,

and in 1880, 3.6.[171] Maternal mortality in Langstaff's rural practice,
already high, became even worse as it reached 29 per 1000 deliveries in the 1870s. In both the 1850s and 1870s obstetrical causes
were among the major causes of death in his practice and, if his
is typical in this respect, may account for why physicians saw
childbearing as threatening.[172] Not all doctors in private practice
had Langstaff's high rates, however. Analysis of James Ross's Toronto practice of over 4700 cases between 1852 and 1877 revealed
a maternal mortality rate of less than 5 of 1000 cases.[173] Hugh
Mackay's Woodstock practice was equally impressive, with a maternal mortality rate of only 0.24 per cent. One rural Quebec
practitioner, however, had a mortality rate of 1.3 per cent.[174] The
University Lying-in Hospital was unable to maintain its earlier low
rate. Between 1867 and 1875 it had a maternal mortality rate of 7
to 8 per 1000 births, although in some years it ranged much higher.
Between 1875 and 1883 it was 12 per 1000 and, as already indicated,
Dr MacCallum blamed the rate increase on sepsis resulting from
'greater interference with the patient.'[175] If true, the interference
did not cease. In 1891 the mortality rate was 18 per 1000.[176] Burnside, too, once had an impressively low mortality rate of 0.63 per
cent.[177] Between 1878 and 1882, however, its rate was 1.7 per cent
and on par with the facility in Montreal. The Ottawa maternity
had a rate of 6.6 per 1000.[178]

Another way of appreciating the danger that childbirth posed
is to calculate what percentage of deaths of women in their childbearing years were actually caused by birth-related complications.
The census figures for Upper Canada in 1850–1 reported 708 women
dying between the ages of fifteen and forty, the prime childbearing years. Deaths that could be linked to childbirth numbered
146 (141 childbed, 3 puerperal fever; and 2 miscarriage),[179] or
approximately 20 per cent. Ten years later the figure was almost
as high – 18 per cent.[180] A similar rate was true for Lower Canada
as well.[181] After mid-century, maternal mortality decreased as a
percentage of deaths in the childbearing years. In 1870–1 the figure
was less than 11 per cent for Ontario, Quebec, New Brunswick,
and Nova Scotia.[182] The rate continued to decline, and by 1890–1
it was just under 8 per cent for the whole country.[183]

It is difficult to know how to interpret the figures for maternal mortality. The census figures were probably unrealistically low given the poor quality of returns. Hospital rates started off low, but by the end of the century were somewhat higher. This may have been the result of many factors: the decline in living standards that the Wards blamed for undermining the health of expectant mothers; the increase in numbers of women these institutions were accepting, which led to increased chances of infection and perhaps decreased care; the end of midwife control and the beginning of physician management with its emphasis on allowing students first-hand practical experience; the higher percentage of their patients undergoing their first pregnancy, which carried higher mortality rates than subsequent ones; the problem of puerperal fever in hospitals; and increased intervention. The one exception to this trend was the Ottawa maternity hospital, but since it largely catered to private patients their health was most likely better; the percentage of first births would not have been high, and the care they received probably exceeded that of the charity patients. Maternal mortality rates in many private practices appeared lower but in some were as high or in Langstaff's practice, a great deal higher than those of the maternity hospitals. Without knowing more about the nature of the various practices, the type of clientele, the training of the doctors concerned, trying to account for the variation would be premature. Percentages, however, do not really reflect the impact of maternal mortality. The real toll was in lives lost and families disrupted. At mid-century one out of every nine children were maternal orphans by the age of ten.[184] One woman in every five who married and started a family did not survive to the end of her child-bearing years.[185] Canadian women knew from their own experience and that of women around them that childbirth could be dangerous if not fatal.

Even though the overwhelming majority of births ended happily, the very real threat of death was the dark side of maternity for women in late nineteenth-century Canada. They knew it and so did their physicians. Compared with the possibility of death in childbirth, the intervention of physicians may not appear to be as extreme as it otherwise would. Physicians, faced with the possibility of their patients dying, were willing to try anything they felt could offset it. So were their patients. By its very nature, medicine in Western society is interventionist. Even in non-Western cultures, medical intervention occurs. Records suggests that native peoples in Canada in the Confederation period resorted to both Caesarian section and the inducement of labour.[186] The issue of intervention is not simply its frequency but how it occurs and what this does to the patient and the practitioner. What intervention meant in the nineteenth-century context was that, increasingly, physicians, not patients, were defining the meaning of childbirth.[187] It was experienced by women but managed by men. Intervention helped make obstetrics into a medical specialty during these years, one of two which focused on the fragility of the female body. The second was gynaecology.

Chapter Eight

The Rise of Gynaecology

In a retrospect of gynaecology written in 1887, Lapthorn Smith, professor of jurisprudence and lecturer on gynaecology at Bishop's College Medical Faculty, waxed eloquent on the advances made in that field. In no other had 'the workers been more active.' Surveying the scene, he could not hide his excitement at the possibilities that were opening up: 'One sees many times a day in Berlin the uterus dilated, the mucous membrane scraped away until one hears the steel scratching on the raw muscle beneath, and then injected with tincture of iodine, and irrigated with sublimate or carbolic solution, without the slightest risk.' Gynaecology had come of age; 'the field is large, almost unlimited' and 'the rewards won by success are larger than in almost any other branch.' Smith patted gynaecologists on the back by smugly pointing out that it attracted able men, with the result that it had quickly moved 'from the position of an uncertain and indefinite science to that of one of the most exact.'[1] And in case the public did not fully appreciate what this meant, George Napheys hammered home the point that so extensive had the knowledge in this field become that only experts – those who gave their 'whole attention' to it – could possibly keep up.[2] The unspoken inference was that only the specialists who could keep up with the field should practise it.

That two medical specializations, obstetrics and gynaecology, focused on women does not mean that men did not have their own 'peculiar' ailments. The 1876–9 casebook of John Helmcken in Victoria is replete with instances of men with problems of the testes and the urinary tract.[3] Alexander Primrose's late nineteenth-century practice reflected similar male ailments – enlarged prostrate, irritated scrotum, penis malformation – which necessitated a variety of medical interventions from circumcision, to vasectomy, to removal of the testicle.[4] Despite the reality of male disorders, no major medical specialty developed that specifically spotlighted men as did obstetrics and gynaecology women. Obstetrics as a specialty recognized an obvious difference in that women gave birth to children and men did not. Gynaecology was predicated on the assumption that woman's sexual/reproductive system was fragile and prone to disorders. It reinforced the concept that women's bodies limited them, not society. There were several reasons for this approach. Because physicians used the male body as the norm they tended to see deviation from it as illness or weakness. The *Emigrants Medical Guide* in 1853 made this clear: 'In prescribing medicines for females, it must be recollected that they are more excitable than men; that the circulation is carried on more rapidly; that the pulse, other things being equal, is more frequent; and that smaller doses will suffice.'[5] Twenty years later, in his medical compendium, Alvin Chase pointed out the specificity of women's bodies, that what 'affects the general system of the male, much more frequently affects the organs peculiar to *her* system only.'[6] As we have already seen, physicians assumed that women were weaker than men. Since the major physiological difference between men and women was the reproductive system, it became the reason for that weakness. Henry Lyman, in his *Practical Home Physician*, told his readers that 'cancer attacks three times as many women as men, and that in one out of every three cases in which the disease occurs in woman it begins in the womb.'[7] Women not only differed from the male norm but their reproductive system was more complex in its design and hence more challenging in its workings. And because of this complexity, more could go wrong with it.[8] The 1867 annual report of the General Hospital in Halifax revealed that of the twenty-eight women admitted for medical reasons, the problems of four – approximately 14 per cent – were due to the fact of their being female or could be interpreted that way (two amenorrhoea, one climacteric disease, one chlorosis).[9] If that reality were not enough, physicians convincingly argued that because their reproductive system dominated women, any disease or disorder of the organs of generation could be visited on any other part of the body.[10] Physicians benefited from making this link, since it reinforced what society already believed and provided a scientific basis for it. This argument no doubt raised the public's awareness of medicine and resulted in the increased credibility and prestige of doctors. Physicians described a need and proposed to meet it – women's bodies were at risk but doctors' skills were such that they could help lessen or at least alleviate the consequences of it.[11] However, caution was needed, for with the expansion of gynaecology as a major medical specialty, physicians were not simply laying claim to be the arbiters of health over just any part of the body but to what they and other Canadians considered the central core of womanhood in late nineteenth-century Canada.

There were at least three indicators of the emergence of gynaecology as a major specialty. The first was the substantial increase in the journal literature published in the field. In the 1890s the *Canada Medical Record* began a separate section on gynaecology in order to keep its readers up to date with the latest advances and to satisfy their interests. Second, Canadian medical schools made gynaecology a required subject. As early as 1861 the first professor of obstetric and diseases of women and children (note the combination of women and children) began teaching at Queen's University. Dr William Gardner became the first gynaecologist appointed to McGill University in the early 1870s. In the academic term 1890–1, instructors at Queen's taught their first gynaecology course separate from obstetrics and in the 1890s the Trinity Medical College curriculum included a gynaecological textbook. Third and more significant than the academic teaching of the subject was its practice. This often went hand in hand with the building of hospitals, for as one historian of Canadian gynaecology has noted it was closely connected to a 'technological, hospital-based medical environment.'[12] The first step was simply to provide facilities for women patients within hospitals. An example of this was in 1863 when the ladies of Victoria set up and ran a ward for women in connection with the Royal [Jubilee] Hospital. Not being able to run it as they wished, the women withdrew their services and established their own infirmary, which remained separate from the hospital until 1869 when the two merged once again. The ladies acquiesced to this merger on the condition that the Royal Hospital maintain a female ward.[13] Although this ward did not specialize in diseases peculiar to women, it was a necessary first step in specialization. The next was to separate those women who were suffering from disorders of their sex. That this was done is evidence by the Halifax Dispensary annual report for 1874, which had a specific medical category for 'Women and Children.' Two years later the report indicated a need for an examining table 'for the purpose of better serving the interests of Gynaecology; and [noted that] additional instruments would greatly facilitate correctness of diagnosis and successful treatment in that branch.'[14] Separation of women into gynaecological wards was the last stage. In 1893 the Doran Wing of the Kingston General Hospital was built with a separate ward for gynaecological cases.[15] Two years later the administrators of the Victoria General Hospital in Halifax were considering establishing a similar division.[16]

These changes revealed a perception on the part of the medical profession and also on the part of women themselves of the need for special treatment for women. At mid-century diseases of the genito-urinary system were among the most prevalent at the Kingston General Hospital since approximately 10 per cent of all patients were so affected, with women being very much over-represented. Moreover, genito-urinary diseases did increase over time; in 1853 they represented approximately 5 per cent of the cases, but by 1866 they were just over 10 per cent.[17] This seemed to be characteristic of other institutions. The annual report of the Woman's Hospital in Montreal for 1878 revealed that the Outdoor Department 'where females suffering from diseases peculiar to women receive medical attendance free of charge' was constantly expanding.[18] This expansion should not be exaggerated, however. At the Halifax Visiting Dispensary between 1868 and 1888 the proportion of patients suffering from 'women's diseases' varied from a low of just under 4 per cent to a high of almost 10 per cent, although seldom did it go beyond 6 per cent.[19] Also, such diseases were never among the most common – bronchitis, dyspepsia, diarrhoea, rheumatism, and constipation were. The Royal Victoria Hospital, Montreal, reflected a much different state of affairs by the end of the century. In 1895 its gynaecological branch treated 13 per cent of all patients and 28 per cent of all women patients. In 1901 this was 10 and 21 per cent, respectively.[20] The higher rates of the Montreal hospital reflected the increase in patients that a department devoted only to gynaecology attracted and the increased availability of treatment that existed in the 1890s compared to earlier decades. Doctors' private caseloads also reflected the importance of gynaecology. Gynaecology and obstetrical cases comprised 18.2 per cent of Dr Hugh Mackay's practice in Woodstock between 1873 and 1879, 16 per cent of Dr Thomas Middleboro's of Owen Sound in 1895–6, and for Dr Alexander Primrose gynaecological patients alone comprised from 3 to 10 per cent of his practice.[21] In Primrose's practice, women represented only 42 per cent of his patients but represented 67 per cent of those suffering from problems of the genito-urinary system.[22]

Advances had been made in the treatment of gynaecological disorders. One of the most spectacular at mid-century was a solution to vesico-vaginal fistula, a rupture of the tissues separating the vagina from the bladder due to difficult labour or poor midwifery treatment. Urine would continually seep through this opening, a constant embarrassment for the women concerned. Although all sorts of remedies were tried, nothing succeeded until J. Marion Sims in the United States, through experimentation on black slave women (sometimes up to thirty procedures on one woman), managed to perfect a technique that by suturing the edges of the opening and inserting a catheter to drain off the urine allowed the wound to heal.[23] The method required skill and patience and not all physicians were able to perform Sims's operation, with the result that other methods continued to be utilized. Doctors at the Halifax Medical Society discussed one case in 1862 where 'from sloughing of the bladder in which by plugging the vagina in a certain way [the doctor] had prevented the passage of urine through the vagina, and the fistulous opening had become much smaller.' Four years later at a meeting of the same society a member reported operating three times on a woman for vesico-vaginal fistula. Unfortunately, he failed to help her.[24] But the fact he had dared to try seemed to be the point he emphasized.

Vesico-vaginal fistula was only one of many problems that women could experience. An examination of the Diseases of Women Casebook for the Montreal General Hospital, University Dispensary, from March 1882 to October 1883 reveals well over fifty different complaints. Among these were ante-flexion, vulvitis, laceration of the perineum, retroversion, catarrh of the cervix, retroflexion, congestion of the endometrium, laceration of the cervix, endometritis, ovarian tumour, vaginitis, leucorrhoea, metrorraghia, degeneration of the cervix, pelvic peritonitis, vesico-vagina fistula, prolapse of the uterus, and ulceration of the vulva.[25] If nothing else, such a list suggests the degree of specialization the profession had reached. Not all within the medical fraternity were pleased about this specialization. For one thing, critics accused specialists of narrowing their focus to the extent that they lost sight of the patient – that is, specialists saw specific organs of the body rather than the whole body. As James Russell, superintendent of the asylum for the insane in Hamilton declared, 'The danger of all specialism is to warp the judgment and contract the mental horizon within the range of its own narrow field of operation.'[26] An example of this was Dr M.A. Curry, obstetrician and gynaecologist at the Victoria General Hospital in Halifax, who at the end of the nineteenth century concentrated on the disorders of the external genitalia only in his gynaecological practice. Internal gynaecological disorders were left to the general surgeons.[27] Such narrowness encouraged its proponents to believe that whatever part of the body they focused on was the most important and the cause of a host of ailments. In his 1868 *Practical Treatise on the Diseases of Women*. Theodore Thomas, himself a gynaecological specialist, acknowledged the truth of this criticism. He admitted that because of the emphasis given to the ovaries in medical literature, doctors looked to them too often as the cause of any form of uterine disease.[28] Almost twenty years later the situation seemed to have become worse. In a wonderful commentary on doctors' penchant for focusing on the uterus as the cause of women's health problems, an article in the 1886 *Canada Lancet* lampooned the profession, taking as its vantage point the perspective of that much maligned organ:

For a long time I have felt that the medical profession was not acting with fairness toward me – that, on the contrary, I am made the object of unjust suspicion and annoying espionage. I am the the victim of constant fault-finding and accusation. Contrary to all rules of law and justice, I am continually called on to prove my innocence – am never allowed the benefit of a plea 'not guilty.' Certain members of your profession have gained the ear of my hostess, and have inculcated a bitter prejudice in her mind against me, so that I am looked on by her, on all occasions and under all circumstances, as the one peccant organ concerning which nothing good could be credited, nothing evil disbelieved.[29]

The reference to the owner of the uterus raised a second problem that some critics had with specialization – it made women into hypochondriacs. The constant emphasis on what could go wrong with their bodies predisposed women to look for and find ailments where none existed.[30]

Whenever experts take over a field, practitioners who have previously worked in it are either eliminated or their prestige diminished. The tension this engenders could account for the cynicism and hostility underlying much of the criticism of gynaecology and gynaecologists. One critic pointedly drew attention to the fact that gynaecology was a very lucrative field.[31] W.S. Muir, a Truro, NS, doctor, sarcastically described the gynaecologist as 'a smart chap from all points of the term, slick at most things, and five times out of eight a money-maker.'[32] There was a sense that specialists had forgotten what real medicine was about, that the general practitioner was the true healer.[33] Certainly, the general practitioner was closer to his patients. On 1 January 1871 the Rev. William Cochrane in his diary wrote a moving account of his dying wife, describing how their doctor had visited five times in one day to help ease her distress.[34] It is difficult to conceive of a specialist being able to provide that kind of support.

Gynaecological specialists were not the only ones who focused on a woman's reproductive/sexual system as the centre of her health problems. Advertisements for patent medicines stressed how frequent disorders of the generative tract were. In the latter decades of the century, medical entrepreneurs made exorbitant claims for the curative powers of their prescriptions. Dr Radway's Regulating Pills were a typical example. The 1872 version of *Radway's Almanac* informed women that the pills could cure a host of ailments including melancholy, hysterics, leucorrhoea, weakening discharges, chlorosis, irregularities, suppression of menses, inflammation of the womb or bladder, and difficult menstruation. That the list of women's diseases was so long underlined the popular perception that women's bodies were somehow weaker than men's and exposed them to different traumas. The 1886 version of the *Almanac* also underscored the reason for the popularity of not only Dr Radway's concoctions but also the whole patent medicine industry to women: 'It is not at all times pleasant or convenient for a lady to consult a physician for every disagreeable or annoying symptom that may occur.'[35] Patent medicines allowed women to avoid embarrassing consultations with male physicians and at the same time permitted them to administer to themselves and take control of their own health. This appeal may help account for those many women who endured ill health for years before they consulted a physician. Until late in the century not many physicians were adept at the treatment of women's diseases, and those who were tended to congregate in urban areas, leaving rural women to consult with their general practitioners or rely on their own expertise.

Women also had access to popular health books published throughout the century. Such texts tended to serve two purposes. One was to allow individuals to treat themselves and the second was to provide a handy reference guide to physicians, most likely general practitioners. Ira Warren's 1865 *Household Physician* gave such detailed descriptions for specific disorders that in some cases women could care for themselves. Warren believed that women should understand their bodies and criticized doctors who kept medical knowledge on female diseases to themselves on the grounds of protecting public morals. His book, then, was an attempt to rectify this situation. For ovaritis he suggested putting six to eight leeches over the diseased ovary and, when the bites healed, to add a blister. This treatment was to continue for five to six months, repeated after every menstruation. While women were able to follow such a course of treatment themselves, his cure for inflammation of the uterine neck suggests that in some cases he expected a physician to be involved. Certainly, few patients would have been able to carry out his direction to 'introduce a speculum, and when the neck of the womb is fairly lodged in its extremity, drop in two or three leeches and allow them to fill.'[36] But if in this instance Warren was addressing physicians, he provided patients with information by which to judge medical treatment given.

The notion that individual women were capable of administering to themselves for some ailments, and would want to do so, continued well into the century. In his 1873 medical recipe book Dr Chase told his women readers its use would 'save the delicacy of exposures, in many instances, and always save the delicacy of conversing with and explaining their various feelings and conditions, to one of the opposite sex.' For general female debility he prescribed taking iron filings and ginger and for leucorrhoea, costiveness, dysmenorrhoea, and for falling womb, the use of a sponge as a pessary.[37] That most of his recipes consisted of both drugs and herbs reveals that home medicine was not restricted to botanic remedies. Indeed, as the century progressed, home medical books became increasingly specific about the drugs prescribed, which indicates that lay people had easier access to them than do twentieth-century Canadians and that physicians had not yet been able to convince lay people that only experts should treat their ailments.[38] R. Pierce's *People's Common Sense Medical Adviser* counselled in 1882 that it was better if women did not consult physicians too often, given their penchant for examining women internally and causing lasting injury to the womb.[39] For many women the first treatment would be home treatment and, only if that failed, would they consult a physician. Home treatment appealed to Canadians because it did not involve anyone else; they were able to preserve their sense of privacy and, in the case of women with disorders of the reproductive/ sexual system. their sense of dignity and decorum. While many physicians were sensitive to this problem, some of the medical procedures that became standard practice during the latter half of the century only served to increase the unease that many women must have felt about consulting a physician. The internal examination pointed out by Pierce was such a procedure.

Early in the century few physicians supported the idea of examining women. Medical lecturers pointed out that 'touching or examining Women indiscriminately would be very improper' and, as a result, rules were needed to guide the practitioner. One of these was to have a nurse examine the patient and to inform the doctor of the woman's condition.[40] Such reservations continued well into the century. In 1850 the *British American Journal of Medical & Physical Science* in a reprinted article warned physicians about being too free in their uterine examinations. It violated the natural modesty of women and, in so doing, broke down their restraint and led them to talk too freely about their own organs. The author pointed to the obvious – examining the vagina was not quite the same as examining the throat.[41] A reviewer of a gynaecology text in the *Medical Chronicle* four years later agreed. Not only would women become immodest and begin talking about the womb but they would even insist on examinations being performed![42] For some women the consequences were much worse, for as Henry MacNaughton-Jones so delicately suggested, 'Next to masturbation, too frequent medical examinations are to be condemned, especially in that type of woman, of the neurotic temperament, who can ill conceal her feelings.'[43] So concerned was Dr D.C. MacCallum of McGill that he not only deplored the breakdown in reserve that 'physical exploration' caused but also questioned whether women should even be taught how their bodies functioned lest it 'blunt that shrinking sensibility and maiden coyness which is so beautiful a feature in the character of the young girl.'[44]

Of special concern at mid-century was the examination of young girls. A physician whose article was reprinted in the 1856 *Medical Chronicle* advised that in cases of amenorrhoea and dysmenorrhoea, 'the treatment in girls ... should in general be confined to the use of external means, such as leeches to the groins and thighs, warm hip-baths, and dry cupping the breasts.' Only when such procedures failed should an 'exploration of the organs' occur.[45] Such sensitivity for young girls was both understandable and commendable but it could sometimes backfire. Hector Peltier, professor at the Montreal School of Medicine, told of a case he had of a young women whose menses had stopped. Being reluctant to give her a vaginal examination he allowed her abdomen to increase in size over the next eight-and-a-half months. As he explained, 'My confidence in the education and moral character of the young lady, kept me, through false delicacy, from asking any question, or making any examination.' The result was that the young women was exposed to insults and the accusation she was pregnant. She was not. As the physician pointed out, a vaginal examination would have allowed him to put such slander to rest.[46] R.P. Howard, professor of theory and practice medicine at McGill College, in 1873 recounted one patient he had seen in 1866 who was weak, emaciated, depressed, and suffered from menorrhagia. Nothing that her physician had done had stemmed the haemorrhage, 'yet from motives of delicacy [he] had not made a vaginal examination.' Despite the woman's unmarried state, Howard did so and discovered a fibrous tumour the size of an egg. He operated to remove it and the woman recovered, regained her health, and began to menstruate regularly.[47] As these cases indicate, physicians were caught between traditional attitudes respecting appropriate behaviour and the demands of their profession, a tension which never totally disappeared.

Gradually the reluctance to examine young women lessened. In his 1861 text, *A Practical Treatise on the Disease of Women*, Friedrich Scanzoni von Lichtenfels felt it necessary to claim he was 'far from wishing to pretend that, in every case where disease of the genital organs is suspected, we should compel patients to submit to an examination which wounds their modesty.' Once this was understood, however, he acknowledged that if the examination were necessary it should be done, modesty or no.[48] For some young women this could be quite traumatic. Mary Ann Perry was sixteen when she came to the Victoria General Hospital, Halifax, in October 1885. She stayed only four days, however, leaving 'very indignant when the House Surgeon attempted to make a vaginal examination.'[49] To offset this kind of reaction doctors devised ways to make it less of an ordeal for the patient. One was to perform the procedure under anaesthesia.[50] When Christie McPherson, a young servant girl, came to the Victoria General Hospital on 22 December 1894 she complained of pains in her breasts and abdomen, vomiting, and leucorrhoeal discharge. Only on 16 January did doctors perform an internal examination, under ether.[51] Although physicians deemed the internal examination necessary in certain cases, they never completely lost their apprehension about it. Indeed, one physician in the *Canada Medical Record* of January 1891 reminded his readers that some referred to a digital examination of a young girl as equivalent to 'moral rape.'[52]

While the focus of concern was on examining young girls or unmarried women, ambivalence and hesitation also existed about examining married women. In his 1882 text Arthur Edis warned that such an examination assaulted the modesty of women, modesty which, as he put it, was 'the best attribute of woman and the surest safeguard of society.' But it was not just the modesty of their patients that physicians had to consider. They also had to be anxious about their own reputation. To ensure the latter, Edis suggested that the physician explain very clearly to the patient why such an examination was necessary and 'to leave entirely to the patient as a general rule, the option of her mother or friend being present in the room during the examination.' He warned, however, that for young, unmarried girls (especially those prone to hysteria), it was 'always a prudent precaution to insist upon the mother or some other discreet married friend being present.'[53] It was prudent not only for the patient but also for the physician, in that he would have a witness that nothing untoward had occurred. Patients were not the only ones who felt vulnerable. False accusations of impropriety were a doctor's nightmare. Even if a woman were willing to be examined, doctors had to be sensitive to her feelings. Dr MacCallum pointed out that some objected to lying on a table and if that was the case, then the doctor 'must ... examine the patient, as best [he] can, either on a bed or a couch.'[54]

The ambivalence that many physicians expressed about internal examinations of married women was reflected in practice. Doctors did not always perform an internal examination for gynaecological problems. Mrs Arthur Dougan came to the University Dispensary of the Montreal General Hospital to consult on the soreness of her genitals and a genital discharge, which she attributed to gonorrhoea contracted from her husband. Her record suggests that doctors did not examine her visually. Some patients made the decision not to be examined themselves, as was the case of Mrs Drew in 1882 at the University Dispensary.[55] Similarly Mrs Seward, who came to the hospital on 1 April 1882 suffering from weakness, loss of appetite, constipation, and menstruation every two weeks accompanied by clots, 'declined to be examined.' Three days later she changed her mind and was diagnosed as suffering from leucorrhoea and laceration of the perineum for which doctors advised hot water douches and carbolic acid to the interior of the uterus.[56] While it is understandable why some women were reluctant to undergo an internal examination and why some physicians hesitated to suggest it even for married women, ignoring its benefits could prove disastrous just as it had for unmarried women. In July 1894 Mabel Donnahue, a woman who at the age of twenty-nine had been married for fourteen years, came to the Victoria General Hospital. Soon after her marriage she had given birth to twins and, as a result, her womb had come down and continued to do so, although she 'was accustomed to shove the womb up herself with a piece of warm flannel.' Unfortunately, it had been down a year without returning to its proper position and for this reason she entered the hospital. While in hospital Mabel died and the post-mortem revealed an incorrect diagnosis of prolapse of the uterus – it was a rectocele into the vagina – that is, a hernial protrusion of part of the rectum. In this case a proper internal examination might have resulted in a correct diagnosis.[57]

By the end of the century, although some qualms remained, most textbooks described the internal examination of women as accepted policy. This was a far cry from the early decades of the century when physicians thought of the genitals of women in a sexual context and therefore did not view them. Even when attending childbirth cases, some physicians had preferred to have midwives or other women examine the patient. While this notion had not totally disappeared, it had lessened as physicians maintained that the genitals were simply a part of the body like any other part. Underlying this shift was a change in the way physicians thought of themselves. When physicians did not 'view' the female body, it was to preserve not only the respectability of the women but also of themselves. When the internal examination became part of normal gynaecological procedure, it signalled that in their professional guise they were physicians, not men. Not that it was easy to keep the two separate. When Rosemary Kennedy, a nineteen-year-old single woman was admitted to the Victoria General Hospital in August 1881, the physician writing her case history could not help noting, 'Dark complexion and very pretty.'[58]

The acceptance of the internal examination also signalled a shift in attitude towards women. The irony of doctors' worrying about the breakdown in women's reserve was that it was physicians' reserve with respect to women that had lessened. This can be seen in other forms of intervention besides the internal examination. For example, the list of medicinal potions inserted into the vagina seems endless: ice, chloroform, belladonna, laudanum, bromide of potassium, iron, sulphuric acid, gallic acid, acetate of lead, port wine, nitric acid, and nitrate of silver among others.[59] Hugh Mackay recorded in his notebook that ergot could be used for a fibroma of the uterus – at times necessitating ten to fifteen daily injections.[60] In 1882 Mrs Benner came to the Montreal General Hospital suffering from inflammation of the womb. She had delivered nine children full term by the time she was thirty-seven. After her last pregnancy she complained of pain at the base of the sacrum and in the left iliac region, leucorrhoea, and urine retention. Diagnosed as suffering from vulvitis and laceration of the perineum, hot water vaginal douches were recommended and carbolic acid applied to the uterine interior.[61] Doctors also used leeches, both externally and, to a much lesser extent, internally.[62] In 1846 Robert MacDonnell, physician to the Montreal General Hospital, reported being the first in Montreal to use electro-galvanism in cases of amenorrhoea and dysmenorrhoea. He placed one pole on the lower part of the spinal column and 'the other button is applied by the patient herself, or by a female attendant, immediately over the os pubis.'[63] Because of the sensitivity to female modesty, the patient became a participant in her own treatment. Electricity in medicine continued to be popular. In 1886 Dr Gardner of the Montreal General Hospital described employing it in pelvic disorders for as often as three times a week for up to three to six months.[64] Doctors also found cauterization of benefit.[65] In his 1861 text Scanzoni von Lichtenfels gave a graphic description of the use of the cautery and the attendant benefits of anaesthesia:

The pain which accompanies the application of the actual cautery to the neck of the womb is nothing, or next to nothing. However, as the very idea of this operation terrifies most patients, it is well not to communicate it to them. The pretext of some little operation should be made, and the iron need not be brought in until, by the inhalation of chloroform, the patients are completely narcotized. When they have returned to themselves, and are persuaded of the harmlessness of the treatment; they may be informed of what has passed. We may, however, add that we have employed the actual cautery several times – the patient, who each time was chloroformized, never suspecting the fact.[66]

Unwittingly, he provides the modern reader with an insight into the ethics of medical practice and attitudes towards patient rights.

If the list of chemicals and other forms of treatment seem daunting to the uninitiated, equally so is the list of instruments that probed the vagina and uterine cavity – speculum, sounds, tents, tenaculums, uterine probes, endoscopes, and exploring needles.[67] It would seem that the physiological make-up of women invited exploration. The benefits of some instruments were obvious. The vagina speculum, which was in use by the 1830s, could help the physician determine the size of the vagina. Since the vagina enlarged after conception this was an aid in diagnosing pregnancy. Similarly the speculum permitted a closer look at the uterus, which changed colour with pregnancy.[68] Any abnormalities could also be located. Despite the evident value of the speculum and other instruments, some physicians questioned the need for so many. One critic sarcastically noted that there seemed to be a great deal of time, effort, and apparatus focused on the womb, an organ only 3 inches long, 2 inches broad, 1 inch thick, and weighing from 1 to $1\frac{1}{2}$ ounces.[69] Nevertheless, the number of instruments continued to increase as physicians made minor changes to those that existed and invented new ones. And once available, instruments tended to be used. Indeed, the internal examination ensured this was the case. As one historian has suggested, 'the field of gynaecology, which was dependent on internal examination, developed more quickly with instrumentation because it allowed increased explorative intimacy and thus, faster and more accurate diagnosis and treatment.'[70]

While critics of the overuse of instruments seldom differentiated among them, they did single out the 'indiscriminate use of pessaries' at the end of the century.[71] At the University Dispensary of the Montreal General Hospital in the early 1880s, a perusal of case records suggests the use of pessaries instead of stitching to treat lacerations.[72] Most frequently used to support the uterus, physicians resorted to them so frequently that, according to one commentator, a 'pessary rage' seemed to be present. Especially annoying was their use by 'amateur gynaecologists' and 'physicians experienced in general practice, but unskilled in gynaecology.'[73] Specialists were once again trying to restrict what other physicians could do in order to assume more control themselves. Unfortunately for the patients, this did not guarantee success. Bella Russell, a young seamstress, entered Victoria General Hospital on 8 May 1882. For three or four years 'her womb came down on her' and, when examined, she was discovered to have a retroflexed uterus. Doctors returned it to its proper position and, no suitable pessary being available, Russell was put to bed and instructed to lie flat. Four days later the uterus had retroflexed again and a pessary was inserted. On 19 May no change had occurred and another pessary was inserted. The next day this pessary slipped out and the uterus was found to be worse than ever, so the doctors removed the pessary. On 29 May Russell left the hospital unimproved.[74] What this example serves to remind us is not the success or failure of a specific treatment but that the patient was the true hero of medicine. Even when treatment did succeed, the cost in separation from family could be extreme. Mrs Ann Duffin was a twenty-eight-year-old married woman from Halifax when she entered the Victoria General Hospital on 29 July 1898 suffering from a lacerated cervix and perineum. On 2 August both were sutured and on 14 August the stitches removed. On 18 September, a tampon (pessary) was inserted and on 10 October it, too, was removed. On 21 October, almost two months after she was admitted, she was finally discharged.[75]

Opponents of instrument intervention raised several arguments encouraging physicians to resort to instruments less often. As already noted, one was to stress the need for expertise in their application.[76] A second was to point out the real danger of physician-induced infection caused by inserting so many sounds, curettes, tents, dilators, and pessaries into the vagina.[77] Dr MacCallum warned that the use of tents had resulted in metritis, peritonitis, pelvic cellulitis, septicaemic fever, and tetanus.[78] Another harkened back to the concerns about the internal examination, that it lessened the modesty of women by having so much attention paid to their reproductive/sexual system. Not considered was how it changed the doctor/patient relationship by placing the physician in a significant position of power. He now knew more about the woman's body than she did herself, for he was able to 'view' parts of it that she did not and, since he had access to the diseased organ itself, he was less dependent on the patient's description of symptoms. Fanny Cowan, aged twenty-eight, came to Dr James

Ross suffering from swelling in the lower part of the abdomen, constant flow from the womb, and pain in her back and sides which moved down her thighs and became more intense at menstruation. After seeing her, Ross wrote, 'No pessary to be used at present. Do no believe she suffers as much as she says.'[79] The actual treatment also placed women in a very dependent situation. Remember Bella Russell who was required to lie flat in bed, totally reliant on those around her, and then who had to have the indignity of pessaries being inserted, removed, and inserted again, all for not. And treatment did not simply involve the patient and what she could do. It affected those around her. Consider R. Pierce and his treatment for vaginismus. He advised that during treatment with a dilator the patient had to live apart from her husband, as did D.C. MacCullum when discussing extreme cases of dysmenorrhoea.[80] Of course physicians had their own pressures with which to cope. C.A. Sibley, a historian of gynaecology in Canada, has postulated, 'If a physician had failed to provide the medical answer, he would have failed to fulfil his male role of benevolent moral steward to the dependent woman. Also, for a man to have been baffled by the organs of a supposedly inferior creature may have caused him personal and professional angst.'[81]

The discussions which took place in the medical literature only provide general outlines of what occurred in gynaecology in Canada. However, Sibley's study of the gynaecological cases in the Kingston General Hospital between 1853 and 1866 gives us a better sense of who the patients were and what form of treatment they were receiving. Patients were predominantly Irish (55 per cent) and this was an over-representation since the general population of Kingston was less than 30 per cent Irish. Compared to non-gynaecological patients, these women seldom entered the hospital from jail or the House of Industry. As would be expected, the predominant age group was twenty-one to forty – that is, women who were in their childbearing years. Indeed, throughout the century, almost two-thirds of the gynaecological patients were in this age category. More interesting are the hints as to actual treatment. Excluding pregnancy and venereal disease cases, just over half of the patients stayed from one to two weeks in the hospital, with the rest remaining from two to four weeks. Sibley linked the relatively long stay to the condition of the patient treated and the treatment given. Many of the patients on entry were in poor health to begin with and had to be strengthened before treatment began. Also, the era from 1853 to 1866 was before gynaecological surgery was safe to perform and non-surgical treatment was the only option; non-surgical treatment tends to be slower than surgical and necessitates a longer stay in the hospital.[82] This, however, should not be exaggerated. At the Royal Jubilee Hospital in Victoria, approximately 65 per cent of patients at the end of the century stayed longer than ten days and long stays were definitely linked to surgical cases, gynaecological being among them.[83] Moreover, treatment at mid-century was less specific than it later became, and the inclination was to apply several treatments rather than one. This, too, would lengthen the stay of the patient.[84]

But what was the actual treatment given to Canadian women? Specific cases suggest that Canadian physicians were not as interventionist as the medical literature feared. Several examples reveal how conservative some Canadian doctors were in their approach to their patients' illnesses and how they tended to combine non-interventionist techniques and common sense. Margaret Mullins, aged twenty-eight and unmarried, became a patient of Dr Gardner of the Montreal General Hospital on 31 May 1888. Diagnosed as having anteversion and cystic ovaries, her prescribed treatment was country air, a change of scene, seabathing, and tonics.[85] Such a regimen would not be suitable for all women, for many could not afford the luxury of such a course of treatment, but Dr Gardner was not alone in appreciating the value of rest and allowing nature to do the healing. The doctors attending the University Dispensary of the Montreal General Hospital during the early 1880s seemed reluctant to send patients to the actual hospital but tried to treat them in such a way that the women could remain at home. When they did send them to the hospital, it was often for a rest. For Millie Sangster who came to them on 9 October 1883 suffering from anteflexion with retroversion and perimetritis, they prescribed hot water vaginal injection, hot poultices to the abdomen, rest in bed, and opium when necessary to relieve the pain.[86] The need to build up a woman's strength seemed to be quite common. Rose Malton entered the Victoria General Hospital on 18 December 1888 suffering from prolapse of the uterus. In 1878 she had given birth to her last child during which 'she had an injury to the organs of generation ... a result of forceps.' As a result, she experienced pain when she urinated, had pain in walking, and a bearing down pain in her back. The first thing doctors did was to put her to bed for two weeks, which the records indicate she enjoyed. Finally on 9 January they inserted a pessary and left it in for fourteen days, and soon after she was discharged.[87] In June 1890 Dr James Ross of Toronto saw Moira Miles, aged twenty-one, whom he diagnosed as suffering from a haematocele of the broad ligament. He treated her with a tonic, warm vaginal douches, and rest in bed. For Barbara Grierson, a nineteen-year-old who had never menstruated and whom he discovered had 'not even an infantile uterus' but who was otherwise healthy, his treatment was 'Leave alone.'[88] The lengthy treatment many women received and which doctors felt necessary may have been one reason women waited so long before seeking alleviation for their ailments. Not many private practitioners would have been skilled in the gynaecological techniques that hospital physicians and specialists deemed essential and not many women could afford a lengthy stay in a hospital, away from work or their families. Perhaps it is not surprising that medical treatment of gynaecological disorders in Canada did not embrace the interventionist apocalypse that some feared. Physicians practising in a particular era are trained under earlier ideologies – that is, physicians practising in the 1880s and 1890s were most likely trained in the 1870s or earlier. This was the era that some critics accused of being non-interventionist to the detriment of the patient. It was the period before antisepsis and the danger of intervention was all too real to these physicians. Even when antisepsis was being touted, not all physicians were convinced that it lessened the danger of intervention.[89] Also, intervention in private practice cost the patient money, and Canadians simply may have been reluctant to pay the cost.

The expansion of gynaecology raised concerns about increasing intervention in medicine and what that meant for patient and physician. Critics worried that internal examinations and emphasis on the sexual/reproductive system would lessen women's modesty. Others feared that physical harm would occur when such intervention was performed by non-specialists, men not trained in gynaecological techniques. In turn, general practitioners were wary about the motivation behind the practice of specialists and concerned about what the expansion of gynaecology or any specialty might mean for their own livelihood. While both groups recognized the danger of intervention and often blamed each other for it, the reality of practice restricted the degree of intervention in many cases. Nevertheless, intervention did occur and was increasing, and became more extreme as evidenced in the rise of gynaecological surgery.

Chapter Nine

Gynaecological Surgery

Not all surgery on the reproductive/sexual system was focused on women. Men, too, were at risk. In July 1862 the minutes of the Halifax Medical Society described a case of a man who had suffered from fungus of the testicle. The treatment – removal of the offending organ.[1] Likewise the annual reports of the Montreal General Hospital more often than not mentioned amputation of the penis and/or testicles. The Surgical Department of the Royal Victoria Hospital, Montreal, in 1895 had among its patients ninety men suffering from problems of the genito-urinary system.[2] But if operations did occur on men, they never reached the numbers of those performed on women; neither did they have the same 'glamour' about them.

Gynaecological surgery was a consequence of the emergence of gynaecology in the nineteenth century and medical advances that made any type of surgery more feasible. In the first half of the nineteenth century surgery was largely limited to minor procedures and amputations. Any more extensive surgical probing of the body resulted in a high mortality rate that discouraged physicians. Part of the reason for this problem was the shock to the patient from the pain associated with the surgery and the sepsis that often ensued due to uncleanliness on the part of the surgical instruments or of the physician himself. With the introduction of anaesthesia the first problem was mitigated. While this eased some of the trauma to the patient, surgery still remained

problematic. Dr Abraham Groves of Fergus, Ont., bemusedly recalled his practice as it was in 1871:

There was no hospital nearer than Toronto, there was not a trained
nurse in Canada, and there were no skilled assistants. Little or nothing
was known about germs. There were no rubber gloves, sterilized gauze,
or absorbent cotton, and silk was the usual material used for sutures
and ligatures.
  My early operative work was done under very primitive conditions.
The operating room was usually the kitchen, there being no other room
large enough in the houses of those days, and either a couple of boards
laid on trestles, or the kitchen table was used as an operating table.
Milk pans were used as basins, sea-sponges for wiping, and horse-hair,
taken directly from the horse's tail, generally the doctor's horse, for
sutures. If the operation had to be done at night a coal-oil lamp supplied the light ... Chloroform was the one anaesthetic. It was dropped
from a bottle with a split cork, the inhaler being a towel.[3]

While physicians believed that Listerism countered the sepsis
problem, even it could not obviate the obstacles faced by rural
practitioners such as Groves. Nevertheless, it and anaesthesia did
provide many physicians with more confidence about undertak-
ing surgical procedures. Hospital records reveal the increase in
surgical admissions. In 1867 the Provincial and City Hospital in
Halifax admitted 121 medical and 106 surgical cases. Twenty years
later surgical cases slightly outnumbered medical cases, 283 compared to 271. By 1897, however, surgical cases numbered 708
whereas medical, only 562.[4] The records of the Montreal General
Hospital indicate a similar shift. After 1882 the hospital made a
distinction between surgeons and physicians and separated patients as to whether they were surgical or medical patients.[5] In
1891–2, 1085 medical and 982 surgical cases were admitted, but in
1900–1 the numbers were 902 and 1222, respectively.[6] Indeed, by
the end of the century surgical cases made up the bulk of admissions to most hospitals.[7]
  Gynaecological surgery followed this general pattern. At mid-

century doctors limited gynaecological operations to surface procedures – 'the removal of polyps, excision of a hypertrophied
clitoris, incision of an imperforate hymen, and attempts at repair
of a third degree perineal laceration.'[8] The Montreal General Hospital in the early 1860s classified tapping an ovarian cyst as a major
operation.[9] More intricate procedures occurred, but rarely. The
advent of anaesthesia changed that – seldom-done procedures became more common and new and innovative operations devised.
The introduction of antiseptic surgery simply intensified the process. The resulting surgery had its own fashion dictates. 'The
uterine displacement craze, when every gynaecologist invented
or modified a pessary for the treatment of backache or pelvic
pain, was followed by a pelvic cellulitis craze which was widely
taken up until it was exploded. Oophorectomy, clitoridectomy,
inflammation of the os and cervix uteri, excision of the uterus
and its appendages, operations for extra-uterine pregnancy and
Caesarian section, all were once prevalent fashions.'[10] Noteworthy
in this process was the central role played by American physicians.
Not to the forefront in scientific theory or in laboratory research,
American physicians came into their own in the number of new
cutting operations they developed and performed.[11] And as in
other areas of medicine, the increase in gynaecological surgery
provoked a heated debate within the medical profession. Generalists criticized specialists, and non-surgeons attacked surgeons;
in turn specialists and surgeons defended their increasing role
within medicine. All seemed to debate the consequences of the
surgery and its impact on women, and, within that discussion,
they used conventional attitudes about women's role and place
in society to justify their positions.

Despite the infrequency of operations, some of those performed
at mid-century were delicate and innovative. Among the more
successful and intriguing was the operation William Hingston described to his colleagues at the Medico-Chirurgical Society of
Montreal in 1866. In this case he fashioned an artificial vagina for
a woman who subsequently married. Her 'possessor,' as he referred to her husband, remained ignorant of the fact 'that the
knife had carved for him a path to enjoyment.'[12] The 1870s and

1880s did not see much change in the status of gynaecological surgery. Non-surgical approaches such as the use of the pessary for retroversion of the uterus and hot vaginal douches for pelvic cellulitis were the norm. Hospitals such as the Victoria General in Halifax and the Montreal General still did not perform many operations and those that were done were minor, such as Tait's operation for laceration of the perineum and Emmet's for laceration of the cervix. References in the Canadian journal literature certainly suggest that Canadian physicians were not knife crazy. In 1886 Lapthorn Smith reported on his visit to various women's hospitals in the United States and how struck he was by the frequency of gynaecological operations. In this case he argued that the results justified the risk and he seemed to be encouraging physicians in Canada to take up the challenge.[13] Of course, it was not always the doctors who were reluctant to operate. Patients could refuse to undergo surgery. Smith described one woman on whom he wanted to operate for prolapse of the uterus but who refused, thereby forcing him to resort to non-surgical treatment, application of electric current. That she was not alone in exerting her wishes was made clear when he grouped her with a class of women for whom he had little sympathy.[14]

The significant increase in gynaecological surgery occurred in the 1890s. At the Victoria General Hospital physicians frequently removed ovarian cysts, although they did not seem to use the cysts as an excuse to remove the ovaries. As we will see, this was not always the case in other practices. In 1898 one-third of all the major operations performed were on women's reproductive system.[15] Gynaecological patients undergoing surgery at the Kingston General Hospital were also more numerous by the late 1890s.[16] Canadian doctors had no trouble keeping up with the advances made in gynaecology. A hysterectomy for uterine fibroids was first successfully performed in 1853. Despite mortality rates of 50 per cent, between 1881 and 1885 the leading surgeons in the Western world operated 400 times.[17] One of these was E.H. Trenholme, professor of midwifery and diseases of women at Bishop's medical faculty in Montreal, who between 1877 and 1889 performed nine of these operations. His mortality rate was in keeping with the rest – he lost five of his patients.[18] Hugh Mackay may not have had much chance to practise surgery but he certainly knew what was occurring elsewhere. For example, in his notebook are references to Tait's amputation of a pregnant uterus taken from the 1 February 1889 issue of the *Canadian Practitioner*.[19] When the Kingston General Hospital's Doran Building for women opened in 1891, it contained an operating room, a sure sign of change in the treatment of women's diseases. Previous to this, operating rooms at Kingston had been known as amputating theatres.[20] The Royal Jubilee Hospital in 1895–6 reported a wide variety of gynaecological surgery performed: ovariotomy, removal of fibroid of the broad ligament, shortening round ligaments, ventrofixation of the uterus, salpingectomy, and trachelorrhapy among others.[21] In the same year, the gynaecological surgery department of the Royal Victoria Hospital reported 408 different procedures performed on 240 patients.[22] It would appear that women had become the canvas on which doctors would practise their art.

Physicians could not help but be aware of the increase in gynaecological surgery. Some blamed the interference in midwifery for creating so many patients for the surgical gynaecologists,[23] patients such as Mme Bouclé who came to the Montreal General Hospital University Dispensary on 8 April 1882. Delivered of a dead child by forceps in 1880, she had never been well since. The diagnosis was a fibroid tumour of the posterior wall, endometritis, and vulvitis.[24] Lawson Tait, a leading British gynaecological surgeon, believed operations were increasing because ovarian disease itself was more prevalent, although he could not explain why this was the case.[25] Operations also replaced other procedures. Lapthorn Smith noted that surgery had taken over from the pessary. In addition, he felt that changes in medical technology, especially the introduction of antisepsis, made surgery safer.[26] Not all were as in awe of the benefits of antisepsis as he was. William Goodell, author of a major textbook on the subject, blamed the increase in surgery on antisepsis which he referred to as a 'spoiler.' It had 'dazzled' gynaecologists so they had become 'too hasty and too radical' in their approach and surgery mad. Moderation was needed.[27] Whether antisepsis actually provided the safety that physicians thought it did has become a debatable point in recent years, but for those who believed in its efficacy it provided a sense of security to engage in surgical techniques which otherwise they might not have had. The rise in surgery was also linked to the development and changing nature of hospitals. By the end of the nineteenth century surgery usually necessitated equipment, assistants, and frequent post-surgical monitoring of patients. Unlike general practitioners, surgeons were reluctant to perform operations in their patients' homes as they had previously done. Patients now had to come to them, to the hospitals. This occurred at the same time that hospitals became less oriented to charity patients and more to paying patients by providing better accommodation for them. Paying patients could afford their stay and to pay for more intricate surgical procedures. Two operations in particular stand out in the late nineteenth century, one because it was seldom performed in Canada and the other because it was performed. Each in its own way provides insight into the nature of medicine in Canada and its treatment of women.

One of the most controversial gynaecological procedures in the nineteenth century was the clitoridectomy, or excision of the clitoris. Its emergence at mid-century was due not to improved medical technology but to the expansion of what physicians and others in society defined as medical problems. Although some had earlier advocated removal of the clitoris in cases of masturbation, in the mid-1860s it became a *cause célèbre* because an English physician, Isaac Baker Brown, was performing it not only to prevent women from masturbating but also to cure certain types of insanity, epilepsy, and hysteria. So upset were his colleagues about this that he lost his membership in the Obstetrical Society of London.[28] Canadians were aware of what Baker Brown was doing, for as early as 1867 the *Canada Medical Journal and Monthly Record* reprinted an editorial from the London *Lancet* reporting on his work. The editorial urged rejection of the procedure, arguing that 'it is simply monstrous and contrary to experience to affirm that [mental] diseases are due in any considerable number of instances to unnatural excitation of the pudic nerve.'[29]

More than thirty years later MacNaughton-Jones, in his text *Points of Practical Interest in Gynecology*, noted that while cauterization of the clitoris could effect a cure for self-abuse, this was due to the effect it had on the woman's mind more than the actual physical affects of the cauterization. He applied this finding to excision of the clitoris and concluded that often self-abuse was a secondary result of neurasthenia, hysteria, or hystero-neurosis and thus clitoridectomy 'can at best, under such circumstances, be experimental' and warned that 'the after-effects on the woman's mind may make her last state worse than the first.'[30] Not all agreed. Henry Garrigues advocated it in cases of masturbation when nothing else worked, when the patient's health was suffering, when her mental faculties were weakening, and when she was contemplating suicide. Dismissing the importance of the clitoris, he offhandedly stated: 'There is no reason why this little bit of flesh should not be removed.'[31]

Although there was some evidence indicating support for the procedure in the literature that Canadian physicians were reading, there was little discussion among Canadian doctors themselves and even less evidence to suggest that Canadian physicians resorted to clitoridectomies in any numbers, unlike their American colleagues who performed it well into the twentieth century.[32] In 1895 one did occur at the Royal Victoria Hospital in Montreal, but this seemed to be a rarity.[33] The hostility of the British medical profession towards it probably had considerable influence, for many physicians practising in this country had been trained in England or Scotland. In addition, the procedure may simply have been too controversial for most physicians to feel sanguine about. Yet if Canadian physicians did not engage in a direct attack on female sexuality as reflected in clitoridectomies, they did, according to some physicians, engage in gynaecological operations to an excessive degree. Many of these operations performed to cure physical disorders often interfered with and sometimes put an end to the very substance of what it meant to be a woman in nineteenth-century Canada – maternity. The most notable among these operations was the ovariotomy.

One of the earliest gynaecological operations, the ovariotomy, as with other forms of surgery, increased significantly in the latter half of the nineteenth century. Dr Ephraim McDowell of Kentucky was the first to perform the surgery in 1809 and by 1830 he had done twelve others. In 1823 the first ovariotomy in Great Britain occurred. However, the results of the early surgery were not encouraging. No successful one was performed in London before 1842 or in Scotland before 1862.[34] Nevertheless, a variation on the ovariotomy, known as Battey's operation, became common in the 1870s. Named after its originator, Robert Battey, a surgeon in Rome, Georgia, it consisted of the removal of normal ovaries to bring about a premature menopause.[35] By 1881 forty-seven surgeons had performed Battey's operation at least 193 times and Battey himself operated on several hundred women between 1870 and 1890.[36] In 1882 Dr Spencer Wells of London claimed he had performed at least 1000 ovariotomies of different kinds and by 1890 his total was over 1200.[37] Dr Lapthorn Smith of Montreal reported in the *Canada Medical and Surgical Journal* of 1886 that in the women's hospitals of New York ovariotomies were daily occurrences.[38]

The high mortality rate for ovariotomies at mid-century limited the number performed. In the 1840s the survival rate was estimated at only 25 to 50 per cent.[39] The *Medical Chronicle* reported in 1856 that one physician who had operated 299 times had lost 120 patients. In all, only 119 cases were successful in both removing the disease and having the patient recover.[40] The high mortality rates, usually a result of peritonitis and septicaemia, continued into the 1860s. Despite this, the numbers performed increased. Theodore Thomas claimed that in 1856, 212 cases had been reported and by 1864, 787 cases.[41] He also pointed out that even with its high rate of mortality, it compared well to other major operations. But the mortality rate remained worrisome. In the *Canada Medical Journal and Monthly Record* for 1871, one physician argued that doctors should be very reluctant to operate as long as the patient remained moderately healthy and comfortable.[42] Such caution was justified in the early 1880s, for the mortality rate for Battey's procedure was still high at 22 per cent,[43] although by 1885 the rate had declined to 14 per cent.[44] Despite the mortality figures, physicians saw ovariotomies as beneficial.

After all, they could now offer some chance of recovery to those women with diseased ovaries who before would have had to endure increasing pain, discomfort, and for some eventual death. This would prove of benefit to those women and also increase the professional stature of physicians. So enthusiastic was the vice-president of King and Queens College of Physicians in Ireland about it that he claimed that ovariotomy 'would alone suffice to stamp our age as one of great progress in the treatment of those affections which are peculiar to women.'[45] Influenced by the success and fame that had accrued to McDowell and Battey, other surgeons tried to improve on their operations. One of the most noteworthy was that developed by Lawson Tait of England. His version consisted of removing not only the ovaries by also the uterine appendages. In the late 1880s he was reporting a mortality rate as low as 2 to 3 per cent, although in some hospitals it was still as high as 25 per cent.[46] The variation indicates the importance of the individual physician performing the operation and may reflect differences in the health of the patients. Many women waited until their health was severely undermined before seeking help; in turn, many physicians were reluctant to operate until the health of their patient was in serious condition. This could only contribute to high mortality rates.

As early as 1864 Canadians were performing ovariotomies.[47] Little is known about the earliest, but on 6 February of that year Dr Robert Craik, professor of chemistry at McGill and consulting physician to the Montreal General Hospital, performed two ovariotomies, one successful and one where the patient died. Especially noteworthy in these ovariotomies was the fact that he used antiseptic precautions, soaking the sponges and ligatures in carbolic acid. This was one of the first examples of the adoption of Listerism in Canada.[48] So rare was the ovariotomy in Canada, however, that when he performed another in 1871 a dozen of his medical friends came to watch. Mrs Garrett was a thirty-seven-year-old mother of four who first consulted Craik in August 1869, complaining of increasing girth without a cessation of the menses. After a vaginal examination, Craik determined that she was suffering from an ovarian tumour of some size. He did not feel that anything but an operation was suitable but was unsure of how soon it should occur given the danger to the patient. He decided to wait and monitor her closely. As long as she was able to carry on normally he was reluctant to proceed, but in May 1871 she began to experience severe pain. The time had come to operate. Assisted by four other physicians, Craik removed the tumour and ovary and Mrs Garrett made a successful recovery.[49] In 1874 Abraham Groves performed an ovariotomy in his general practice[50] and one year later E.H. Trenholme performed Battey's operation or a double ovariotomy on a thirty-two-year-old married woman with no children. The operation was a success and Trenholme proceeded to advocate it for fibroids of the uterus when 'excision of the uterus is impracticable.'[51] In the same year, he performed a second such operation on a twenty-eight-year-old married woman with two children.[52] In 1878 he reported doing another which included removal of the uterus. Six years later he reported six more cases, all single women, one of whom he operated on in hopes of alleviating her insanity.[53] He was fairly satisfied with the results of the operation, although he believed that combining ovariotomies with removal of the fallopian tubes (Tait's operation) was still on trial, since 'the data for its performance and the exact class of cases where we can safely predict a successful issue are not sufficiently established.'[54]

By the late 1880s the number of ovariotomies performed in this country was increasing. In 1886 William Gardner performed sixteen ovariotomies and eleven removals of uterine appendages (Tait's operation), two hysterectomies, and three removals of the uterus, claiming only one death among the thirty-two operations. He operated not under antiseptic conditions but under clean conditions.[55] In 1887 twenty-four Tait's operations were performed in Toronto by at least seven or eight different physicians.[56] After this date ovariotomies in their multiple variations became so frequent that numbers were no longer reported in the medical press. However, the annual reports of hospitals give some hint of frequency. For 1884–5 the Montreal General reported four ovariotomies and one oophorectomy, whereas for 1900–1 the numbers were three ovariotomies, five oophorectomies, one double ovariotomy, one double oophorectomy, six double oophero-salpingectomies, two single oophero-salpingectomies, two single salpingo-oophorectomies, and two double salpingo-oophorectomies plus four hysterectomies.[57] At the Royal Victoria Hospital in Montreal, twenty hysterectomies, four ovariotomies, fourteen single salpingo-oophorectomies, and twenty-seven double salpingo-oophorectomies were performed in 1895.[58] In 1887 the Victoria General Hospital in Halifax was very conservative in its treatment. Ruby Granger, aged thirty-two, entered on 2 July of that year suffering from an ovarian cyst. It had been tapped two weeks previously and one-and-a-half buckets of liquid removed, but the swelling of her abdomen reoccurred. On 7 July doctors tapped the cyst again and removed thirteen quarts of liquid; on 12 August they removed fourteen quarts and on 17 September, nine quarts. They finally discharged Ruby on 19 September – unimproved.[59] There was no indication that doctors considered an ovariotomy. This conservatism still existed in 1894, for the Medical Board of the Victoria General Hospital in Halifax reported only three ovariotomies and two hysterectomies. However, in 1899 these surgical procedures had increased to twenty-six ovariotomies and three hysterectomies.[60] Ovariotomies had become the most common major surgical procedure performed in the hospital. At the Provincial Royal Jubilee Hospital in Victoria for the year 1895–6 doctors performed twenty-three ovariotomies, the second most common surgical procedures of any kind listed. Only curettage of the endometrium of the uterus occurred more.[61]

Although the number of ovariotomies was increasing, it remained a major operation and physicians stressed that the indicators for such surgery were limited. In his 1868 text Theodore Thomas made it clear that a physician was justified in performing an ovariotomy solely to remove 'solid and polycystic tumors which are curable by no other method, and to extirpate those of unilocular form which have resisted all other procedures.'[62] In 1877 the *Canada Lancet* published an article whose author insisted that ovariotomy should occur only when there was a tumour impairing the life of the patient.[63] The indicators for Battey's procedure seemed equally severe. The purpose of the operation was not the removal of diseased ovaries *per se* but bringing to a halt menstruation – that is, introducing premature menopause. Clearly this was a serious step and physicians were understandably cautious. Battey himself claimed he only removed a woman's ovaries if he could answer affirmatively to three questions: 'Is the condition to be remedied a grave one ... Is it incurable by other and less radical means ... [and] Is it curable by the arrest of ovulation or change of life?'[64] When doctors described the patients they operated on, they emphasized the suffering the women endured before the surgery. Dr Trenholme, in justifying his decision to perform an early double ovariotomy, related that his patient's life had 'become perfectly intolerable, so much so, that death would be joyously welcomed as a relief to her agony.'[65] He also noted he had tried every other form of treatment with no success.[66] Physicians continued to stress the need for caution into the 1880s. Arthur Edis recommended Battey's operation only when life was becoming unbearable for the patient.[67] Dr Gardner, in the *Canada Medical and Surgical Journal*, agreed – Battey's operation was not an alternative to cure but a last resort. However, he sounded a note of unease; he feared, despite such a warning that 'the operation opens a door for wide-spread abuse.'[68] Because Tait's variation was even more extreme than Battey's operation, doctors voiced similar caution regarding it.[69]

Medical indications were not the only criteria for deciding to operate, although they were the main ones. One historian of the 'normal ovariotomy' in the United States has argued that most patients were either middle- and upper-class women or women who had been institutionalized.[70] The literature Canadian physicians were reading and that which they wrote themselves suggested that ovariotomies were also performed on poor women since they had to earn their living and could not afford to undergo some of the lengthy treatment that might have been an alternative to surgery.[71] Dr Trenholme in discussing a St Catharine's, Ont., woman reported that 'as she had received no benefit by treatment, and being a poor girl, who was obliged to work for her living, which she was unable to do, the ovaries and tubes were removed in the usual way on 2nd July 1883. The recovery was rapid and perfect. She has returned to the duties of her station.'[72] Likewise, Dr Adam Wright, professor of obstetrics at the University of Toronto, was concerned about the interference that nervous diseases connected to menstrual disorders caused poor working women.[73] At least two authors of medical texts expressed similar sentiments. Garrigues suggested to students, 'It is necessary to know something about the financial resources of the patient. In the poor recourse to more radical measures is often imperative, while those who possess adequate means may be benefited by a less vigorous but more protracted treatment.'[74] Macnaughton-Jones made a similar point.[75] These physicians were responding to an economic reality both they and their patients had to face.

In addition to the economic circumstances of patients' lives as a determinant of surgery, moral and psychological deviation prodded some physicians to operate. In the United States especially, many physicians justified ovariotomies to control female sexuality.[76] Canadian physicians were more reticent about this and little literature exists on the topic. An 1876 *Canada Lancet* article reported that even Battey was careful to argue that his operation was not a solution for nymphomania. The fate of Isaac Baker Brown had not been forgotten! As noted in chapter 4, William Goodell in the *Canada Lancet* of 1894 reported one of his cases where he removed the ovaries of a woman who feared becoming promiscuous since her sex feeling was so strong before her monthly periods.[77] But such articles were rare. Less rare was discussion of psychological indicators for ovariotomy.

As early as 1878 Goodell advocated the use of Battey's operation for the cure of insanity and in his 1890 text he guardedly noted that 'in carefully selected cases, it will prove the sole means of curing many mental and physical disorders of menstrual life.'[78] But Goodell was not the only major figure to espouse this cure. Lawson Tait had apparently resorted to ovariotomy to provide relief from epilepsy.[79] Dr Trenholme, one of the pioneers in the field of gynaecological surgery in Canada and indeed the Western world, also felt that the ovariotomy had possibilities in the area of mental disorders.[80] In *The Canada Medical Record* of 1884 he reported he had performed Tait's operation on a woman for the cure of mania. The apparent success he had with this case led him to argue that 'there is still much to be done in this line, and I am anxious to see what may be achieved in the way of castration of insane male subjects.'[81] There is no indication that this was ever done. One year later he seemed less optimistic. He discussed a case of a patient in the London, Ontario, Asylum who had had her ovaries removed with no change to her mental condition. She later had her tubes removed and died. This case suggested that great caution had to be taken and that the procedure was not a panacea for insane women. He concluded that removal of ovaries and tubes should be done in cases where there was imperfect sexual development to the degree that 'nervous energy is diverted and expended in fruitless attempts to perfect its growth' and where the sexual system of the woman dominated her mental life. In those two instances, he wistfully queried, 'may we not hope that the cessation of this controlling force will be followed by a calm and such a change in behaviour as the results of castration in the lower animals would lead us to expect.'[82] Those involved in such surgery expressed the need for care and caution, but the fear of many within the profession was that once operations for non-pathological conditions were accepted, abuses could occur. Indeed, even attempting to cure physical abnormalities, they charged, could lead to excessive surgery.

Battey himself was wary and warned that his procedure was being abused, especially in American insane asylums.[83] Similar concerns were expressed in Canadian medical journals. In 1884 the *Canada Medical and Surgical Journal* published an over-view of gynaecology in which one of the physicians quoted thought that the frequency of ovariotomies should be examined.[84] Two years later Adam Wright admitted he had removed normal ovaries in the case of a nervous disorder but excused it by saying the life of his patient was otherwise unbearable. Once he had justified his own surgery, he protested against what he saw as the tendency to perform the procedure 'in all cases of serious dysmenorrhoea, the so-called menstrual epilepsy, hystero-epilepsy, and various forms of mental disease.' By 1890 some physicians were arguing that operations on ovaries had become a craze within the profession and accused gynaecologists of performing needless surgery.[85] For one physician, the fundamental principles had been overturned: 'In general surgery conservation of tissue holds as a basic principle and its great aim is the extirpation of injured with the least cost to healthy substance. But in the pelvis it would almost seem as if a malthusian spectre were at work luring on the not unwilling fingers to the destruction of vital centres.'[86] Compounding the problem of frequency was the conviction among some that ovariotomies (and its multiple variations) were still experimental.[87] In a paper on dysmenorrhoea, read before the Toronto Medical Society, J. Algernon Temple, professor of obstetrics and diseases of women and children at Trinity Medical College, acknowledged that ovaries were being removed in cases of tumours and fibroids. But he was uneasy: 'I have not satisfied myself as to the complete justifiability of this operation. I suppose ... there are some cases demanding it. As yet I have not met with them.'[88] And as William Goodell reminded his colleagues, 'far more women perish from the operation of removing the tubes and ovaries than from their diseases themselves.'[89] Of added concern was the fact that doctors did not really know what the functions of the ovaries were and hence could not accurately anticipate the repercussions of the surgery. Well into the 1890s the medical profession remained confused about the relationship between menstruation and the ovaries.[90] This was evident in an 1898 article in the *Dominion Medical Monthly and Ontario Medical Journal*. The author, who advocated a more conservative approach, quoted one authority that 'it is *probable* that the ovaries, like the liver and thyroid gland, modify the blood circulating through them, and add to the blood some peculiar product of their metabolism.'[91] It is rather disconcerting to think that physicians did not know the function of the organs so many of them were removing.

If some physicians were vague about the function of ovaries, others were equally so with respect to when surgery should occur – despite the very precise indicators that many proposed when the operation first appeared on the scene. Critics did not believe all doctors took enough care in determining the need for surgery.

Innovators such as Lawson Tait may have; unfortunately, their disciples were not equally careful 'in their discrimination of the cases which actually require this radical cure.'[92] But such critics were not necessarily advocates of the women patients. Most who performed the surgery discussed at length the pain and misery their patients had experienced before surgery. Some opponents questioned that – not the physician's belief in the pain but the reality of the pain. One argued that neurotic women, especially, often exaggerated the ovarian pain they felt. For him, pain was not a sufficient indicator for surgery.[93] As James Ross, gynaecologist to the Toronto General Hospital, summarized the situation, 'The axiom seems to have become: "If a woman has indefinite pains or pelvic symptoms that you cannot account for, take out her ovaries."' Certainly the problem of defining the limits of pain a patient should endure was a difficult one and one that was largely subjective. Equally subjective for Dr Hingston of Montreal were symptoms expressed by hysterics – they were simply not trustworthy.[94] In these cases, doctors did not perceive women as adequate judges of their own bodies.

Operating for pathological symptoms was not without its own difficulties. Physicians did not always understand the female body, nor were they always able to distinguish between healthy and diseased states. Dr Gardner of the Montreal General Hospital reported one authority who claimed that the normal ovary, as physicians envisioned it, simply did not exist. Gardner agreed to a certain extent, maintaining that ovariotomies had been abused, 'women ... needlessly mutilated, and that certain conditions of ovaries and tubes thus removed are not pathological, but really physiological.'[95] To offset the criticisms that were developing about the removal of normal ovaries, Battey insisted that the normal ones he had removed were in fact diseased, even though when he removed them he had thought they were normal. It is unclear whether he thought such logic would exonerate him, but when one of the leading experts in the field admitted he could not always tell a healthy ovary from a diseased one it raises the question of who could? Referring to an operation he performed on 3 November 1885, Dr Adam Wright made the predicament of the physician clear. He described a young woman, 'Miss —, one of our most efficient and intelligent nurses,' who since the age of twenty-one had had severe pelvic pains accompanying menstruation. By 1885 they were so bad she 'was confined to bed from ten to twelve days out of every 28.' The pains usually started over the left ovary and at times she was in 'an unconscious or semi-unconscious condition.' According to Wright, 'there was evidently a large element of hysteria in the patient's condition.' Eventually she was unable to work and implored one of his colleagues to remove her tubes and ovaries. Assisting in the operation on 3 November 1885 Dr Wright described what he saw: 'The left ovary was large, and I think, more cystic than it should be, although, I must confess that I am frequently unable to draw the line between a diseased and normal ovary.'[96] Such an admission would have done little to provide the patient with confidence if she had known of it. But it did underline the fact that the critics of ovariotomies had reason to believe that physicians often operated for symptoms that were ill defined and vague.

More disturbing than the fact that many doctors could not distinguish between healthy and diseased ovaries was the willingness of some to remove what they believed to be healthy tissue. In 1884 the *Canada Medical and Surgical Journal* reported one German physician who favoured not only the removal of a diseased ovary but also that of the second as well. He viewed the removal of the remaining normal ovary as preventive medicine since if one ovary was diseased, the second would most likely become so. Three years later the same journal published the views of Montreal's Dr Gardner on the topic. He admitted that there was no known way for a surgeon to determine whether an apparently harmless second ovary would eventually demand a second operation. To make matters worse, he pointed out that not all abnormal ovaries – those either enlarged or cystic – were 'commencing ovarian tumors,' or he did not think they were. He acknowledged that some surgeons automatically removed the second ovary if the woman was nearing or had already reached menopause but that in young women, who still hoped to bear children, he recognized that the decision was more fraught with problems.[97] Even those advocating conservatism in surgery were not immune to the allure of 'preventive surgery.' In an attempt to limit the number of operations that were occurring, William Goodell advised in cases of ovariotomies never taking out a healthy organ (in this case the uterine appendages) unless menopause had already been established or unless there was evidence of a uterine fibroid, uterine disease, or insanity in the patient which made it undesirable for her to have children.[98] Although he was an advocate of conservatism in surgery, Goodell's willingness to remove a healthy ovary simply because the woman had reached menopause suggests he had a very functionalist approach to medicine. If the organ had outlived its usefulness, take it out. Uterine fibroids did not always require surgery and the all-encompassing term 'uterine disease' would not have encouraged caution. As for the removal of healthy appendages because the patient was insane, it suggested less the sphere of medical therapeutics and more the arena of genetic control.

Physicians continued to stress that ovariotomy was a last resort despite the fact or perhaps because of the fact that its incidence continued to increase.[99] In 1885 the *Canadian Practitioner* reprinted an article which urged doctors to be patient in treating uterine fibroids and not to assume that an ovariotomy was in order, estimating that only in 10 per cent of cases was surgery warranted. James Ross added his voice, arguing that many women suffered from problems connected with the ovaries and tubes without damaging their health and that the fatality among such women was overrated. As we have already seen, many women had so-called abnormalities because of childbirth injuries and, while many may have required surgery, certainly the majority did not. Advocates of conservatism advised doctors to remove only the diseased ovary and leave as much healthy tissue behind as possible.[100] Preferably, they should try non-surgical treatments first. Critics pointed out the need for physicians to use restraint and not subject women to possibly life-threatening surgery until they had tried other treatments and failed. As the article in the 1885 *Canadian Practitioner* urged: 'Patient waiting, palliation, and temporizing are required; the result is more slowly attained, a brilliant successful laparotomy [for the tumour only] is not proclaimed in societies and journals, but the ultimate condition of the patient is every way preferable, for she has undergone no mutilation.'[101] Certainly many Canadian physicians seemed to agree. Wright, who pioneered the operation in Toronto, stressed that non-surgical treatment should always be tried first. Even Lapthorn Smith of Bishop's College believed that the more rational approach to re-place the pessary was not operative procedures but an attempt to rebuild the health of the system and the abdominal and pelvic muscles by less radical means.[102]

Despite all the caution, there was still a sense that removal of ovaries was occurring too frequently. In the 1899 *Dominion Medical Monthly* Dr G.R. Cruickshank from Windsor, Ont., referred to the aggressive approach of surgeons and gynaecologists. As a general practitioner 'whose patients are pretty comfortable without such radical measures,' he could only 'conclude that the uterus is made the scape-goat for the shortcomings of all other organs.'[103] And at least two articles could not help but point out that the male reproductive/sexual system did not come in for such atten-tion or for such radical treatment. The authors wondered if phy-sicians were more prone to operate on their women patients because of the challenge the complexity of the female repro-ductive/sexual system presented. As one delicately phrased it, if the older term 'testes muliebus' was still used instead of 'ovaries,' then more conservative treatment would probably follow since 'the conservatism with which the male organs are treated would have been reflected upon the gynaecological field.'[104] Dr James Russell of Hamilton was even more blunt: 'Happy, thrice happy, should man be because of the simplicity of his genital outfit and its meager attraction for the operation of surgical science. Had nature decreed him to wear his genitals within the abdominal cavity, he too, might have been compelled to suffer surgical martyrdom.'[105]

Underlying the concern of many critics of ovariotomies was the effect of the operation on the patient. Just as a vaginal examination differed from an examination of the throat, so too did the removal of ovaries differ from removal of the tonsils. E.H. Trenholme re-

ferred to the procedure as spaying.[106] Others referred to it as
castration.[107] Dr MacCallum of McGill in his lecture 'On Women's
Medical Problems' made it very clear that the ovaries were 'the
analagies [sic] of the testes in the male and the essential organs
of generation in the female.'[108] If both ovaries were removed, the
woman could no longer bear children; if only one was removed
her chances of bearing children decreased. For some, such interference was a moral issue and for others, such as Montreal's
Dr Hingston, it 'was a crime against society, and ... interfered with
the interests of the state.'[109] William Gardner, describing his own
experience in surgery, acknowledged the difficulty he had in
removing both ovaries when the patient was young.[110] In the judgment of another physician, 'an unmarried girl who has her ovaries
removed has no right to enter marriage.'[111] Marriage was for the
procreation of children and without the ability to bear children,
sexual intercourse, even within the marriage relationship, made
the woman a prostitute. Such harsh views reflected the widespread belief that female sexuality existed not for the woman's
pleasure but for the perpetuation of the species. Without the
ability to bear children, some felt that a woman was not quite
whole, that she was less of a woman. In a rather extreme analogy
Goodell made it clear that he and most physicians and 'all laymen'
viewed women deprived of their ovaries as 'unsexed.' 'No women
would marry a eunuch, and few men would wed a woman deprived of her ovaries.'[112] Ignoring the fact that physiologically a
eunuch and a woman without her ovaries are hardly equivalent
states, what such a perspective underlines is the utilitarian view
many had of women. Women existed to bear children; without
that ability there was no reason for them to marry or for anyone
to want to marry them.

Patient records suggest that physicians acted on the above beliefs. Susan McIntyre, forty-five and single, came to the Victoria
General Hospital from Cape Breton in June 1896 suffering from
an ovarian cyst. Although a cyst was found only on her right ovary,
both ovaries were removed, perhaps because she was single and
approaching menopause. Mrs Maly, aged fifty-nine and a widow,
was admitted to the Victoria General Hospital on 11 September

1900. She had an ovarian cyst on the left ovary and it and the ovary were removed. The right ovary was found to be cystic and en-larged and it too was removed. It is possible that the physician in charge did not see the removal of both ovaries as a problem because Mrs Maly was a widow and already past menopause; her childbearing years had already ended.[113] This is given credence by the experience of Miss Beth Crowell, aged seventeen, who entered the hospital six days later. She was suffering from en-dometritis, erosion of the cervix, antiflexion, and a slight enlarge-ment of the fundus. When operated on, doctors discovered that the right ovary was cystic and they removed it. The left ovary was a bit cystic as well but, unlike the cases of Susan McIntyre and Mrs Maly, doctors only punctured and stitched it. The physician in charge had left her with the possibility of having children. One cannot help but draw the conclusion this was because Beth Crow-ell was young and approaching her childbearing years.[114]

Those advocating ovariotomies could not deny that the surgery interfered with childbearing. Beyond this, however, they main-tained there were no lasting ill effects. Battey argued that women undergoing a successful ovariotomy experienced improved health and had their femininity or sexuality unimpaired.[115] In his 1890 text *Lessons in Gynaecology*, Goodell agreed that removal of ovaries did not unduly affect women.[116] By 1894, however, he was not so sure. In an article published in the *Canadian Practitioner* he admitted that 'the number of cases of insanity following oöphorectomy is large.' He also acknowledged that by bringing about artificial menopause, which is what a double ovariotomy did, the effects of menopause were extended. The latter would not appear to be serious except when the symptoms of menopause are remembered – hot flashes, perspirations, skin tingling, gastro-intestinal disturbances, and nerves.[117] But although Goodell con-ceded that the operation directed women to 'old-maidhood,' they were not to worry. After all, 'their breasts do not flatten or wither up; they do not become obese; abnormal growths of hair do not appear on the face or on the body,' and their voice does not deepen.[118] Whether any woman would be comforted by this rather backhanded assurance is questionable, especially when other physicians were not as sure.

Theodore Thomas advised the readers of his text that, when the ovaries were removed, a woman became more masculine – her breasts flattened, the voice and her features became more masculine, and a beard appeared on her face.[119] When he examined a woman with no vagina or uterus, Dr Ogden, lecturer on midwifery and the diseases of women at the Toronto School of Medicine, speculated on the existence of ovaries: 'From the well developed breasts, the state of the mons veneris, and the occasional experience of strong sexual desires, combined with the usual feminine voice and instincts, one would be inclined to think the ovaries were present *somewhere*.'[120] And even Goodell, who argued there were no real effects on women (other than premature menopause), when faced with 'a splendid specimen of female humanity ... shrank from mutilating' her.[121] The ovaries were what made women female.[122] At least one practitioner went further. In 1890 Dr Ross of Toronto argued that removal of the ovaries interfered with women's 'intellectual capabilities and diminishes their intellectual calibre.' This was serious, not just for the woman concerned but for her husband who no longer had a true companion.[123] In an attempt to settle the question of whether removal of the ovaries did affect the physical aspects of women, Dr Charles Penrose argued a middle ground. For those women who had reached adulthood with their secondary sex characteristics intact, removal of the ovaries would have little impact. For young women not fully developed, removal of the ovaries would prevent that development, although it would not necessarily make them masculine.[124]

More was at stake, however, than the physical appearance of women and their ability to bear children. The impact of ovariotomies on a woman's sexual feelings was an issue. We have already seen that physicians disagreed over how strong women's sexual feelings were. Because some referred to the removal of ovaries as castration, there was the suggestion that ovariotomies unsexed women. Understandably, Battey denied this outcome.[125] So did William Goodell. He pointed out in clinical terms that 'the seat of sexuality in woman has long been sought for, but in vain. The clitoris has been amputated, the nymphae have been excised, and the ovaries removed, yet the sexual desire has remained unquenched.' Then switching to a more poetic bent: 'The seat has not been found, because sexuality is not a member or an organ, but a sense – a sense dependent on the sexual apparatus, not for its being, but merely for its fruition.' Proof of this for him was that women continued to experience sexual desire after menopause (after the ovaries ceased to function) and that some women had been known to masturbate before puberty (before the ovaries began to function).[126] Nevertheless, Goodell was not consistent about this belief and associated the operation with mental disturbances not only because of the shock of the operation but as a result of the emotional environment surrounding the woman – that is, women who had had their ovaries removed brooded about being unsexed. And women had every right to worry. Even Goodell came to believe that because removal of the ovaries brought about menopause, it lessened and eventually deadened woman's sexual instinct. Of course this was not all that significant since, without the ability to bear children, what was the point of women having any sexual feelings? But he did acknowledge that for young married women this could present a problem and lead to domestic unhappiness. In addition, some women experienced pain during intercourse as a result of castration. He told of one woman who did but 'with true womanly devotion she has studiously kept her husband in ignorance of these facts.'[127] His admiration for this woman was clear, but less clear was any sympathy for the fact she was not receiving any sexual satisfaction. For Goodell, the removal of sexuality was not the problem, but the repercussions of it on the marital relationship. The author of one article reprinted in the *Canadian Practitioner* was quite perturbed by sexuality becoming an issue. The question of whether ovariotomies decreased a woman's ability to experience sexual feelings distorted woman's true character. She was not a creature of lust but of procreation. The issue of sexuality simply 'appeal[ed] to the lower elements of human nature.'[128] Other doctors, while believing that interference in sexual feeling was a possible consequence of ovariotomies, did not see it as a problem. As noted in chapter 4, James Ross was convinced that 50 per cent of women did not have sexual feelings anyway.[129] In his text, Penrose was perhaps more honest than most when he admitted he did not know what the consequences of the operation were. In some cases sexual desire was destroyed while in others it increased by restoring a woman to health.[130] Such a view did not provide much assurance for those women who underwent the procedure.

Concern for patients was not the only factor that generated the debate over ovariotomies. Antagonism towards gynaecological surgeons played a role. In a letter to the editor of the *Canada Medical and Surgical Journal* signed 'A General Surgeon,' the author accused gynaecologists of taking over what was once the domain of the general surgeon and of trying to establish a place for themselves within the field of medical surgery. Trying to regain the status general surgeons once had, he reminded his readers they had been the first ovariotomists and hinted there was no reason why they should not remain the only ones. If gynaecologists were left to perform surgery, he envisioned a truly terrible fate: 'I see a vision in the future of the special organs belonging to the male in the ruthless and sacrilegious hands of the ubiquitous gynaecologist, who is continually, like Alexander, seeking new worlds to conquer. Then, alas! will come the deluge, for the testicles will be much easier to remove than ovaries.' The editor of the journal was not worried. He believed that abdominal surgery, as a new specialty, signified progress. He certainly did not have a high opinion of those who practised general surgery, for he took up the argument of the testicles coming under the knife and, instead of getting indignant about this prospect, rather dismissingly wrote that removal of the testicles could safely be left to the general surgeon since the procedure was so simple. Rejecting the point that the first ovariotomists were generalists (and therefore should remain so), he ended his rebuttal by reminding the 'general surgeon' that 'all great men were babies once.'[131] His voice was not alone in defence of specialization within surgery. Six years later the editor of the *Canada Medical Record* pointed out that surgery necessitated training and that the women who were being needlessly mutilated were not those operated on by gynaecological surgeons but by physicians who had not had extensive instruction and who operated with little understanding of what the necessary indicators for surgery were.[132]

Several themes are evident in the original exchange. One is the hostility of the general surgeon towards the gynaecologist becoming involved in surgery. In this case, it is not the surgery *per se* that offends him but the competition. Second is his perception that gynaecological surgeons operate too frequently. The worst prospect that the general surgeon could think of was not the trauma that surgical mutilation caused women but that the gynaecologists might focus their attention on men. Clearly as a male he identified more with men than with women and could appreciate an assault on male sexuality whereas he had difficulty doing the same with respect to female sexuality. The third theme was raised by the editor. He believed in the need for specialization and that only specialists could perform the intricate surgery necessary in abdominal cases. If the general surgeon had hostility towards such specialists, specialists in turn had contempt for the abilities of general surgeons. The medical profession was in no way unified.

James Russell of Hamilton did not see the problem as being specialization or even surgery. He viewed extremes in medicine as the norm. Looking back on the century in 1898, he noted that before antiseptic surgery 'the uterus was mercilessly treated to all sorts of local applications, including dilation, curettement, cauterization, douches, and the application of pessaries of all shapes and sizes.' With the introduction of asepsis, nothing had really changed. One form of treatment had simply replaced another. Now 'the abdominal cavity has become the happy hunting ground of the surgeon, and the very impunity with which it may be eviscerated or mutilated is a strong incentive to the specialist in search of surgical glorification to ply his art.'[133] While not denying the lure of personal reputation, Dr Cruikshank of Windsor noted that the surgeons were not alone in promoting surgery. The public was enthralled by it and the patients themselves demanded it. Still he felt that physicians should be able to resist such pressure and he had only contempt for those 'pseudo-gynaecologists' whom he placed 'in three classes: The fellows who repair lacerations, those who take out ovaries and those who take out everything.'[134] For physicians on both sides of the controversy, access to patients was a major issue. Gynaecological surgeons expressed concern for patient safety in an effort to assume exclusive control over surgery. General surgeons and others who wanted to moderate intervention made a similar argument. Concern for the patient, however, had its limitations. Constrained by the gender roles of the time, physicians rarely viewed or treated women as other than beings whose sole purpose was to bear children.

The history of ovariotomies in the nineteenth century demonstrates what occurs with new medical procedures. Those who introduce a technique claim much for it. Others, attracted by the claims of success and the excitement surrounding it, adopt it but are not always able to replicate the success rate of the originators. They also find there are limitations to the procedure and, in some cases, the cure is worse than the disease. A reaction against the procedure takes place and caution and moderation are urged. But in the case of ovariotomies even more than this was occurring. We cannot overlook the fact that it was an operation performed on women and that the indicators for it were such as to encourage surgery. Many physicians were concerned about this trend and about the physical consequences for their patients. Even more, they worried about the impact an ovariotomy would have on a woman's social role. Similarly their anxiety with respect to the operation's impact on female sexuality seldom addressed the right of the woman to individual pleasure but her marital/procreative function. More disturbing was the use of the operation for the cure of mental illness.[135] That women were more prone to such disorders was conventional wisdom in the late nineteenth century. Physicians and laymen alike saw women as more emotional than men, more prone to nervous disorders, and in need of control. Increasingly the medical profession became involved in providing that control.

Chapter Ten

Women and Mental Health

'Every physician who has been in practice for any length of time must have come across cases of bed-ridden women, whose lives were being hopelessly wasted, and who were useless members of society; and such physicians must, as I have, felt humiliated by the sight, and more or less disappointed with medicine as a science and an art.'[1] With these words Dr A. Halliday of Stewiacke, NS, expressed the frustration that many physicians experienced when faced with patients suffering from no obvious physical ailments but from what was, in their opinion, more nebulous nervous complaints. And they feared the problem was increasing as the pressures and challenges of modern society took their toll.[2] As already noted, doctors often disapproved of the emphasis the educational system placed on intellectual development to the detriment of physical health. This was of special concern with respect to young women entering puberty. Similarly, the emphasis that modern life placed on intellectual pursuits disturbed the natural equilibrium between mind and body in adults. The signs were there for everyone to see – the increase in men and women suffering from all types of nervous ailments but, particularly in the latter part of the century, from neurasthenia. Considered to be a disease of modern life, and at one time referred to as the American disease, neurasthenia was characterized by a lack of energy and moderate depression. Everyone was at risk – the young, the old, the rich, the poor, men and women – but doctors felt especially vulnerable were those merchants and society ladies

'whose education and mode of life have given too great a preponderance to the functions of the nervous system.'[3] Man's nervousness was a response to his importance in world affairs and
woman's to her emergence from the home and participation in
wider society.[4]

Not all physicians considered 'progress' to be the culprit. In
keeping with their training, some argued that nervous disorders
were really the result of physical problems. The *Canada Medical
Record* in 1875 reported that weakness of the arteries could lead
to nervous complaints, whereas a review of George M. Beard's
Sexual Neurasthenia suggested that in some cases they were the
consequence of disorders of the genitals. The 1891–2 Annual Report of the Montreal General Hospital listed neurasthenia among
its gynaecological diseases. The records of the Victoria General
Hospital for the year 1893–4 indicate that social factors, other than
the fast pace of modern life, could result in nervous complaints.
Mrs Caroline Furness from New Glasgow entered the hospital on
19 February 1894. She was forty-one years of age, with four children
between the ages of ten and fifteen and had been a widow for
nine years. She had worked hard to support her children but two
years previously her appetite failed, and she became sleepless,
nervous, irritable, and despondent. Her own doctor made light
of her troubles and so she had come to the hospital in Halifax.
Meeting with some sympathy, she was given medication and,
retroflexion of the uterus being discerned, had a pessary inserted.
She was also given several massages. Diagnosed as neurasthenic,
the doctors treated her with kindness and took her symptoms
seriously, which, considering her experience with her own physician, she must have appreciated.[5] What her history indicates is
a woman who was suffering from 'nerves,' most likely caused by
the exhaustion of constantly struggling to make ends meet in order
to keep her family together. Working men, too, experienced similar pressure but, despite doctors' recognition of this, the medical
literature stressed the greater susceptibility of women. An article
published in the *Sanitary Journal* in February 1876 referred to
the numerous women who took 'nervines and opiates ... to quiet
their nerves.' The *Canada Medical Record* in 1879 quoted William

Goodell as asserting that 'every physician' was interested in the problem because '*nerve tire* is so common a disorder in our over-taught, over-sensitive, and over-sedentary women.' An item in the 1897 *Montreal Medical Journal* focused on the female reproductive function as the primary factor:

When we remember the great disturbances which mark the advent and departure of the reproductive era of a woman's life; the profound changes taking place during ovulation, menstruation, pregnancy, labour, and lactation; the subtle and complex activities of her psychical life in her various diastaltic functions; it is not remarkable that neuroses should manifest themselves, particularly in relation to her reproductive mechanism. That they are increasing, *pari passu* with the advance in our higher civilization, cannot be denied. Among the poor, the inducing factors were overwork, overworry, ill-regulated and poor nutrition; among the well-to-do, educational strain, over-indulgence, the stress of life, and emotional excitement.[6]

Once again, women because they were female were at risk. This was particularly true in the case of hysteria and to a lesser extent insanity. The former makes sense from the perspective of the nineteenth century since most doctors viewed hysteria as a female disease. But insanity was an illness experienced by both sexes and yet it, too, was seen through the lens of gender.

Today hysteria is defined as 'a form of psychoneurosis in which the individual converts anxiety created by emotional conflict into physical symptoms that have no organic basis ... The term hysteria is also used to describe a state of tension or excitement in which there is a temporary loss of control over the emotions.'[7] The late nineteenth-century medical profession would not have accepted the first aspect of this definition, but it certainly did the latter. Lack of control over the emotions was the predominant characteristic of hysteria. Historians agree that most individuals deemed hysterical in the late nineteenth century were women, although they disagree why this was the case. Feminist historians have argued that hysteria was a psychological response to the limitations placed on women's lives. The family was changing and so was women's place in it. Added to this pressure was the lack of alternative roles for women outside the home. Hysteria in such a context became an option or tactic offering 'particular women ... a chance to redefine or restructure their place within the family.'[8] As Elaine Showalter has postulated, hysteria was 'an unconscious form of feminist protest, the counterpart of the attack on patriarchal values carried out by the women's movement.'[9] If so, it was a response of the powerless. Hysterics could manipulate their families and assert their own needs only in a passively aggressive way.[10] While not denying the impact of hysterics' actions, Edward Shorter disagrees with the psychological interpretation of its origins. He maintains that hysteria was not a psychological response to women's reality but a mistaken diagnosis of a physical ailment. He suggests that much of the hysteria of the nineteenth century was the result of uterine infection. Because it was difficult to diagnose and because many of the symptoms were similar to those of hysteria, doctors tended to confuse the two. Hysterical women, then, were suffering from a physical ailment.[11] The problem with both these interpretations is that neither can be easily substantiated. Historians arguing that hysteria was a psychological response have little proof to offer. The motivation of such women hysterics was subconscious and virtually impossible for historians to probe. Shorter's hypothesis is not much better, for he does not offer concrete evidence to prove misdiagnosis. But if cause is difficult to pinpoint, medical attitudes about and treatment of hysteria are not. Because hysteria was a condition with which few Canadians could cope, many turned to the medical profession for assistance and advice. What advice they received confirmed them in their predisposition to view women as dominated by their bodies more so than men.

It is difficult to know how prevalent hysteria was. Those who sought aid most likely preferred private consultations with physicians and many of these records have been lost. Those not able to afford private physicians would have gone to hospitals and, fortunately, many of their records remain.[12] In 1857 the Halifax Visiting Dispensary treated twenty cases of hysteria, in 1868, twenty-four cases, in 1874, eight cases, and in 1878, seventeen cases. Between 1882 and 1888 the Provincial and City Hospital in Halifax saw eleven cases. Over the next ten years there was a total of fifty-three cases of hysteria and ninety-nine cases of neurasthenia. The Montreal General Hospital in 1865 reported eight cases of hysteria, five of whom died; between 1871 and 1881 it listed 137 cases.[13] What these records indicate is that hysteria was common enough to be of general interest to physicians and that it was one of the most frequently reported nervous disorders. Judging from the literature that Canadian physicians were writing and reading, they *perceived* hysteria to be an ailment that all physicians would sooner or later encounter in their practices and consequently worthy of discussion. What they also indicate is that most of the patients were women. The nomenclature itself suggests the long tradition of associating hysteria with women, for the Greek root word means womb or uterus. Although a few physicians acknowledged that hysteria could occur in males[14] and, indeed, one recommended treatment for it was compression of the testicles,[15] the consensus was that hysteria was essentially a female disorder. As the *Canada Lancet* of 1880 noted, physicians, when faced with male hysteria, tended to call it by a different name, 'there being an unwillingness to apply the term hysteria to males.'[16] William Goodell even went so far as to claim that all women were liable to hysteria.[17] The willingness of physicians to associate hysteria with women was linked to its symptoms – lack of control over the emotions. According to nineteenth-century perceptions, women were more emotional than men and thus were more likely than men to succumb to hysterical fits. Hysteria in women was simply a normal condition that had become extreme. In men, such a condition went against the very nature of being male and would have been viewed as much more serious and in fact deviant.

Despite the symptoms of hysteria being a parody of female characteristics, some of the perceived causes were attributable to both sexes. Dr Arthur Edis, in his *Diseases of Women*, blamed poor childhood training, especially among the affluent, 'in whom emotionalism is intensified at the expense of reason and self-control by injudicious training in childhood, and the subsequent pampering that ill fits them for the trials of life.'[18] Although Edis specifically had the education of women in mind, that of men was almost as problematic in that it overworked the brain and caused mental fatigue. Similarly heredity, indulgence, overwork, financial worries, and domestic difficulties were all factors that were not necessarily gender based.[19] But most doctors did not see these as central. The primary cause of hysteria was the physical or biological reality of being female. The consensus was that puberty triggered its onset.[20] Perhaps no one was more clear about this than Richard Maurice Bucke, superintendent of the insane asylum in London, Ont. Viewing youth as a period of stress for both men and women, he believed that each exhibited the stress differently. For men 'it is the age of bad poetry' but for women it was the age 'of hysteria.'[21] Puberty brought the reproductive/ sexual system of women into play and it was this system that differentiated the male from the female. If hysteria occurred largely in women, it followed it was rooted in those areas where her body differed from man's. In his 1848 text Thomas Watson noted that hysteria only occurred in women during the years of menstruation, particularly when they experienced some menstrual dysfunction.[22] Two decades later Henry Guernsey in his homeopathic text agreed. Between puberty and menopause women were at risk because of their exposure to the excitement of sexual intercourse and childbirth. Central in causation were the ovaries. As Guernsey made clear. 'The uterus ... has usually been considered the seat of Hysteria ... but the *ovaries, as head-centre of the sexual system*, must now be regarded as the real ... fountain head of all hysterical affections.'[23] That doctors assumed women were more susceptible to hysteria than men is not surprising when the medical perception of women's bodies is remembered. Physicians continually evaluated health using the male norm. As R. Pierce phrased it, woman was 'man modified.'[24] The physiological differences between men and women affected the emotions and determined that the two sexes would remain separate – in the case of hysteria in a pathological way. This remained the belief throughout the century.[25]

While there was no way for women to avoid a predisposition to hysteria since it was centred in the physiological make-up of being female, certain conditions did exacerbate it. As seen, Guernsey believed that sexual excitement and childbirth could trigger it. Arthur Edis argued that 'the wives of incompetent husbands, and barren women, as well as widows and old maids, are frequent victims of the hysteric malady.'[26] Henry Lyman, Pye Henry Chavasse, and Hamilton Ayers in their popular health manuals agreed that childless women were especially susceptible. According to Lyman, by denying 'the natural culmination of a woman's life' – maternity – such women had 'no other object in life which may divert their attention.'[27] Just as a woman's body deprived of the experience of pregnancy might rebel and form tumours, it could just as easily divert its unused energy into hysterical fits. The lesson to be drawn was clear – women should have children. Lyman's disapproval of these hysterics was matched by the Trinity College Medical School lecture notes taken by Archibald Mc-Curdy. They reminded him that 'young, vigorous girls – actively employed seldom or never have this disease; but the indolent and luxurious are prone to it.'[28] Guernsey pointed out that 'egotism, especially in married females as opposed to their husbands, is the most prominent and the only constant moral symptom of Hysteria.' Their illness dominated their households, placed their needs and demands uppermost, and destroyed 'domestic peace, harmony and affection.'[29] Such 'self-love' denied the natural role of women and went against the norms of proper behaviour. Both were in themselves evidence of deviancy and 'disease' and accounted for the underlying tone of hostility and frustration when hysteria was discussed. The characteristics of the hysteric were at odds with the ideal concept of womanhood.

Equally annoying for physicians was that the symptoms of hysteria made the ailment difficult to diagnose, for they took forms that could be associated with a host of other diseases.[30] At times, doctors could take advantage of this uncertainty by using hysteria as a diagnosis to cover those instances when a patient complained of discomfort, for which doctors could find no cause. In 1882 two women entered the Montreal General Hospital complaining of pains either in the head or in the back. When doctors failed to locate the origin of the pains, they entered a diagnosis of hysteria.[31] On 31 May 1894 Bernice McKenzie entered the Victoria General Hospital. Single and twenty-nine years of age, she complained of headaches, a pain in her back, and general weakness. Her case history revealed she had been born in Annapolis and had always lived there. Never strong, she had tubercular glands when young that had suppurated and caused her trouble for several years. She had also had an eye infection. Menstruating at fourteen, she had suffered from dysmenorrhoea; when a doctor informed her four years before that her os was constricted, she had been treated with little effect. Her menstrual flow was now more profuse but accompanied by pain and the passing of clots. She also suffered from a leuchorrhoeal discharge. Seven days after entering the hospital doctors applied the 'battery' to her, as they did again the next day. On 9 June she developed a headache and experienced dizziness. On 22 June she had the same pain in her back that had brought her to the hospital. Perhaps frustrated by the lack of progress in the case, the doctors diagnosed her as hysterical and discharged her on 26 June.[32]

The ability of hysteria to take on so many different symptoms led some physicians to consider it a 'feigned' disease. Lyman was willing to admit that in some cases physical 'derangement of the sexual organs' was the origin, but he felt that in many cases 'hysteria is a purely mental disorder, the result of a lack of balance between the emotions and the will.'[33] Others agreed. Susan Eckert entered the Victoria General Hospital in May 1885 suffering from leucorrhoea, retroflexion of the uterus, and a dragging feeling about the pelvis. When treatment was not successful, her doctor concluded that the symptoms in her legs and back were hysterical and decided to put a plaster of Paris jacket on her for 'moral effect' and to apply electricity.[34] So common was the belief that hysteria was somehow a counterfeit disease that A Manual of Nursing, published in 1898, had to emphasize the point it was 'a real malady' and 'not employed to denote mere simulation of symptoms, or for imposture, as it frequently is by the public.'[35] As revealed by the actual cases in the Montreal and Halifax hospitals and the unwillingness of some to accept hysteria's reality, hysteria was an ailment doctors had difficulty treating. This could only add to their frustration, especially since physicians treated most patients in their own homes where their inability to bring about a cure would be all too evident. Postulating that hysteria was feigned placed the blame for lack of cure on the patient and absolved the doctor of any responsibility. Of course, this approach would impress neither the patient nor her family who had to deal with the reality of her symptoms whether there was a reality to her disease or not. Perhaps for this reason, doctors seemed willing to try almost anything in their attempts to bring about a satisfactory resolution.

Considering the reluctance of some to accept hysteria as a disease, it is not surprising that doctors resorted to the use of placebos in dealing with it. In the 1880 *Canada Lancet*, William Goodell reported: 'I am in the habit of regarding a hysterical woman in the same light as a skittish, unmanageable horse; and just as I catch the one by means of a handful of oats, so I do not hesitate to entrap the woman by much the same means. I remember one instance, in which I assured the husband of a hysterical woman that the drug I was giving – assafoetida – had a very powerful odor and had come from a very great distance. I have no doubt that he thought I had sent all the way to the Orient after it, and gave his wife to understand accordingly; certainly my words acted like a charm in that case.'[36] His lack of sympathy with his patient is indicated by comparing her to a horse, while his use of the word 'entrap' suggests his inability to see hysteria as a disease that was real. Hysteria presented a challenge he had to outwit, not cure. Placebos were not the only form of treatment attempted. Since hysteria's symptoms were so general and varied, treatments were as well. Indeed, they seemed to follow the general development of medical therapeutics more than any change in perception of the complaint. Early in the century, William Buchan advocated bleeding and blistering hysterical patients as well as giving them opium.[37] Perkins Bull in his history of Canadian medicine also mentions the use of blistering for hysteria. He notes: 'Among the substances used to produce a blistering effect were turpentine, mustard, cayenne pepper, strong vinegar, liquid ammonia, and cantharides. More often ... especially at times of emergency, boiling water was used, a cloth soaked in cold water serving to limit the area of flesh on which the torture was inflicted.'[38] Such therapy was in keeping with the heroic tradition of medicine at the time. Eschewing the medicinal approach, others advised more botanic remedies. The 1839 *Family Physician and the Farmer's Companion* suggested a concoction of 'hysop, skunk cabbage root, and Solomen seal root' made into a strong syrup to which ginger was added. The patient was to take this every morning and before she went to bed.[39] At mid-century one manual described a wide choice of treatment: a dash of cold water on the face; burned feathers to the nostrils; ether to the temples; or a turpentine injection.[40] More novel was Eugene Becklard's recommendation of marriage. In addition to curing hysteria, marriage apparently cured nymphomania, uterine epilepsy, uterine cholics, virgin convulsions, and bad complextion.[41] Normal behaviour (marriage) cured abnormal behaviour (disease). After mid-century, treatments became more specific. In his medical casebook Hugh Mackay noted that the use of monobromide of camphor had been recommended in the *Canada Lancet* of 1873.[42]

Since so many physicians believed that nervous disorders in women were connected to the reproductive/sexual system, some tried therapy that focused on that system. This occurred after mid-century, when the morality of a male physician's treating a woman's sexual appendages had become more accepted. William Goodell carefully explained that when faced with a hysterical young girl he put 'at once firm pressure in the neighbourhood of both ovaries,' noting this was most likely to quiet the patient immediately. He also advised giving her an emetic, arguing that while it was working the woman had no chance to be anything else but nauseated. The third method suggested was to place ice on the nape of the neck.[43] The latter would produce a shock to the woman's nervous system and bring about a cessation of the attack. Similarly, at the Montreal General Hospital when one patient experienced a hysterical fit, doctors applied a cold douche.[44] Fortunately for their patients, Canadian physicians seldom went as far as others in their quest for a cure. As we have already noted, in 1867 the London Obstetrical Society reported that Isaac Baker

Brown had used clitoridectomy in cases of hysteria.[45] The *Canada Lancet* observed in 1883 that another treatment was cauterization of the clitoris.[46] In the *Canada and Medical Journal* of 1881 a review of treatment elsewhere put forward the efficacy of female castration as a cure.[47] However, there is little evidence that doctors in Canada favoured any of these treatments for hysteria.[48]

Another approach advocated by American physicians and noted in the Canadian medical press was that of Weir Mitchell, a Philadelphia practitioner. The *Canada Lancet* published an article in 1883 endorsing Mitchell's treatment, which consisted of removing the patient from her home and providing a rest cure for her. Massage and electricity therapy to produce muscular waste was used in addition to excessive feeding, so that the entire nervous system could be nourished.[49] Some of the texts that Canadian physicians were reading also recommended this approach.[50] Practicalities, however, probably prevented its becoming popular in Canada. Unlike Americans, Canadians did not have available to them the same variety of health spas that were necessary if the patient were to be treated away from her home. Such spas were expensive and this, too, may have prevented many physicians from advising such therapy for their patients. American feminist historians would view this as a positive situation, for they have argued that Mitchell's treatment exemplified the control doctors exerted over their female patients. The focus of therapy was removing the patient from all other influence but that of the physician and its goal was to make the patient a passive recipient of medical care.[51] There is no denying that physicians exerted control over their patients in an attempt to help them. George Napheys, in *The Physical Life of Woman*, described a case in which a group of young girls, who were exhibiting hysterical symptoms, were cured by having a doctor threaten to burn them.[52] That the physician had enough authority to convince the girls he could and would do such a thing is in itself disturbing but indicates the influence physicians were able to exert in many of their doctor-patient relationships. Dr Halliday stressed how important it was to gain the patient's confidence and to convince her that medical science could cure her. 'In such cases the physician has to assume the role of instructor, and has to advise with regard to her moral as well as her physical constitution.' This he claimed he had been able to do with a Miss C, who for thirty years had remained in bed. With firm assurances that Halliday could enable her to walk again, she placed herself in his hands and underwent the specific therapy he prescribed.[53] Such influence or control was part of the 'moral-pastoral' responsibility physicians were assuming throughout the century and which by the end of the century they had largely achieved.[54]

The perception and treatment of hysteria in women followed that of other diseases. Physicians connected the illness to the reproductive system and weaknesses within that system. In such cases physicians were sympathetic to the patient, for there was a concrete cause of the hysterical manifestation they could understand and treat. About hysteria not caused by obvious physical abnormalities, physicians were more ambivalent. But in whatever guise, hysteria was a foreign ailment because it was a female ailment. The domination of woman by her reproductive system was a given. If disordered, there was no telling where it would end. Henry Howard, medical attendant to the Longue Point Lunatic Asylum, thought he knew: 'Some disordered state of the digestive or uterine organs, producing irritation of some part of the ganglionic system, causes hysteria, which is followed by irritation of the cerebellum, producing moral insanity, which develops itself in strong sexual desire, in time this irritation spreads to the cells of the cerebrum, and the consequence is violent mania.'[55]

The superintendent of the lunatic asylum in Saint John would have agreed. Between 1875 and 1900 thirty-four cases of hysterical mania had been admitted, thirty-one of them manifested in women.[56] That hysteria could lead to mania or worse was a frightening thought. It certainly was for the family of Susan Blandford. Blandford was a dressmaker, single, and twenty-seven years old when first admitted to the Toronto Asylum in April 1888. According to her physician, he had attended her four years previously for a nervous system disorder which he described as an excited form of hysteria consisting of insomnia, restlessness, and a disposition to sit up all night. He had seen her since that time and had watched her condition deteriorate to the point where she refused to speak, was intolerably dirty, and continually paced, wringing her hands and at times laughing to herself. According to her brother, she had been an intelligent 'girl' until she took to late hours and excessive novel reading. From this developed hysteria and a delusion that a young man was in love with her. Her brother described her as generally quiet but that fits of anger occurred frequently during which she used 'filthy' language. She wore nothing but a wrapper, boots, and stockings all year round and even slept in the wrapper she had not removed for over eight months. He added that she refused to eat with her family or go outside, and that she never washed any part of herself except her hands and these only occasionally. Her father stated he was afraid to be alone with her since she threatened him and had already 'knocked him down and stomped on him.' By the time Susan entered the asylum she was no longer suffering from hysteria but was classified as the victim of dementia.[57]

Nineteenth-century Canadians were very aware of people like Susan Blandford and how little could be done for them. No more serious mental disorder than insanity existed. Whereas those suffering from general nervousness and neurasthenia could still function in society and hysterics could live at home with few restrictions on their actions, the insane faced physical confinement more often than not behind the walls of an asylum. Superintendents of these asylums continually discussed what they felt were the most important causes of insanity. In 1865 Joseph Workman, superintendent of the Toronto Asylum from 1854 to 1875, argued that the real causes of insanity – that is, those that were more than symptoms – were the puerperal state, injuries to the head, masturbation, exposure to cold, and exposure to the sun.[58] All were physical in nature, a not surprising conclusion considering that Workman and other asylum doctors were trained to cure physical disease. While Workman may have believed these to be *the* causes of insanity, he listed others, as required by the province, in his annual reports. Five classifications existed: moral, physical, hereditary, congenital, and unknown. Under moral causes were domestic trouble, religious excitement, love affairs, business troubles, and mental worry. Intemperance in both drink and sexual matters, overwork, sunstroke, accident, pregnancy, brain disease, and fevers were illustrative of what went under physical causes. Heredity stood on its own as did congenital causes. Both were used in conjunction with one of the other more specific causes listed, and those in the asylum field considered them predisposing as opposed to exciting causes of insanity.[59] Alienists, doctors who specialized in working with the insane, recognized that both women and men could suffer from insanity and often for the same reasons. They also acknowledged that some causes of insanity were gender linked and that others were sex specific. However, they tended to emphasize the repercussions of common causes on women more than on men, to reveal their own expectations of normative behaviour when discussing gender-linked causes, and to continue their belief in the inherent frailty of woman's body when faced with sex-specific causation.

Although in the listed causes of insanity religion was equally significant for the two sexes, the tendency was to focus on women more than men. For example, Workman admitted the relationship between religious melancholy and the 'abnormal condition of the generative organs in *both* scxes,' but he made a point of emphasizing the threat to asylum medical staff in dealing with such women. According to him, they often transferred their religious zeal in a sexually aggressive way upon their attending physicians.[60] While this clearly reflected the lack of women physicians within the asylum system on whom male patients could centre their attention, Workman never discussed what happened to the male patients who, from his description, must have become equally aggressive. Whether for practical or ideological reasons, he did not view religiously aggressive men in the asylum as a problem. Similarly, asylum officials perceived hereditary insanity as more problematic in women than in men.

In theory, heredity should affect both men and women equally, but the perception at the time was that it did not. Based on a 10 per cent sampling of all patients admitted to the Toronto Asylum in the years 1841–1900, there was a slight over-representation of heredity as a cause among women compared with men.[61] Families may have been more willing to acknowledge a hereditary taint in their female than in their male relatives, fearing that once discharged such a label might inhibit the men's ability to earn a living. Also, in the context of the time, it was easier to acknowledge weakness with respect to women than it was for men. Generally, however, families were reluctant to admit an hereditary predisposition for either sex, since it not only reflected on the individual insane person but on the family as a whole. Asylum officials did not share this reticence and railed against the idea of the insane marrying.[62] But, when they went beyond generalities, what they focused on was the problem of insane women marrying and bearing children. Frances Winter was typical. A thirty-two-year-old woman who came to the Toronto Asylum on 2 July 1899, she was married with five children and exhibited strong symptoms of mania. She was suspicious that her relatives were trying to harm her and, according to her husband's testimony, she had been insane since the birth of their first child, being either despondent or excited, manifesting insane jealousy, breaking windows, smashing furniture, taking no interest in her husband or children, leaving home without notice, and threatening to do serious injury to her husband and children to the extent of pouring boiling water on her husband and wishing her children were dead. Winter had already been in an asylum twice before and the attending physician noted she had been allowed to leave and to bear children. In a rather exasperated tone he wrote that these children would probably inherit her insanity.[63] While heredity likewise worked through the male line, there is little, if any, mention that male patients would leave the asylum and father children.[64] The emphasis on women is perhaps understandable when the belief in maternal impressions on the fetus is remembered. Workman's successor at the Toronto Asylum, Daniel Clark, when trying to account for why not all great men had equally great offspring, felt the explanation lay in 'how much maternal influence affects offspring, especially if mediocrity is joined to towering genius, and children partake of the similitude of the former.'[65]

The predisposition of asylum officials to connect certain causes of insanity to women more than men, as in the case of religion and heredity, was very much influenced by medical perception of gender roles. This was also the case when they focused on epilepsy. Alienists viewed epileptic insanity as incurable and noted that it was more prevalent among women than among men.[66] *The Practical Home Physician* of 1884 speculated that the cause of epilepsy was abuse of alcohol, sexual excesses, venereal excess, masturbation, and lead poisoning, although the author did not feel that masturbation and venereal excess were as frequent causes as many believed.[67] As for women suffering more from epilepsy than men, several physicians accounted for this by linking it to ovarian irritation, irritation of uterus, or menstrual irregularities.[68] This focus is intriguing. Epilepsy was not a cause of insanity frequently reported in the Toronto Asylum. The 10 per cent sampling of the patient records reveals only twenty-six patients, seventeen men and nine women, whose cause of insanity was deemed to be epilepsy. This represents only 3 per cent of the total patients and 5 per cent of those whose cause was recorded. The concentration on such a small number probably reflects the problems such patients presented, for superintendents viewed epileptics as dangerous and noisy individuals who experienced fits they could not control. What is more curious is that doctors perceived that epilepsy was more frequent among women when indeed this was not the case either in asylums or in the wider society.[69] The lack of control exhibited by epileptics may be the answer. Victorians would be less willing to tolerate this in women than in men and would have been more sensitive to it when it occurred in women. Also, by connecting the cause of epilepsy to female sex-based disorders of the reproductive/sexual system, physicians were suggesting that epilepsy was a possibility for many women whereas the largely male gender-based causes of epilepsy did not imperil the male sex in the same way.

While doctors did not emphasize male gender-based causes of insanity with respect to epilepsy, they did when discussing intemperance and masturbation as direct causes of mental illness. Most believed that intemperance was a major cause of insanity.[70]

What was worse, drunkards caused insanity in others – the sins of the fathers being visited on their children. Workman even suggested that 'drunken husbands contribute largely to the filling up of our female wards.'[71] Insanity in men could also stem from intemperate use of tobacco and drugs.[72] Certainly intemperance of any sort was a significant factor in perceived disease causation. In 1858 Workman estimated that 10 per cent of the patients in the Toronto Asylum were there because of intemperate habits and characterized these as 'the most miserable, and the most pitiable, of all which find their way into insane hospitals.' The vast majority of these were men.[73] The figure declined somewhat and, by the 1890s, a survey of patient records reveals it was only 6.3 per cent, perhaps because what had once been seen as a cause of insanity was now a symptom. Nevertheless, the association between men and intemperance remained. Over 70 per cent of the patients entering the Toronto Asylum in the nineteenth century because of intemperance (of any sort) were men.[74] This probably reflected the reality of the times. Men had greater access to alcohol and, given the social mores of the time, women's drinking was not acceptable behaviour. Nonetheless, women were admitted who clearly had alcohol problems. Mercy Thomas, wife of a shoemaker, at age forty first entered the Toronto Asylum on 25 February 1841. Her case file indicates that she exhibited a violent and abusive spirit towards her family and her 'keepers' and that she was of intemperate habits. On 5 April she was discharged, on 29 May readmitted, on 15 July discharged, on 31 July readmitted, on 29 September discharged, on 22 October readmitted, on 13 November discharged, on 10 May 1842 readmitted, and on 8 June discharged. It is difficult to avoid concluding that she and her family used the asylum as a place for her to dry out.[75]

If the association between women and intemperance was weak, that between women and masturbation was even more tenuous. Alienists at mid-century and beyond considered masturbation an important cause of insanity in men, not women.[76] It wasted seminal fluid and decreased vital force, thus weakening the system. Workman believed such cases were generally hopeless and found it awkward and embarrassing 'to be prevented by delicacy from assigning ... reasons' for this to the friends and relatives of such patients.[77] He believed that, as a cause of insanity, masturbation was an 'evil of horrific magnitude.' Almost one-third of his male patients masturbated, and a small percentage of his female patients. While he acknowledged the possibility that masturbation could be a symptom of insanity as well as a cause, at mid-century he emphasized the causal side.[78] But whether cause or effect, the linkage with men was there. Only rarely did physicians discuss masturbation leading to insanity in women. The connection physicians made between men and masturbation came from their assumption that men were more sexually active than women. In 1877 Clark described a typical case of what he referred to as 'an enshrouded moral pestilence.' The man 'is retired in his disposition; to an unusual extent he is fond of solitude: his habits, it may be, lead him to loathe and shun the company of the opposite sex; his former loquacity has been succeeded by taciturnity ... He has a pale and bleached looking countenance with possibly a hectic flush on one or both cheeks.'[79] Clark's perception was that masturbators were generally withdrawn, reclusive, and not attracted to the opposite sex. Such traits were deviant for men in the nineteenth century and it is understandable why Clark focused on them as signs of illness. Earlier in the century Workman was taken aback by a male patient who was 'excessively addicted to masturbation' and did not have 'the sly, stealthy, and cast-down aspect of this class of lunatics' but was 'active, noisy, an inveterate whistler, and quarrelsome.'[80] Although Workman did not realize it, this was the way in which physicians described women who masturbated. Susan Blandford whose dementia doctors believed developed out of hysteria certainly did not exhibit the predominant characteristics of withdrawal that seemed to signal self-abuse in men. Yet after describing her more manic symptoms, one of the certifying physicians confided: 'I am strongly suspicious that she masturbates.' Like Blandford, Amelia Hiller had aggressive symptoms of insanity. In her case the cause of her melancholy was not seen as masturbation, although it was a factor. Hiller was nineteen years old when first admitted to the asylum in January 1880. Her mother said she had been 'odd' for at least three or four years, refusing to do light work around the house. More recently she had begun to tear her clothing off and to become very violent. According to one certifying physician who had known her for several years, she had several symptoms suggesting 'impropriety of personal misuse of herself' to which she had admitted. Mary Hall entered the asylum on 17 December 1893. One doctor suggested the underlying cause of her mania was masturbation. Apparently her friends told the certifying physician she would call out to men passing the house and invite them to come in and see her. That physician also noted that she appeared to have a strong desire for intercourse or self-abuse.[81] As the description of male and female masturbators indicates, masturbation resulted in uncharacteristic behaviour. In men it led to sexual passivity, in women it could lead to aggressiveness, sexual and otherwise. In either case, the expectations were gender based.

Not surprisingly, physicians linked all sex-specific causes of insanity to women. Men were the norm and in those areas where the female body deviated from the male, practitioners located additional causes of insanity. As MacNaughton-Jones made clear in his turn-of-the-century textbook:

Such terminological divisions in the classification of insanity as ... 'ovarian,' 'climacteric,' 'old maids,' show the recognition by psychologists of such influences. We are not now considering such morbid mental conditions as are consequences of pregnancy, labour, and lactation. These phases of adolescence and the menopause are, as I have said elsewhere, weaker links in the chain of the woman's life, which, when its strength is tested by any exceptional strain, either by the influence of the environment of her social position and surrounding circumstances, her calling, or accidental occurrences, yield through some pre-existing flaw, and the sudden snap ensues.[82]

Menstruation put an extra stress on the body that many physicians felt not all women could sustain without breaking down. So sure of this was one author of an early nineteenth-century text that he declared 'the insanity of females is always aggravated at the period of menstruation.'[83] Late in the century Dr Hobbs of the London,

Ontario, asylum still argued that a woman's mood shifted during menstruation and concluded that people should not be surprised if insanity sometimes ensued.[84] No woman was immune – the ovaries affected the intellect whether they were healthy or not. According to Tyler Smith, the ovaries 'appear to be an exciting cause of insanity in unmarried females, in the puerperal state, and at the catamenial climacteric.' Indeed, during menstruation, 'the temper is disturbed in women of irritable constitution – in some women almost to madness.'[85] While not all would perhaps go that far, physicians did feel that women were vulnerable because of their reproductive/sexual system.[86] Richard Bucke thought so when he argued that any utero-ovarian disease was 'capable of acting as a cause of insanity.'[87] And that risk continued throughout menopause. In one article reprinted in the *Dominion Medical Monthly*, the author linked different insane classifications to menopausal women, describing the symptoms for each. For example, mania in such individuals was 'characterized by hallucinations, sexual excitement, violence, phantastic ideas and obscene behavior. It is usually met with in widows, old maids of not very high morals, and, generally speaking, in persons with unsatisfied sexual cravings, or in such who have committed excesses in venery.'[88] In this case, although the insanity was being blamed on a physiological process, it exhibited itself in women who for one reason or another were not conforming to the female norm of being married – in the situation of the widow through no fault of her own, but for the rest seemingly through their own transgressions.

Of most concern to physicians was childbirth, because of the energy it demanded and the emotional toll it took. Such a view was not unwarranted. Puerperal insanity did exist, often caused by puerperal fever, other childbirth complications, and post-partum depression. Approximately 10 per cent of the women whose cases were studied and whose cause of insanity was known entered because of problems linked to childbirth, excluding miscarriage and lactation. Emily Connors was a typical case. She took cold after bearing her fifth child at the age of thirty-three and began accusing her husband of infidelity and of trying to poison her. She attempted to kill herself and her infant, her husband and the nurse. One examining physician thought it was important enough to mention she had no secret vice. Admitted in December 1870, Connors was discharged as recovered the following September. Catherine Furness, aged twenty-six, married with one living child and one dead one, had given birth to a healthy baby girl at the end of June 1877. Shortly after, she exhibited 'the usual symptoms' of puerperal mania – sleeplessness, restlessness, talkativeness. She would not look at her baby and at times claimed it had drowned and she did not care. She imagined her husband had been changed into a horse and her daughter into a cow. Admitted on 11 July, she died only three months later of heart disease. Whether the cause of her death was related to her insanity is unknown. Certainly the attending physicians in the asylum did not suggest any link. Neither did they in the case of Jane MacNaughton, who entered in June 1850 suffering from puerperal fever and who died one month later of consumption of the lungs.[89] If there was a bright side to puerperal insanity it was that it was often curable. On the dark side was not being able to prevent it and the fear it could be transmitted to the new-born child. Workman was incensed by one patient who regularly became insane just after childbirth. She would enter the asylum, become well, be discharged, and then return home and become pregnant again. He looked forward to her reaching menopause but in the meantime was concerned about the mental health of her children. At no time in his diatribe against this woman did he blame her husband for sharing his wife's bed.[90]

Physicians made the connection between childbirth and insanity in women very clear[91] and warned medical students to prepare themselves for the eventuality of puerperal mania when attending childbirth cases. Kenneth Fenwick, in his textbook on obstetrics, estimated that 3 to 5 per cent of all women admitted to insane asylums suffered from puerperal mania or that one out of every thousand women who gave birth became insane.[92] But unlike men who masturbated, women were hard-pressed to avoid childbirth. If they did, according to medical convention, they became susceptible to all the physical diseases that denying their natural role in society would cause, including insanity. Recently historians have suggested that woman's bodies were not the ultimate culprit of insanity in women; rather, the pressures of women's role in society were to blame.[93] Women in their domestic situation experienced intense stress. They had to bear, raise, and care for their children and, as the century advanced, this meant not only providing for their physical well-being but also for their emotional well-being, a seemingly never-ending task. In addition, they had to provide similar care to their husbands and kin. They had an incredible amount of physical labour to do in running a household and, for farm women, there was often added the problem of extreme isolation. Moreover, through their own expectations and those of others, women were vulnerable to emotional crises within the family. Mrs Ross entered the Nova Scotia Hospital for the insane in June 1871 suffering from monomania. She was deemed sane except 'that since the loss of a child in January last she has been haunted with the idea that the child's death was attributable to want of care on her part.'[94] Some physicians were sensitive to this problem. Letitia Youmans, when visiting the asylum in London, Ontario, remarked on the number of farm women in it due, according to the superintendent, to 'hard toil and monotonous mode of living.'[95] Dr Hall in the *Christian Guardian* of February 1872 reported that the causes of insanity in women were known and could be eliminated. He felt the two main ones were anxiety about making a living and the married state. For the first, he advised parents to train their daughters for an occupation, and for the second he urged husbands to be more sympathetic towards their wives.[96] In his 1895 text Alexander Skene queried why a normal function such as childbearing should lead to insanity. His answer was one with which many present-day mothers could agree: 'too many other duties are usually imposed upon women during the age of reproduction.'[97]

Such voices were in a minority. Most commentators felt that woman's body was simply prone to disease, including insanity. In one autopsy performed at Toronto, Workman discerned that the woman had had a 'chronic enlargement of the uterus, and ... varicose state of the spermatic vein.' He could not help but wonder if this condition was somehow linked to her epileptic insanity.[98] A few years later, in another post-mortem, he found an ovarian tumour and again queried: 'What morbid affinity subsisted, during life, between this woman's peculiar habits and the diseased uterine appendages.'[99] Workman was not alone in this. Experts on the diseases of women often blamed insanity on uterine disorders.[100] The process at work was again reflex action.[101] Richard Bucke of the London Insane Asylum spent a great deal of time working out the reasons for the specific link between women and insanity. He, too, believed in reflex action but his explanation was more detailed than most. He subscribed to the theory that those functions which had undergone the most change most recently were at risk. These were the 'sensuous-intellectual-moral' attributes linked to the cerebro-spinal and the great sympathetic system. The latter determined the moral or emotional nature of individuals and was particularly important in maintaining mental health. Bucke believed that the organs most closely tied to this system were the stomach, heart, liver, kidneys, supra-renal glands, the testes, ovaries, and the uterus, among others. Any disorder in them could result in emotional imbalance. While the sympathetic system existed in both men and women, Bucke and others believed it was more highly developed in women. Women had two organs linked to it missing in men – their well-developed mammary glands and their uterus. Further evidence was women's greater capacity for love and faith than men possessed, both of which Bucke associated with a higher development of the sympathetic system. Dr Hobbs, Bucke's medical assistant, made explicit the importance of this connection: 'the brain is intimately connected with the uterus and its appendages through the great sympathetic system.'[102] But prevention was not as simple as eliminating the physical disease. One of the concerns of those who questioned the frequency of ovariotomies was their belief that removal of the ovaries had been known to result in insanity.

Not all physicians were convinced that the female body was the source of insanity in women. They argued that their colleagues spent too much time blaming the reproductive/sexual system and pointed out that a woman's life did not revolve around her uterus.[103] Only if she were already experiencing mental illness could physiological functions exacerbate it.[104] But while such physicians may have asked for a degree of common sense in ascribing causes of insanity in women, they were not always sympathetic to women. In an article reprinted in the *Canadian Journal of Medicine and Surgery*, J.J. Morrissey of New York dismissed 'pathological conditions of the uterus' as being central to women's insanity. Of more influence was 'the habit of introspection with which many women are unfortunately afflicted, the proneness to magnify the lesser evils of domestic life, [and] the irritability associated with maternal cases.'[105] Insanity was the fault of the woman. In addition, Morrissey had not really rejected the earlier focus on the uterus. While maintaining that the neuropsychoses originated in the nervous system, he admitted that puberty, adolescence, the puerperum, menstruation, and menopause caused imbalance in it.

The records of the Toronto Asylum in the nineteenth century reflect the connection that physicians made between insanity in women and the female body. Almost one-quarter of the women entering Toronto, whose cause of insanity was known, did so because of female-related causes: childbirth, lactation, miscarriage, menstrual disorders, uterine disorders, and the like. That physicians focused on such causes was to be expected. The association was part of orthodox medicine and conformed to perceptions of physical-disease causation in women. So strong was this belief that women internalized it. Irina Lower, a patient in Toronto, firmly believed she suffered from 'female trouble' such as falling of the womb. Although there was no evidence she had prolapse of the uterus, asylum physicians in the patient register entered uterine or ovarian irritation as a possible cause of her insanity.[106] When physicians associated the cause of insanity to normal physiological changes in women's bodies or to disorders of the reproductive/sexual system to which they believed women were predisposed, they somehow suggested that women as a whole were susceptible to insanity. They acknowledged that certain causes of insanity were more likely to be experienced by men but they linked these to men's social role in society. Men were more sexually active than women; among the causes of male insanity was masturbation. Men were not as morally pure as women; among the causes of male insanity was intemperance. But while men may have been more sexual and less morally upright than women, these were attributes that men could through exertion of will overcome. Through self-control men could stop masturbating and drinking. But self-control was not going to help women. Women not only suffered from all the causes of insanity that men did (even masturbation and intemperance) but in addition suffered because of the complexity and demands of their reproductive system. These were causes that no amount of self-control could overcome. Even in insanity, doctors saw women as victims and prisoners of their own bodies. As such, the asylums must have been overflowing with the female insane, but, based on a study of the Toronto Asylum records, this was simply not the case.

For most of the nineteenth century, Toronto Asylum officials allocated equal numbers of beds to men and women.[107] Only in the decade of the 1840s and carrying through into the 1850s did men significantly outnumber women. Joseph Workman, superintendent of the asylum, suggested this was because insane women were less dangerous than insane men and could be cared for at home.[108] Most likely this discrepancy was a result of the conditions that existed in the Toronto institution, which in the 1840s was a converted jail, and the unwillingness of families and officials to send women to live in such a place. By the end of the 1850s this no longer seemed to be the case; the new institution had opened and had proved itself, so that when the century is examined as a whole the percentage of male and female patients was essentially even. Workman, struck by this apparent equality of insanity among men and women, questioned: 'When we consider how very different, in the two sexes, are the disturbing agencies, in which insanity is usually ascribed, can its equal incidence be a matter of accident, or even the result of compensating diversities of agency? How many of the ascribed causes of insanity, may be but the first manifestations of the malady itself?'[109] He did not hazard a guess and continued to view the causes of insanity as different for men and women.

The equal representation of women and men in the asylum is intriguing, especially since in the general population insane men outnumbered insane women.[110] Part of the explanation for this discrepancy is the difference in how women, compared with men, entered the asylum. Individuals could be admitted to the asylum either by means of a medical certificate or through a lieutenant-governor's warrant. The first assumed that the family of the insane would call in two or three physicians who, if agreed on the diagnosis of insanity, would sign the appropriate certificates allowing the committal of the individual to an asylum if there were a vacancy. The warrant procedure circumvented the family and allowed lunatics considered dangerous to be placed in jail. Once deemed insane (after medical examination), the prisoner remained in jail until moved to an asylum under a lieutenant-governor's warrant.[111] Warrant patients had priority over certificate cases because of their supposedly dangerous nature,[112] with the result that families often declared a person to be dangerous in order to assure committal to an asylum through the warrant system. Such a situation distorted the admission regulations, but even the asylum officials acquiesced in it. In 1886 the brother of Angela Saunders enquired about having his sister admitted to the Toronto Asylum. Superintendent Daniel Clark responded by saying there was no vacancy in the asylum but that if she were troublesome, the best chance the family had of getting her admitted was to commit her to a jail as a dangerous lunatic.[113] The case of Saunders was atypical only in that she was a woman. Most warrant cases were men. Of the 248 individuals admitted to Toronto by warrant between 1867 and 1875, fully 216 were men and only thirty-two were women.[114] Between 1841 and 1899 there were 1780 warrant cases, of whom only 598 were women.[115] Women's insanity was less violent than men's and, as a result, they did not come to the attention of the authorities to the same extent. Also, much of male violence occurred outside the home and was more public than that of women who, because of their domestic responsibilities, often focused their hostility on the family. While families may have been reluctant to commit their insane male relatives to an asylum fearing that committal could ruin the man's future earning power, that decision was taken out of their hands in the case of the truly dangerous insane. It may be, too, that it was more difficult to convince authorities that a woman was as dangerous as a man, or that the idea of a woman in a jail was unpalatable. Whatever the reason, delays in the warrant system meant that some of these cases had to remain in jail pending admission and, unfortunately, the stay could be extensive considering the overcrowded condition of the asylum.[116] This may help account for why, although there were more male insane than female insane, there were equal numbers in the asylum. Some of the male insane were incarcerated in jails.

Beyond explaining the numbers of insane in the asylum and suggesting the location of others outside the asylum, the difference in committal procedures between men and women is difficult to interpret. If Canadians saw the asylum as a place for cure, committal of their female relatives was a sign they cared. If families saw the asylum as a place of incarceration, it suggests the families were willing to rid themselves of the burden represented by the female insane more than the male. But even this may not suggest an uncaring attitude as much as a practical one. Because women, more than men, would be present in the household, they could be more disruptive, especially if there was no other adult within the family to care for them. In such a situation the family may not have had any other choice. Whatever the reason, the result was that women avoided the humiliation of a jail committal and were treated as ill rather than as criminal.

The women who entered the asylum differed from the men in other respects as well. One was age, although significant differences between men and women were only evident in the 1890s and among those over the age of sixty. While women over sixty were slightly more numerous than men in that category throughout the century, almost 45 per cent of all the elderly women who entered the asylum did so in the last decade whereas for men it was approximately 24 per cent.[117] Unfortunately, historians know very little about the experience of the elderly in Canada during these years so it is difficult to speculate why the numbers of elderly women seemed to be increasing. Women had longer life expectancies than men and there were simply more women over the age of sixty than men. Life for such women could be difficult, especially when they were ill. If widowed, a woman would be dependent on her children to care for her; if married her husband might simply be unable to do so without assistance. Amelia Kennar was seventy-two years of age when she first entered the Toronto Asylum on 30 November 1893. Apparently her insanity was hereditary and was characterized by her being restless, sleepless, experiencing memory loss, and being unable to agree with a servant for more than two or three days. At one time she chased a servant out of the house with a walking stick. Assuming that her husband was older, he may not have been able to care for her.[118] In the case of older single women their lack of family may have necessitated their entry.

More crucial than age in differentiating the female from the male insane was marital status. In the Toronto Asylum, patients whose records were studied were equally divided between married and single at approximately 46 per cent each. The rest of the asylum inhabitants were either widowed or their spouses had deserted them.[119] While there were no real differences between the numbers of married and single patients within the asylum, there were significant differences between which patients were married and which were single. From the beginning of the asylum's history more married woman than single entered the asylum, and more single than married men entered. The annual report for the asylum in 1864 surveyed the admissions to the asylum since 1841. Of the 1646 men admitted, 731 were married or widowed and 915 were single. For the 1468 women admitted, the figures were 950 married or widowed and 518 single.[120] This trend continued for the rest of the century and for other asylums within the province.[121] The male patients in the Toronto Asylum over the century were divided among married, single, and widowed at approximately 41, 54, and 4 per cent, respectively. For the women patients, it was 51, 40, and 8 per cent.[122] Evident in these figures was the dominance of women in the widowed category. Although just over one-half of the patients in the asylum were women, more than 67 per cent of the widowed patients were women.

The differences in marital status between the two sexes intrigued asylum officials and others and their attempts to explain them reveal a great deal about the social norms of the time. In his 1858 report, Workman explained the preponderance of married women by noting that women married younger than men, hence there were simply more married women than men in certain age groups. Thus Workman was sensitive to the particular demographic or life-cycle experience of women. While Workman's perception was true, this does not explain why women still outnumbered men in the asylum when all the age groups were considered as a whole. Interestingly, Workman suggested another reason that would help explain this phenomenon. Not only did women marry younger than men but they sometimes married men who were not good husbands. 'Were all women sure of getting good husbands,' Workman declared, he would 'have no hesitation in advising them, if they required any suggestion ... to exchange single comfort for married bliss.'[123] Contrary to his reasoning about bad husbands causing insanity in their wives, Workman never suggests that wives were to blame for their husbands' insanity. The next year Workman returned to the subject. He argued that marriage was basically conducive to sanity but, to explain the large numbers of married women in the asylum, he again mentioned women marrying at a young age. What was new in his argument was the way in which he accounted for the dominance of single men, whose presence in the asylum supported his contention that marriage was healthy. According to Workman, masturbation was the culprit. Single men masturbated more than married men.[124] What was worse, masturbation led to an incurable form of insanity. In 1860 when the numbers of single men and married women admitted to the asylum seemed abnormally low he was careful not to perceive this as a new trend; rather it was accidental and 'no proof of improved morals in the former, or in the husbands of the latter.'[125]

In 1862 Workman continued his discussion and again referred to the plight of women with drunken husbands. But this time he also listed additional problems women experienced from which men were exempt: gestation, parturition, lactation, uterine disorder, want of sleep, defective nourishment, and bad air.[126] The extensive nature of the list reveals a sensitivity on Workman's part to the pressures women faced in their day-to-day lives. Blaming the stresses placed on women by the natural functioning of their reproductive system was in keeping with the beliefs of the medical profession in general, but his acknowledgment of lack of sleep, poor nourishment, and not enough fresh air recognized the social reality of being a woman in nineteenth-century society. Women tended not to get enough sleep because of the demands of childcare. They often cut back on the food they consumed in order to ensure that their husbands and children had enough to eat. In addition, because of their domestic responsibilities, women, especially in urban centres, would be less likely than their spouses to get enough fresh air. Although Workman recognized that married women seemed predisposed to insanity, he was reluctant to associate that with marriage *per se*. Rather it was marriage to a bad husband or because of the accompanying problems incidental to marriage that gave rise to mental illness. The idea that marriage was good for men but bad for women was a difficult concept to accept. Nevertheless, Workman came close when he argued that celibacy in women after the age of thirty would ensure sanity. His advice to men: if they wanted to marry women exempt from insanity, marry women over the age of thirty.[127]

Workman remained fascinated by the marital breakdown of his patients. Determined to explain it, at least to his own satisfaction, he tried a new approach. In his annual report for 1864 he denied that married women were over-represented in the asylum; rather they were under-represented when compared with the population at large.[128] Unfortunately for his argument he was not examining comparable groups. He made his calculations based on the number of women between the ages of thirty and forty years in the general population of Ontario in 1860–1, an age when the highest percentage of women would be married. He then compared this to the female population of the asylum as a whole for the years 1841 to 1864. In addition, his figures for 1860–1 did not correspond with the census figures. Nevertheless, even using his own statistics there was an over-representation of married women in the asylum.[129] Age was a factor: asylum records reveal that married women were over-represented up to the age of forty, but after that age married men were over-represented.[130] Approximately 35 per cent of the male patients were between the ages of twenty and thirty whereas only 30 per cent of the women patients were. This would ensure a large number of single men in the asylum. Almost 30 per cent of the women patients were between thirty and forty years whereas only 24 per cent of the men patients were. This would ensure a large number of married women in the asylum. However, age does not explain the total discrepancy because, relative to the general adult population, married women were still over-represented. Perhaps realizing the unrealiability of his calculations, Workman in 1873 returned to his earlier arguments and made one of his last statements on the subject: 'Prudent old bachelors and venerable maidens sometimes inquire whether marriage conduces to insanity. Reversal of the terms of their question would render the answer much less difficult. Looking, however, at the ... figures, and disregarding, as figure-head men too often do, all their elemental relations, it would seem that, as far as liability to insanity is concerned, marriage is very dangerous to women, and single life very dangerous to men, whilst married men and single women enjoy comparative immunity.'[131]

Workman was not alone in being intrigued by the marital differences of asylum patients. Richard Bucke also tried to account for them. Looking at the patients somewhat differently but picking up one of Workman's arguments, Bucke believed that in the London Asylum single women, especially older ones, were greatly over-represented, a situation he found quite remarkable. After all, everyone knew that the childbearing responsibilities of women often led to insanity and thus one might expect many more married women to be in the asylum than there actually were. His conclusion was to imply that middle-aged and elderly women who had remained single had somehow missed out on their natural role in life and insanity was the result.[132] Unlike Workman, he did not appear to be sensitive to the social problems of women in society. He certainly seemed unwilling to entertain the idea that for many single women, life was extraordinarily harsh, not because they had rejected their natural role in life by not marrying but because society was incapable of allowing them to lead full and productive lives. At the end of the century the surgeon of the London Asylum, Dr Hobbs, seemed to reverse Bucke's claims. No longer was the emphasis on trying to prove that single women were over-represented. Hobbs clearly acknowledged that unmarried men and married women outnumbered others within the asylum. His explanation harkened back to Workman. Men were insane as a result of masturbation and women because of problems linked to their reproductive responsibilities.[133] To these two factors British Columbia's Ernest Hall added abuse of alcohol to explain unmarried male insanity and venereal disease to explain both unmarried male and married female insanity.[134]

Overlooked by all commentators was the practical problem presented to the family when the wife and mother became ill. Men more than women worked in paid employment outside the home. In the event of their wives becoming ill, they had few places to turn. Because they were working, they did not qualify for charity to help them take care of their wives at home and, because they worked, they were unable to do it themselves. For such men, the asylum may have been the only alternative. The husband of Eliza Henley certainly thought so. Suffering from mania, Henley entered the Toronto Asylum on 22 November 1866 at the age of thirty-six. She had six living children and had the delusion that someone was going to shoot her and her family or set fire to the house. She had threatened to poison herself or cut her own throat and, when excited, she became quite violent. Before her committal, her husband wrote to Workman explaining why he felt it necessary to take such a step. Since his wife's illness he had moved closer to his place of work so he could occasionally run up to the house and check on her when she became excited. He had removed his daughter from where she was working to look after her mother, but the girl was only sixteen and could not control her. Trying to find a woman to do so was even more difficult, since he had found that people had strange ideas about the insane. Even if he had been able to find someone, Eliza had made it clear she would not tolerate her. Perhaps it was just as well he could not locate anyone, for he could not afford to pay her since he earned only $1 a day and this meagre income had to support him, his wife, and the five children who still lived at home. To make the situation worse, he worked nights but found he had to stay at home every other night for Eliza would not sleep without him. Being absent from work meant the family finances were in a crisis state. Clearly there was little else this man could be expected to do. He felt comfortable in writing to Workman and being so frank because he had been a former attendant at the asylum.[135] While others would not have been so forthcoming, Henley's plight probably represented that of many men when their wives became ill. Although married women whose husbands became ill would be in a very tenuous situation financially, they became candidates for charity and help from family and friends. And because they were unlikely to be in paid employment outside the home, they could care for their husbands rather than resorting to the asylum.

The attempts of physicians to explain the marital status of women in asylums reveals more about medical attitudes towards women than it does about the female insane themselves. Once again the perception was that the female body, in those areas where it differed from the male, was weak and prone to illness, even mental illness. Neither were doctors alone in their willingness to emphasize women's frailty. For whatever reason, the families of insane women seemed more likely to commit their relatives to an asylum than families of insane men. Consequently, even in an illness which both sexes experienced, there were gender differences. This was especially evident in the perceived causes of insanity. Evident as well was the tendency to apply sex-specific causes of insanity to women and thus emphasize the close relationship that was thought to exist between a woman's reproductive system and her mind. This was also apparent in the discussion of hysteria, a mental disorder from which doctors believed only women could suffer. Not only was woman's body at risk because of her femaleness, but also her mind. And as already seen in the case of hysteria, curing the mind sometimes necessitated curing the body. Not surprisingly, a similar approach was followed in the medical treatment of the insane, except with them the stakes were higher. Diagnosis of insanity could lead to incarceration in an asylum, which the best medical opinion of the day considered the only suitable environment for recovery.

Chapter Eleven

Insane Women: Their Symptoms and Treatment

Martha Blodgett suffered from mania. Married with three children, two of whom had died of diphtheria, Martha was convinced her children were murdered and mutilated and talked on this and 'kindred subjects.' She was incapable of being reasoned with and, if the attempt were made, she became violent. The attending physician had even been obliged to use restraint by tying her hands to prevent her from breaking windows. Anne Burton was classified as melancholic. A thirty-seven-year-old farmer's daughter, she was unable or unwilling to talk on any subject. She neglected her appearance and feared that something dreadful was going to happen. She was not violent but had tried to drown herself. Amelia Ryan did not have that kind of energy. A fifty-four-year-old widow, the cause of her dementia was grief over her husband's death combined with mental exhaustion occasioned by caring for him while ill. She had a 'lost state of mind,' extreme melancholia, want of thought, and and did not appear to be aware of her surroundings.[1] As the descriptions of these women reveal, the symptoms of insanity could be quite varied. Nevertheless, they were the central fact of the disease. Symptoms not only determined whether a person was going to be incarcerated but to a certain extent dictated what treatment that individual received once committed to the asylum. Considering the gender role division that existed in late nineteenth-century society, it is not surprising that symptoms of insanity were often gender based despite the fact that insanity was an illness to which both sexes were vulnerable. While this often led to a gender-based treatment, at times physicians determined that sex-specific therapeutics were indicated. Unfortunately, women bore the brunt of the most extreme of these treatments.

The nineteenth century recognized three major classifications of insanity – mania, melancholia, and dementia. Despite what we have noted about the differences in perceived causation of insanity in men and women, there was little reflection of this in classification. Of the 862 patients whose cases were studied in the Toronto Asylum (1841–1900), physicians assigned the designation of mania to at least three-quarters of both the men and the women. Although women suffered from melancholia more than men, approximately 18 per cent compared to 15 per cent, the difference was negligible.[2] The classification of patients, however, tells little about the specific characteristics of insanity that prompted committal. A person suffering from mania could be a person who laughed inordinately or someone who was homicidal. In either case, the individual had lost control over his or her actions, but those actions were hardly equivalent. A closer look at specific symptoms reveals that the similarities between men and women as reflected in classification were illusionary. Gender played a central role in how physicians assessed symptoms of insanity.

One aspect of the insane that examining physicians mentioned was how they looked, whether they were clean or dirty, whether they had a vacant expression or a certain look of the eye. While there was no correlation between the kind of comment made on appearance and the sex of the individual, physicians commented much more on the appearance of women than of men. Of those patients whose appearance generated notice from the examining physicians, just over 62 per cent were women and 37 per cent were men.[3] Physicians clearly believed that appearance was significant to note in women. In the latter decades of the century, the domestic image of women had reached its peak. Respectability and the semblance of it was a woman's prized possession. Once lost, it could never be regained. Deviation from it could have devastating effects and a woman's refusal to conform without reason could only indicate illness. Utter inattention to dress and appearance was something that both certifying physicians mentioned about Susan Crearar, a farmer's wife. She not only ignored herself but also the condition of the house, and left her children 'entirely uncared for' as well.[4] Appearance for a man was not as central. Society was willing to countenance more varied activity on the part of men than of women, and this may have extended to physical appearance as well. Deviating from a respectable appearance may not have been as significant for men as for women, considering the other symptoms of insanity that men exhibited. For example, insane men were more violent than insane women and a description of male appearance when their violent paroxysms had already been described would be somewhat irrelevant for the purposes of diagnosis and ensuring a committal to the asylum. In the case of women, whose insanity was revealed in less dramatic ways, any information, such as appearance, would help to create a more complete picture of the illness. What appearance suggests then is not that women looked more insane than men but that their other symptoms were such as to be unconvincing of either insanity or the need for committal.

More symptomatic of insanity than appearance was excitement, the behaviour associated with mania. It included inordinate laughing, crying, talking, praying, jumping, and the like. At least one-quarter of all patients studied exhibited such characteristics. In addition, another 14 per cent were incoherent, a state which could very well be considered a form of excitement.[5] Many physicians viewed women as more excitable than men. When Sally Bedford, aged twenty-two, entered the asylum on 26 February 1884, the accompanying documentation stated she talked a great deal 'even for one of her sex.'[6] Workman himself referred to the noisiness of the female wards in one of his early reports, as did the inspector of asylums in 1868 and 1878.[7] That both the superintendent and inspector felt called upon to mention the fact suggests that such verbal display was out of keeping with accepted female behaviour.[8] But this should have been expected in an asylum. Most patients were in an asylum because they did not conform to accepted behaviour. While women may have *seemed* noisier than men, they were not any more excitable. Only 121 women compared with 102 men were excited, and women were only slightly more incoherent.[9]

Closely aligned to general excitement were specific actions that called attention to the insane – such as swearing, refusing food, refusing to work, drinking, quarrelling, wandering, and sexual impropriety. Almost 38 per cent of the patients acted in a way that caused notice.[10] Asylum officials seldom referred to any differences between the actions of insane men and women once they were admitted. In 1869 Workman discussed the relationship between religious melancholy and certain deviant acts and language. Women outnumbered men in this regard but, as Workman pointed out, this may have been the result of such actions being so incongruous in women that they attracted attention.[11] Although Workman and his successors did not spend much time discussing differences in the actions of the male insane compared with the female insane, differences did exist. Of the eight cases involving refusal to work in those patients studied, five of them were women.[12] Susan Crearar who neglected her own appearance also neglected her home and family. Born in Ireland and entering the asylum from jail on 10 June 1876, Fanny Pollock was twenty-five years of age with two children. In the description of her insanity, mention was made of her sitting all day, singing and crying. She threatened to kill her oldest child and, while she never actually attempted to hurt anyone or herself, she had expressed a desire to jump into water. In addition, she heard voices and saw the dead who she believed were trying to poison her. Fanny, then, was potentially dangerous, suicidal, and paranoid, and she hallucinated. As if that were not enough in her history to be considered indicative of abnormal behaviour, the phrase 'does not do housework' was added to her case notes.[13] A woman refusing to do her household tasks was disruptive to the family and made it impossible for family life to continue. A man refusing to work placed a family in economic jeopardy, but the day-to-day living arrangements may not have altered significantly unless he exhibited other symptoms of insanity, in which case they, rather than the refusal to work, were considered of more moment. What this reveals is the centrality of women's work in the home and *her* willingness to do it as the cohesive bond. It is not coincidental that all five of the women whose unwillingness to work was mentioned were married. Perhaps the situation of Margaret Youmans illustrates this best. Married with four children, Youmans was forty-eight years old when she entered the asylum on 11 April 1893. Classified as melancholic, her case history revealed a quiet woman who took no interest in her surroundings, with an 'absence of all care and attention to her household duties.' Other than this she exhibited few characteristics worthy of notice. Whether her family was unwilling to cope with someone who would not work is unknown, but Youmans herself would demand little care. What is particularly heart wrenching about her case is that thirteen days after her committal she died of marasmus, a wasting away from diet deficiency which she must have had before her incarceration.[14] It is difficult not to conclude that her family was trying to get rid of her.

Because the actions of the insane were so varied, I have summarized them into five major categories: unsocial acts (swears, untidy, spits, eats and drinks filth), sexual acts (masturbates, erotic, sits indecently, strips), acts relating to food (drinks, refuses to eat), restless (wanders, sleepless, runs away), and other (idiocy, imbecility, wicked). Of those patients whose actions were mentioned, approximately 14 per cent were said to engage in unsocial, sexual, food-related, or other acts, and 43 per cent were restless. What is intriguing is that there was a significant correlation between the type of action and the sex of the patient. The most clearly defined differences occurred in the categories of sexual and unsocial acts; 68 per cent of patients whose deviant behaviour was sexual were men. The differences in sexual actions reflect the social norms of the time. Men could engage in sexual release more than women. Even insane women had internalized this taboo to the point that, for many, this was not an option. This is in direct opposition to Elaine Showalter's work on English asylums in which she concludes that 'uncontrolled sexuality seemed the major, almost defining symptom of insanity in women.'[15] Other unsocial acts did not suffer from as extreme a taboo and it was in this category that women dominated, since they represented

63 per cent of the offenders. Most of these women had resorted to swearing.[16] Whether this means they actually swore more than men or that such language was unusual in a woman and thus worthy of comment is unclear. Whatever the reason, swearing was viewed as a symptom of insanity worthy of note in women more than men.

Equally indicative of social expectations of women and the way they internalized them were the delusions insane women experienced. Delusions among the insane were quite varied. Merry Tomlinson believed her other children were plotting against her youngest son; Anna Berensen feared some person had injured her character and fancied she saw the Devil performing miracles. Margaret Carruthers was convinced she had sold herself to the 'old devil,' given up God, and was consequently damned.[17] Although the details of the delusions could be quite specific to the individual, most delusions of the patients studied fell under six general categories: delusions of grandeur (25 per cent), delusions of seeing and hearing (9 per cent), religious delusions (28 per cent), domestic delusions (5 per cent), sexual delusions (3 per cent), and those whose delusions were not described but just indicated (24 per cent). Of the patients in the asylum, approximately one-third suffered from delusions (excluding paranoia) of one kind or another. And as in the case of actions, men and women differed significantly in the type of delusions they experienced. Of those suffering from delusions, women more than men had delusions revolving around home and family (76 per cent compared with 23 per cent), seeing and hearing (77 per cent compared with 22 per cent), and sexual delusions (89 per cent compared with 11 per cent). Men, in contrast, dominated delusions of grandeur (71 per cent).[18]

Delusions of grandeur suggest that the individual has a strong and positive self-image. That men experienced such delusions more than women simply underlined the fact that in nineteenth-century Canadian society men had status, opportunities, and prestige. Fred Wallace, a twenty-one-year-old Quaker farmer, entered the Toronto Asylum on 7 January 1898 suffering from mania. One of the characteristics of his insanity was his fancy he was born a genius and had received honours from the Queen. He was even a 'greater personage than Lord Salisbury.' He could do anything and everything and had been 'lionized' all over the country when people found out who he was. As his case notes summarize him, 'He is very locquacious and pleased with himself.'[19] One reason men may have had more grandiose delusions is that they more than women suffered from general paresis (insanity caused by venereal disease), which was typically characterized by 'golden' delusions. Nonetheless, men accepted the way in which the world measured success; what their delusions offered them was the opportunity to see themselves as successful according to those terms. For insane women this did not appear to be as possible. Even in insanity, women had difficulty creating a positive self-image for themselves. Not surprisingly, their delusions tended to be of the domestic kind and reflected their established role in society. Contrary to men's grandiose and happy inventions, women's delusions were often unhappy ones revolving around concern for family. Melody Burton, for example, believed that her children had been shot and her home burned.[20] Even women's tendency for delusions of seeing and hearing reflected their more passive status in society, for such delusions allowed them to retreat into a world of their own that had little connection with the reality of the world in which they had to live. Their dominance of sexual delusions was not significant simply because the numbers this represented were too small. One debilitating form of delusion experienced by 30 per cent of the patients examined was what contemporary society refers to as paranoia.[21] For the person suffering from paranoia life is frightening. Some feared they were going to be murdered or poisoned; others were suspicious of those closest to them. Still others feared for one reason or another they were damned. For those living with such individuals, life was difficult and frustrating. The constant effort to reassure and cajole could eventually take its toll. It did not seem to matter whether the person was male or female, the paranoid delusions were intriguingly similar. Both sexes equally feared being poisoned or murdered and, despite the emphasis in the historical literature on the importance of religion for women, both sexes were equally concerned about being damned. Where the differences between the two existed was that women more than men experienced paranoia. Almost 59 per cent of those feeling threatened were women whereas less than 42 per cent were men. This divergence again emphasized the lack of power that many women felt they had over their own lives and their consequent feelings of vulnerability.

This vulnerability, however, should not be exaggerated. Women could and did exert their frustrations in very visible ways, sometimes to the point of violence. Indeed, violence was probably the most important single symptom of insanity. From 1841 to 1875 over 50 per cent of the patients studied had exhibited signs of violence before committal. Some individuals took out their anger against the furniture in their homes, throwing, breaking, or burning it. Others tore their clothing. Some were very aggressive against others, including their families, friends, or strangers, and used a vast array of means – hands, axes, knives, guns, fire, feet, sticks, and even a spittoon. Still others focused their violence on themselves, attempting to drown themselves, cut their throats, or taking a hammer to their skulls. As is evident, the acts of violence fell into three basic categories: violence to property, violence to others, and violence against self. Of the three, violence to property was the least significant both in how often it was mentioned and in the seriousness of its repercussions. Only about 11 per cent of the Toronto patients examined were violent to property in any way. However, women more than men had a tendency to be violent to property. Although women were just over 50 per cent of those in the asylum, they represented 64 per cent of those patients whose acts of aggression were against property.[22] Amelia Rosard's husband, Theodore, seemed to feel that Amelia's destructive tendencies were more than he could put up with and augured more dangerous behaviour to come. She was forty-five years of age with eight children. The record accompanying her from jail indicated that she believed someone was in the basement who was dangerous. Formerly industrious and careful, both as a wife and mother, Amelia had become restless, complaining, and unwilling to stay at home. The deposition by Theodore claimed that Amelia had begun to smoke and, since that time, her behaviour had become worse. She broke his grindstone and he was convinced she did so on purpose. She burned out his churn, which had soft soap in it and which his daughter was going to clean so they could churn butter in it. Amelia also burned feathers that the family had been saving. In Theodore's words, 'I have been afraid she might set the place on fire and afraid she might hurt the children. My reasons I am afraid she might hurt the children because she is crazy.'[23]

Women's violence to property may have reflected their physical weakness compared with men, the fact that if they expressed their anger against people they stood a good chance of being hurt themselves. It might also be that the social norms concerning the non-aggressive nature of women were sufficiently influential to mean that when women committed aggressive acts, they were often harmless to others. But we should not overestimate this behaviour. Approximately 40 per cent of the patients in the asylum had exhibited aggressive behaviour towards other individuals and, of these patients, 40 per cent were women. While an under-representation compared with their presence in the asylum population, the proportion was high considering the social pressures on women not to be violent.[24] Despite the willingness of many women to attack family and non-family members, the perception of this violence in the records was not strong. The descriptions of male violence are more detailed and colourful, characteristics that provide an aura of reality to their violence more than women's. Nonetheless, some descriptions of women's violence could be quite graphic. Ann Goddard, a labourer's wife, aged forty with three children, was described as careless and indifferent, sometimes singing, at other times crying. She had injured her children by shaking them and had even struck one of them on the head with an axe. Europa Bennett, aged thirty-eight, entered the Toronto Asylum for the second time on 21 September 1871 suffering from 'erotic mania.' That she had given birth to two illegitimate children may account for the diagnosis. Bennett was described as talking, singing, and wakeful except for one day a week when she became dull, sleepy, and quiet. She was in the habit of tearing her clothes off and, as the record very obliquely commented, it was 'not known if she has secret habit but it is suspected.' If all that were not enough, she frequently attacked her sister with sticks and chairs. Janet Dyard, too, had many symptoms other than violence. One certificate of insanity described her as restless, in constant movement, and with false ideas about strangers and their intentions towards her husband's property. She imagined they wished him to die and their sons to marry her in order to have the tools in her husband's shop. Her husband claimed she had threatened the life of a customer with an axe, had struck him with a bar of steel, and had threatened a young girl who had called at the house. She had also become negligent of herself and the house.

While for these women the reasons for their violence were unclear, for others it was evident. Elsie Donovan struck her mother only when the mother tried to prevent her from going out. Marjorie Keller physically resisted when her family made attempts to keep her at home. In both instances the women were exerting their will and were being met with opposition. Whether their attempts to overcome their restrictions seemed more serious because they were women is impossible to know. Their efforts certainly would not be in accordance with accepted feminine behaviour.[25] Resorting to suicide might be given that it was violence directed towards self, but asylum figures certainly do not substantiate this interpretation. Men and women were equally disposed to attempted suicide.[26]

Whether a woman or man would be placed in an asylum for violent tendencies or any other symptom of mental instability was dependent on a range of factors. Seldom was one symptom enough to convince family or authorities. Even violence, if unaccompanied by other symptoms, was likely to result in a prison term rather than an asylum stay. But persons exhibiting the same signs of insanity may not have been treated identically. So much depended on their personal situation and history. Women who had been previously admitted to an asylum seemed to be more prominent over time than men. In the 1870s, 16 per cent of men and almost 13 per cent of the women had been under asylum care

before they entered the Toronto facility. By the 1890s it was almost
19 and 27 per cent, respectively.[27] Whether this indicates a willingness to commit women more frequently to an asylum than
men is unknown. Since women tended to enter through the certificate or family system rather than the warrant system, their
patient files may simply have been more complete owing to information provided by family members. Unfortunately, we know
very little about the families of insane women or men. But one
fact should be noted. The existence of a family was a mixed
blessing. For the four women deserted by their husbands and the
nine widows among the patients mentioned in the 1842 Annual
Report, being alone made them vulnerable to admission to an
asylum when they began to show some indications of mental
disorder. Even when family existed, they were not always able to
care for their sick relations. Maggie Matthews had had several
attacks of insanity and had always recovered at home, but on 30
April 1852 she entered the asylum because a family crisis prevented
her son from caring for her. It is unlikely that the husband of
Annie Scollard would have been willing to care for her, since, in
a confidential letter to Workman, Scollard's physician made it
very clear that her husband was lazy, unemployed a lot, and had
left her alone a good deal. Certainly the asylum was a refuge for
Martha Harris, a physically abused wife. The certificate of insanity
described her as incoherent and holding conversation with the
angels. According to her husband, she talked to her dead son and
claimed she saw him. She also believed that another son in Michigan had taken away some of her property. The doctor examining
her went on to write that Harris imagined a great many persons
wanted to injure her. Whether true or not, one person wanted to,
for in her medical history one of her examining physicians wrote:
'I believe from what I can learn that the cause is more likely due
to absence from her husband and son as well. The former had
been in the habit of pounding her, on the head and has laid her
scalp open with a butcher knife.' To Edwina Timberlake, too,
strapped down at home, the asylum with its commitment to non-
restraint would seem like deliverance.[28] Just being in the safe

environment provided by the asylum could be of benefit to these women.

Once in the asylum, the care given to women was only as good as the staff providing it. The superintendent and his medical assistants were practising physicians but this did not mean they had any specific training in treating the insane. In the latter half of the century, most alienists tried to follow a regime of moral treatment – that is, surrounding the insane with a comfortable and pleasing environment in which their bodily needs would be met and their psychological wants responded to with kindness and understanding. Little training was required for the staff, except a willingness to attend to patients in a humane way. Of more relevance for women in the asylum was that all the medical personnel were men. On one level this may not have been disquieting since it reflected the reality women patients faced outside the asylum, but it may have restricted their willingness to discuss physical symptoms with those in charge. Certainly some physicians were uneasy about women sharing intimate details about their bodies with the opposite sex. An examining physician of Rachel Petersen made it clear he considered her willingness to discuss the laceration on her womb with anyone of 'either sex' indicative of her unbalanced state of mind.[29] While doctors would not have applied the same criteria to women patients confiding in their medical advisers, the women themselves may very well have done so, not necessarily making a distinction between male physicians and other men.

Although the superintendents and medical officers of the asylum had medical licences indicating a modicum of education, the qualifications of other asylum workers are less known. Yet these individuals, particularly the attendants, really determined what the quality of life was like for insane women within the asylum walls, since they more than anyone had most contact with them. If judged by their conditions of work, the care provided by the attendants must have been minimal. In 1851 there were only nine female and ten male attendants to care for 131 women and 136 men patients both day and night.[30] The crowded conditions only made this situation worse. In 1854 the asylum designed for 250 had only one-half the planned space but already 373 patients, and such overcrowding continued for the rest of the century.[31] Patients had to learn how to cope with this, and so did the staff. Overcrowding intensified the work expected from attendants, but even those with some semblance of authority had little relief from their labour. For example, the matron of the Toronto Asylum had not had a holiday for ten years when she finally took one in 1865.[32]

Work in the asylum was segregated according to sex. Women attendants took care of women patients. The only exception was in the London Asylum, where Richard Bucke introduced female attendants onto the male wards in the hopes of regulating male behaviour. The experiment was initially an apparent success, for even the inspector noted the difference after the first woman began to work there: 'Since this lady's coming to the Asylum, a greater tidiness in person, a greater activity in employment, and a general brightening of the condition of those in the male wards is perceptible.' The men were so determined to make a good impression on their new attendant that fifty to sixty of them had begun to work in the asylum, something they had until that time refused to do.[33] To counter any suggestion of impropriety concerning women taking care of healthy, albeit insane men, Bucke only allowed widows to work on the male wards.[34] While women attendants (if they were widowed) could work on both male and female wards in London, this was probably the only advantage, if it were an advantage, the women asylum workers had. They were very much underpaid compared with their male colleagues. Ordinary attendants on the female superior wards in Toronto received $9 a month, whereas the comparable male salary was $20 a month.[35] Even when the women did the same kind of job for the same patients they were paid less. In the London Asylum, Bucke admitted that women attendants on male wards received only £30 sterling a year, whereas men attendants received £50 sterling.[36] Not only were women attendants paid a minimal salary, but the salary scale within the asylum denied the value of the work they did. At mid-century, even the laundress was paid as much as and sometimes more than those women taking care of patients.[37] Not surprisingly, the turnover rate for women workers was high. In 1870 Workman complained how often they left to get married.[38] But no wonder they saw marriage as a way out. At the asylum pay was minimal, hours long, and the work hard and sometimes dangerous. Why should women forgo a home of their own for a job that gave them little recognition of their worth? They would certainly forgo marriage if they remained, for married women (except widows) were not allowed to work in the asylum.[39] The high turnover among women attendants had repercussions on their charges. Women patients did not experience continuity in those who cared for them and, because attendants did not stay long, they developed little expertise in providing that care.

Since asylum officials did not know how to cure insanity, treatment was largely custodial – supplying adequate food, clothing, and shelter. While both women and men received these basics, some discrepancy existed between what extras women and men received. To encourage male patients to work in the asylum, superintendents sometimes resorted to a reward system, offering the men alcohol or tobacco. It is unlikely, given the moral climate of the time, they would have been able to offer such amenities to women; indeed they did not seem to offer any amenities to them in exchange for work done. Perhaps the idea of men getting paid for work and women not getting paid was so much a part of social norms that the uneven treatment was not even noticed. The climate of gender difference, however, could sometimes act in women's favour. In 1881 the inspector noted that few pillows were available on the ordinary wards in the Toronto Asylum and ordered that pillows should be supplied to all the women.[40] Women patients also seemed to be better off in regards to personal hygiene, probably owing to a belief that women were more fastidious than men. In Toronto a spray bathroom for women was inaugurated in 1896. The men had to wait two more years for theirs.[41]

One of the major innovations of moral treatment was the removal of mechanical restraint. While asylum officials replaced mechanical restraint with psychological restraint, especially closer surveillance, the absence of mechanical restraint in the asylum from the patient's viewpoint must have been a welcome relief. The inspector of asylums in Ontario was particularly committed to non-restraint and pressed his superintendents to follow it as much as possible. For women this was especially important for, as the inspector noted in 1881, more restraint seemed to be used on the female side of the Toronto Asylum than on the male side. In that year, three crib beds (small confined beds in which the individual could scarcely move) were in use in the women's section but none in the men's.[42] The same situation existed at the London Asylum. According to Bucke, try as he and his colleagues might to keep women out of restraints they could not: 'Insane women on the whole are more unmanageable than insane men.'[43] Why this was the case is difficult to determine. There was little to suggest that women were more violent than men in the asylum, although the perception was they were more excitable. Nevertheless, violence could erupt on the female wards. On 1 April 1884 one woman in the Toronto refractory ward killed another woman with whom she shared a room.[44] Compared with male attendants, female attendants may not have been able to cope with such behaviour, even on a reduced scale, and as a consequence may have resorted to restraint more often.

If, as Bucke suggested, women were less manageable in the asylum, their resistance might have been related to the work and activities provided them. The complementary side of non-restraint was work therapy. By providing insane patients with some activity, superintendents hoped to dissipate some of the energy the patients had and which, in times past, had necessitated mechanical fetters. Work was part of creating a normal environment for the insane, for sane people worked; consequently, superintendents considered willingness to work on the part of patients a sign of their recovery. It also indicated that, if released, the patient could be able to support herself or himself and not be an economic burden to family or society. Not all patients were willing or even able to work. In response to those who judged an asylum by how many patients were working, Workman in his 1868 report defensively claimed that he allowed patients, especially women, to lie down when they wanted to because it conserved their strength and 'soothes their mental distress.'[45] The question is why he was more willing to allow women to lie down than men. Was it because he viewed them as weaker and more prone to collapse? Or was it because he did not view women's domestic work in the asylum as real work? For those patients willing to work, the work they did in the asylum was gender specific. Men performed outdoor labour and women were employed in domestic activities. In addition, the work of women patients was not as varied as that of men. At the London Asylum men could work on the farm, in the garden, in the horse and cow stables; they could work with the carpenter, mason, painter, tailor, engineer, baker, and butcher. They could milk cows or tend pigs. Work was available for them in the dining-room, kitchen, and laundry. They could sew or knit, they could make and mend shoes, boots, and slippers, seat chairs with cane and reed, and make mats. They could involve themselves with tinsmithing, blacksmithing, locksmithing, upholstering, clerking, bedmaking, sweeping, scrubbing, sawing and splitting wood, shovelling coal, grading land, making roads, working in the store, or picking hair for mattresses. For the women there was sewing, knitting, bedmaking, sweeping, scrubbing, milking, picking hair for mattresses, gathering fruits and vegetables, and working in the kitchen, dining, and laundry rooms.[46] The difference in the lists may account for why men in the asylum seemed to put in more work days. They simply had more choice of jobs.[47] And the jobs they did took them outside the asylum's main building either into shops or barns or working out of doors. Women's work kept them largely tied to the asylum. Even the inspector recognized this reality when in 1879 he observed that farm and garden work provided the most liberty to patients. Ignored was the fact that women were denied this liberty or that they might even want it.[48]

While providing something for the patients to do was certainly a good idea, for some the work they did seemed to go beyond therapy. Susan Crosbie, aged thirty, entered the asylum on 2 April 1892. Exhibiting signs of restlessness and sleeplessness, she claimed that her brother and 'lots of others' had intercourse with her during the night but that she was asleep and did not wake up. In 1909, when she was forty-eight, her record indicates she was a good worker and 'scrubs and helps in the dining room' despite the fact she was not very strong. At the age of sixty-eight she was still in the asylum and was still scrubbing floors. What therapeutic value such work had is difficult to gauge, although its exploitive nature is not. Some patients were aware of this. Mary Ashcroft was forty-three, married with four children, when she entered the Toronto Asylum on 21 February 1894. According to her husband, she had suffered from hallucinations for five years and believed her neighbours were operating on her nerves by means of a galvanic current or electric batteries. She felt persecuted and had gone to a detective seeking help from those annoying her. She had also repeatedly struck both her daughter and her husband. On 3 June 1911 she was discharged on probation and, while she was not cured, was considered harmless. After her discharge both she and her husband wrote to the asylum doctors keeping them informed of her progress (or lack of). In one of those letters she referred to the work she had done while she had been in the asylum and pointed out she should have been paid more for it.[49]

Linked to work therapy and to keep patients busy, asylum authorities also provided them with recreational activities. In this area men again seemed to have been favoured. There were certainly a raft of outdoor engagements for men that was forbidden to women. In 1879 the inspector called for even more outdoor activity for the Toronto patients – 'cricket, ball, skittles, quoits, racing, etc., for the men, frequent pic-nics, occasional drives and other outdoor amusements for the men and women together.'[50] He made no mention of amusements specifically designed for women. This oversight perhaps reflects the male bureaucracy of the asylum system and their inability to identify women's need and desire for outdoor recreation. When the Toronto Asylum lost the grounds on which its farm had stood, Superintendent Clark argued that his male patients required a gymnasium or a bowling alley because the remaining land was too limited for exercise. He did not seem to feel his women patients might equally have needed access to spacious grounds.[51] Indoor recreation, too, was gender based. Clark was proud of an 1100-volume library that existed in the Toronto Asylum. Although open to all patients, the male insane used it more.[52] This was not because they read more but because they had more leisure time than women. Their work was largely outdoor, so when the light went from the day their time was their own and, in winter, the weather curtailed the amount of labour they could do. But women's sewing and other domestic chores continued rain or shine. Even in the asylum, women's work was never done.

While the partial elimination of restraint and the introduction of work therapy were tangible changes that had occurred, the life of the asylum revolved around custodial issues, primarily keeping the patients safe. For women patients this meant separation from the male insane and from male attendants. Sexual abuse was not common but it was not unknown. On 11 January 1857 James Magar, porter at the Toronto Asylum, wrote to the *Globe* enclosing a letter he had sent to Workman accusing the steward of the asylum of having 'been guilty of seducing and having illicit communication with a patient.' To the visiting commissioners of the asylum he reported: 'That the female lunatic patients were exposed to improper intercourse by the Steward, George McCullough, who allowed Thomas Pearce, a patient ... to go at his pleasure through the female wards.' The provincial secretary ordered an investigation and the visiting commissioners determined that the charges were 'utterly without foundation and completely void of truth, so far as establishing any criminal charge against the Steward or any other person in the Asylum.'[53] To guard against sexual transgressions, the rules and regulations of the Toronto Asylum by the 1870s made it clear that 'no male attendant shall ever enter a corridor occupied by female patients, and no female attendant shall ever enter a corridor occupied by male patients except by permission of the Medical Superintendent.'[54] Some even suggested separating women and men into their own asylums. While Workman did not approve of this, Clark was willing to consider the idea. He saw that by removing men from the asylum the women insane would have more liberty. They would be able to roam the grounds without risk of impropriety or, as he so delicately phrased it, 'without the liability of the augmentations of morbid sexual susceptibilities.'[55] The danger, however, was to more than women's susceptibilities. To his consternation, Richard Bucke at London was well aware of this problem. On 14 July 1884 one of his patients, Mary Stapleton, 'was found by Mr. Spickwell, in the act of buttoning her drawers, and patient Grant Hartwell suspiciously near her: she admitted that patient had connection with her.'[56] But separate asylums were not to be and Bucke, Clark, and other superintendents had to continue to guard women patients as best they could against the patients' own expression of sexual activity and possible sexual exploitation of them by others. They were not always successful. In 1886 Owen McIlroy, a former Toronto attendant who had been fired for abusing a patient, attended a dance at the asylum where his sister was a cook. While there, McIlroy had intercourse with one of the women patients. Charged with rape, he was acquitted when it was discovered that the patient suffered from erotomania.[57] Even if insane, women were expected to maintain the proper norms of sexual behaviour.

Elaine Showalter has argued that many of the limitations of asylum life could be attractive to women. They had amusements rather than hard work. For middle-class women the emphasis on chaperons, restriction, enforced sexlessness, limited occupation, and subjugation to authority all reflected the reality of their lives outside the asylum.[58] Even assuming this was true in the English context to which Showalter was referring, it does not reflect the experience of women in the Toronto Asylum or elsewhere in Canada. The records indicate that many of the women worked very hard and what amusements there were seemed designed more for men than for women. Enforced sexlessness was certainly the norm in the asylum but, as seen, this did not always protect the women from sexual assault.

Some women remained in the asylum until they died. Others stayed until they recovered or were considered suitable for discharge. For the former, the asylum was a custodial institution, for the latter a curative hospital. After at least ten years experience, Workman felt that women tended to stay in the asylum for longer periods than men because of having 'been admitted in the chronic stage of insanity [more] than ... males.'[59] In 1874 he was still maintaining that women stayed longer but explained it differently. Women did not succumb to fatal brain disease as much as men and thus survived longer in the asylum. Unlike men, women were accustomed to the inactive, indoor life of the asylum and adapted to it much better. In addition, the ravages of alcohol were not visited on them to the same extent.[60] The inspector carried Workman's observations to their logical conclusion in the next year and advocated that greater accommodation for the female insane be made.[61] Statistics for the century bear out Workman's perception. Approximately 60 per cent of men whose cases were studied stayed less than one year. The comparable figure for women was about 55 per cent.[62] Of course, a short stay in the asylum does not necessarily mean that the patient was cured and discharged. A patient who entered the asylum and died soon after would have had a brief incarceration. How the patient left the asylum may be more telling than how long the patient remained. Three major ways of leaving the asylum existed. First, the superintendent could grant the patient a probationary leave; this would allow the family and the asylum to determine whether the patient could cope with the outside world and be deserving of a permanent discharge. Second, the patient could be granted a permanent discharge; discharge, however, cannot be equated with cure, for patients could be discharged cured, improved, or unimproved. Third, death was the final way of leaving the asylum.

Authorities did not introduce probations for the Toronto patients until 1872,[63] but once adopted they proved very popular. Clark especially thought they were suitable for women suffering from puerperal mania. Such women 'become home-sick when the mania subsides, and feeling keenly their position have natural longings for liberty to go among friends and relatives.'[64] Certainly officials granted more women probations than men. Of the patients whose records were examined, twenty-nine women received them whereas only fourteen men did. Because more women than men in the asylum were married they had a home to go to during their probation. Neither was women's insanity characterized by violence to the same extent as men's. Superintendents who granted the probations and the families of the insane who had to oversee the patient during the probationary period may also have assumed that female violence, when it did manifest itself, could more easily be controlled.

Of more interest than probations were discharge rates, for they indicated how successful the asylum was in returning people to society. For the period 1841 to 1900, approximately 36 per cent of the Toronto patients studied had been discharged cured, 10 per cent had been discharged improved, approximately 15 per cent had been transferred to different institutions, and just over one-quarter had died. The remaining either escaped from the asylum or were discharged with no indication in what condition. This means that, in all, 46 per cent left the asylum improved.[65] Workman believed that asylum statistics suggested insanity was more curable in men than in women, and accounted for this by arguing that women entered the asylum very often in a chronic state of their illness whereas men entered sooner, before they reached that stage.[66] While this may have been true in the early years, for the century as a whole there was no significant difference in discharge rates between men and women (nor was there any evidence that women entered the asylum later in their illness than men). Women were discharged unimproved marginally more than men, perhaps because even when ill they were easier to control at home. This was particularly the case in the 1890s when crowded conditions may have prompted the superintendent to discharge anyone who could be dealt with outside the asylum in order to make room for those who could not.[67] It may also have been because women were committed more through the family. Warrant patients could not be discharged unless they were well and safe to be at liberty. Family committals could be released at any point at the insistence of family and friends. Other than this, the only difference was that men had a propensity to escape from the asylum more than women. Escaping or attempting to do so indicated a reluctance to accept authority and may be why women were not highly represented among those who escaped. Women's willingness to accept authority was part of their socialization process and thus they, more than men, would have been less likely to question their incarceration.[68] Since men had more opportunity than women to be outside, their chances of escaping were also better and, because of the skills needed to avoid capture, more men than women were successful at it.

All asylum officials were sensitive to deaths that occurred in the asylum. Death removed the possibility of cure and potentially suggested that asylum care itself had somehow been deficient. But death was something with which superintendents and their medical assistants were familiar. Here was something concrete they could explain. For these reasons they kept careful records on the number of patients who died each year and the cause of their death. In 1864 Workman noted that more men died from general paresis than women. In turn, women tended to die from tuberculosis, although he did not fully understand why this was the case.[69] While he stressed the importance of exercise and fresh air for health, he did not link women's susceptibility to tuberculosis with their lack of access to either compared with men. Of course this was not unique to the asylum. In any event, Workman felt TB was 'the compensative death factor against General Paresis in men.'[70] So closely did he associate paresis with men that when two women apparently died from it in 1861, Workman did not believe they were true cases.[71] Daniel Clark, too, felt that any woman's death from general paresis was highly unusual.[72] Even in cause of death, the gender distinction between men and women was maintained. Of the patients examined, thirty-two women died of TB and eighteen men; twenty-three men died of general paresis and only one woman. The only other major difference in cause of death was that eleven women died of marasmus and only five men. Since marasmus was a wasting disease caused by poor nutrition, it lends credence to the theory that women often neglected their own health for the sake of others in the family. Although there may have been differences in the causes of death, there was little in the rate at which men and women died. At one point Workman believed that the nature of insanity for men and women was different. For women, insanity was 'a reflex disturbance of the brain,' whereas for men it involved 'cerebral lesion,' resulting in a higher mortality rate for men.[73]

By 1873 his experience in the asylum had convinced him otherwise. Both men and women had similar death rates, which convinced him of the basic similarity of their insanity.[74]

While the world of the asylum was not an attractive one for
either men or women, in some respects entry into the asylum
may have been less traumatic for women. Historians have discussed the domestication of madness, viewing the asylum as a
home and the superintendent as a patriarchal father.[75] For women
this situation was really not all that different from the world outside the asylum. They were already accustomed to being dependent.[76] For men, however, such a situation removed their
autonomy, their sense of power. Asylum care also reflected other
facets of the world in which women lived. Women had fewer
opportunities in the asylum to choose what work they wanted.
The choices for men were much greater, just as they were in paid
employment outside the asylum. And unlike men, women were
accustomed to working without pay. In many respects the asylum
simply continued the life with which women were already familiar. This was the rationale behind moral treatment – to duplicate the values of the outside world and persuade patients to
accept them. An active therapy it was not and perhaps for this
reason some working among the insane looked to what was happening in the wider world of medicine to help them in their
efforts to cure the insane. Not surprisingly, women were the focus. The rise of gynaecology was reflected within the walls of the
asylum.

Edna Slater was a thirty-year-old servant, single with two children when she entered the asylum in London, Ontario, on 4 September 1890. She imagined that people were annoying her and,
as a consequence, exhibited 'violent fits of passion.' Such fits
must have been sporadic for while in jail awaiting committal she
had been calm, well-behaved, and helpful. On 13 January 1892 her
case notes reveal she was calm and might have been let out of
the asylum if she had had anyone to care for her, but she did not.
Three years later she was reported in good health but had become
violent towards the other patients. On 15 November 1895 her case
file stated: 'Having complained of having some uterine or other

similar trouble was ... sent to Main Building Infirmary for special treatments and operation.' While her case history does not reveal the type of operation, elsewhere in the records it is clear that she underwent curettage and amputation of the cervix.[77] Edna was not alone in undergoing such major surgery. Many women in the asylum became the focus of a procedure designed to cure not only their physical disorders but their insanity.

As we have seen, the care asylum officials provided to insane men and women was more or less similar. What differences existed revolved around the traditional work roles of the two sexes – men worked outside, women worked inside. Medical treatment tended to focus on curing physical ailments because in actual fact there was no 'medical' treatment for insanity. In the London Asylum, however, the superintendent, Richard Maurice Bucke, was not satisfied with this attitude. At the end of the nineteenth century he instituted gynaecological surgery as an active therapeutic. Such surgery reflected the strides that gynaecology had made in being accepted by the medical profession as well as the desire of asylum physicians to offer the most up-to-date medical techniques to their patients and to be seen to be part of an active profession. Nor was it surprising that those who worked with the insane might connect the removal of gynaecological disorders with alleviation of insanity. It was a truism that a close relationship existed between disorders of the reproductive system and mental instability. If doctors could remove the physical disease, perhaps the mental one would disappear.[78] As already seen, Bucke's philosophical and medical beliefs predisposed him to connect gynaecological disease and insanity in women. He believed that the sympathetic nervous system was larger in women than in men and that the health of this system was closely connected to mental stability. He also believed, like many others, that gynaecological disease could, though reflex action, disturb the sympathetic nervous system. As Bucke made clear, 'there exists between the female sexual organs and the great nerve centres a closer relation than between these last and any other of the bodily organs.'[79] In April 1893 patient sQ at the London Asylum underwent 'a very radical operation' for uterine disease. At the end of several months she began to improve mentally and continued to do so over two years. Despite the fact it had taken SQ two years to recover, Bucke and his surgeon in charge, Dr A.T. Hobbs, believed they had discovered a potential aid to restoring some insane women to normalcy. So convinced were they that from 8 April 1895 Hobbs was on leave in New York to study gynaecological surgery.[80] On his return and, under Bucke's authority, he began to examine women patients in the asylum and to perform operations, 'many of the gravest character' on them. In his 1895 annual report to the inspector, Bucke made his first public mention of the surgery, listing nineteen patients on whom Hobbs had operated.[81]

As was clear, the first step in determining the need for surgery was to perform a pelvic examination. When any woman resisted, the doctors placed her under anaesthesia and continued the examination undisturbed.[82] Despite the controversy that still existed in Canada about the morality of internal examinations and the concern when such examinations were done on patients under anaesthesia, neither Hobbs nor Bucke publicly viewed it as an issue. The extraordinary results of the examinations probably dispelled any qualms the two men may have had about examining insane women in such an intimate way. In his annual report for 1896, Bucke noted that of the fifty-four women they first examined, fifty-two, or 96 per cent, had 'been found to be suffering from disease of the uterus, ovaries or both.'[83] Subsequent examinations confirmed this high frequency of gynaecological disorders in their women patients. Hobbs in 1898 reported he had examined 136 patients out of 750 women patients in the asylum, and of these 126 had had pelvic disease of some kind and 121 of them required surgery. He concluded 'that perhaps one-sixth if not one-fourth of all the women in asylums for insane are there because of the special infirmities of their sex and the disasters and penalties of their lives as wives and mothers.'[84] The operations performed at London varied in type and severity. In his 1896 report, Bucke listed 107 surgical procedures, ranging from curettage to abdominal hysterectomy, performed on forty-seven patients.[85] Hobbs pointed out that the tendency to operate was likely greater in an asylum situation where normal medical procedures on the insane were at times difficult if not impossible to carry out. Nevertheless, both he and Bucke were very careful to maintain that the operations at London only occurred to alleviate physical distress.[86] One of the women operated on was Georgia Prentice. Certified insane on 10 May 1893, Georgia was a thirty-three-year-old mother of three who, after the death of her father, began displaying emotional instability. She ran out into the street partly dressed, had no regard for her appearance, and neglected her domestic duties. She had threatened and even attempted to kill her children. Prentice did not settle into the asylum well. On 22 May she attempted to escape and on 3 June succeeded but was returned. By November she had become less anxious to leave and had become more tidy and industrious. On 2 January 1894 she was in good health, similarly on 1 January 1895. At some point diagnosed as having a subinvoluted uterus with endometritis and a cystic and hypertrophied cervix, she underwent surgery on 8 December 1896. She recovered physically from the operation but remained in the asylum until she died in 1921.[87]

While it may be true that physical disease indicated the need for the operations, what both Hobbs and Bucke stress in their writing and the aspect that is stressed in the debate over the surgery was the mental recovery of the patients. For Bucke the logic was evident: 'Many insane women have disease of the uterus, ovaries, or both ... Such disease can nearly always, in the present state of surgical science, be removed by operative interference, and ... The removal of such disease is nearly always followed by marked improvement in the physical health of the patient, and very commonly by equally marked improvement in her mental condition.'[88] The danger of the last claim was to predispose physicians to operate on insane women more than they might otherwise do. Although in the above quote Bucke took a moderate tone, he did not always do so. He believed he had found an answer to insanity among women and he exhibited a missionary zeal in spreading the news of his discovery. He not only enthused about the surgery in his annual reports but also in articles that he and Hobbs wrote for Canadian medical journals. Even more significant, in terms of audience, was his article published in the 1898

American Medico-Psychological Association Proceedings, in which he made it very clear 'that the removal of the pelvic disease by operation is often followed by relief or cure of the mental alienation.'[89]

Over time, Bucke and Hobbs kept the medical public up to date about the results of the surgery. Looking back in 1899, Hobbs estimated he had had a 38.5 per cent mental recovery rate, a 26 per cent improvement rate, with 33 per cent of the patients having experienced no improvement and 2.5 per cent of the patients having died.[90] For Hobbs, the physical recovery of his patients had become a given. What really absorbed his interest and made the results of the operations so important and worth publishing was the mental improvement of those women on whom he operated. Bucke was equally excited by the effects of the surgery on the mental health of his patients and, like Hobbs, explained them in a way that any asylum superintendent would understand and appreciate – recovery rates. He calculated that between 1892 and 1895 male and female recovery rates in the London Asylum were approximately even at 34 and 37 per cent, respectively. Between 1896 and 1899, however, the rates diverged, with the male rate remaining relatively constant at 35 per cent but with the women's rate increasing to 51 per cent. The reason for the discrepancy – the sexual surgery that had begun in earnest in 1895.[91]

Once Bucke had proven to his own satisfaction that the operations were a success, he tried to analyse the reasons in more detail. He concluded that type of disease was closely linked to the results of the surgery: 'Diseases of ovaries and tubes have the most influence upon the mental health of the patient, that is, the most influence in the causation of insanity.' This focus on ovaries as central to women's health (whether physical or mental) was widely accepted within the medical profession. Next in significance was disease of the uterus and cervix, followed by uterine tumours and lacerations of the perineum. Diseases such as hernias and tumours of the non-generative system had little if any effect in causing mental disturbances. To Bucke this hierarchy was not a surprise. After all, 'the ovaries and tubes ... [were] the most vital, the most highly organized, the most intimately associated with

the mental and spiritual life, of all the organs under consideration.'[92] In the ovary, the endometrium, and the cervix 'centres
the life of the woman as such.' The reproductive glands secreted
material to the blood, which when the ovaries were diseased
became poisonous and caused havoc to a woman's health.[93]

Explaining why the operations led to mental recovery in some
patients was straightforward compared with explaining why the
operations failed to have any effect in other patients. Jennie Munro
was a case in point. When operated on in 1897 she had been in
the asylum for thirteen years. Admitted when she was only twenty-
two years old, she was already the mother of three children. Before entering the asylum she had become 'flighty' and thought of
herself as a prophetess. She was afraid of being killed by her
husband and friends and was deemed dangerous to herself and
others. The supposed cause of her insanity was 'domestic infel-
icity.' In the asylum she was quite excitable and on 7 May 1884,
shortly after her arrival, claimed she was 'in family way.' However,
there had been no visible increase in her size and so her statement
was not considered significant. Her husband brought clothing to
her and at one time had also smuggled in a flask of brandy with
which to bribe the attendant to let her post letters. On 29 May
she tried to cut off her hand, claiming that the Bible directed that
if your right hand offended, you should cut it off. On 1 June her
pregnancy was confirmed and on 25 July she gave birth to a baby
girl who, three months later, was sent to the Infants Home 'for
safekeeping' where she died the following month. Munro remained excitable and, when doctors diagnosed a large and cystic
cervix and subinvoluted uterus that bled easily, they operated on
9 March 1897. Jennie underwent an abdominal hysterectomy, removal of an ovarian cyst as well as a fibroid tumor. She recovered
her physical health but did not improve mentally. She remained
in the asylum and died in 1927.[94] Bucke could only conjecture
about the failure of surgery to help women like Munro. He speculated that if organic disease was already present in the central
nervous system, then no operation to remove gynaecological
problems was going to help in the mental recovery of the patient.
All that surgery could succeed in doing would be to improve the

physical condition of the woman. Bucke also hypothesized that improvement would not occur in cases 'where the brain has undergone ineradicable changes from long continued assaults on the nervous system by the irritation set up and the depreciation of the general health following the pelvic disease.'[95]

So convinced was Bucke that the operations were a positive tool in the treatment of insane women that he encouraged Hobbs to return to New York in 1900 to purchase instruments needed to continue the surgery.[96] Shortly after his return, Dr Hobbs resigned his post for health reasons and to enter private practice. Hobbs had performed all the surgery at the asylum and, faced with the prospect of losing him, Bucke appealed to the government, urging the importance of continuing the work. Not only had it saved some fifty women from spending the rest of their lives in an asylum but, in an argument designed to appeal to a budget-conscious government, Bucke pointed out that 'we have collected here a great mass of instruments and other apparatus; have trained our nurses and have things now in perfect shape for the work; not to go on now would be to lose all this.'[97] Investment in the operations had been made; to quit would be financially irresponsible. Although the operations did not altogether cease after Hobbs left, the number did decrease. In 1902 Bucke died as a result of a fall from his veranda and this further restricted the number of operations performed. Hobbs as surgeon and Bucke as superintendent were the two men most enthusiastic about the surgery. Without them there was no one willing to continue the operations with the same zeal.

The logic underlying the surgery performed at London was not unique to Bucke and Hobbs. As indicated in the discussion on ovariotomies, some physicians were willing to concede that gynaecological surgery might help in the treatment of the insane. Shortly after the operations began in London, Dr R.W. Smith, resident physician at Orchard House Asylum for the Insane in Hamilton, told of an insane woman who was given thyroid extract in a last attempt to cure her before removing her ovaries (despite the fact that the ovaries appeared to be normal). In this case the extract worked but the willingness to operate in such a case suggests that neither Bucke nor Hobbs were out of step with their medical colleagues.[98] Perhaps the most enthusiastic supporter of the surgery was Dr Ernest Hall from Victoria, BC. Like many others, he believed that insanity was the result of physical disease and, in the case of gynaecological disorders, was caused by reflex action on the brain. Cure the disorder and you cure the insanity. And like Bucke, he had an explanation worked out to explain why the operations did not always succeed in bringing about sanity – the damage to the brain caused by the gynaecological disorder had become permanent.[99] So assured was Hall by the logic of this and impressed by the work being done by Hobbs and others, he persuaded the medical superintendent of the BC Provincial Asylum to allow him to perform similar surgery. Because the asylum was not equipped for this, he had to convince hospitals to accept his patients. As he described the situation, 'After a few cases had been operated on in private houses, the Sisters of St Anne kindly extended to me the privileges of the hospital, but the city, or Jubilee Hospital, still pursues its course of "impious stubbornness."' In detailing his work, Hall noted how important it was to save as much healthy tissue as possible and how rarely he removed both ovaries. This placation of critics of ovariotomies aside, the details of his cases reveal otherwise. Of twelve women operated on, he removed the cervix, ovaries, or both appendages from nine, essentially ending their ability to bear children.[100]

Not all physicians supported what was being done at the London Asylum. For one, MacNaughton-Jones in his 1901 text wondered about the efficacy of pelvic examinations of all insane women.[101] In truth, Bucke and Hobbs did not examine all their women patients. They only examined those women who exhibited visible signs of pelvic disease, which accounts for why they continually turned up such high rates of disease in the women they examined – they were looking at a preselected sample, not that they always made this clear in their writings or when they gave papers at conferences. After one such paper given before the American Medico-Psychological Association, Dr Woodson, an American physician, struck by the high disease rate in the women whom Bucke examined, queried what this suggested about the health of Canadian women. Upset by what he interpreted as a slur on Canadian womanhood, Dr James Russell from the Hamilton Asylum rose to 'object to the idea Dr Woodson has expressed about the Canadian woman. I think that the physical as well as the mental type of the Canadian women [sic] is in every way equal to that of the American women. (Applause.) And I deny most emphatically that they are more subject to disease of the generative organs than the American women.'[102] Russell was one of Bucke's most vocal critics and at this meeting made it clear he sided with those espousing conservative treatment of the female insane. Of more concern to some physicians than the incidence of disease in Canadian women was the fear that too many physicians were performing gynaecological surgery in the hopes of curing nervous disorders.[103] Could gynaecological problems really account for insanity in women? When cases were examined it was evident that reasons other than physical could account for women's insanity – the death of a child, financial trouble, the death of a brother, or overwork.[104] More problematic was the difficulty physicians had in duplicating the mental recovery rates claimed by Bucke. Until others could duplicate the work being done in London, the results of the operations would be questioned.

One criticism with a modern ring was that gynaecological surgery on women to cure mental disorders was sexist, although the term itself was not used. Only a few physicians raised this issue but it was one that lurked beneath the surface of much of the debate over any kind of sexual surgery. In 1885 the *Canada Medical and Surgical Journal* reported that the International Medical Congress had deemed removing ovaries for nervous disorders was not acceptable, just as it was not acceptable to remove the testicles from insane men.[105] Dr Russell of Hamilton was clearly uneasy about the surgery being done on women at London. Responding to Bucke's description, he sarcastically referred to the attraction that such surgery had: 'Men not only seem to love to operate on these poor organs, but love to discuss the subject as well.' He blamed postgraduate medical schools for encouraging their students in this 'meddlesome surgery and cruelty to the female who is suspected of uterine disease.' From Bucke's report, he concluded one would think that uterine disease was a major cause of insanity, yet 'experience in asylum work is this, that the ratio of insanity between the sexes is about equal. We do not hear of any such battle royal over the male organ and its appendages.'[106] Because of the nature of their reproductive system, women offered a challenge to physicians that men did not. To none of this criticism did Bucke respond. Ernest Hall, however, was prepared to engage in debate on the issue of equal treatment for men and women in the asylum. He agreed it was not right to focus on women's genitalia and ignore men's – the sexual system of men was linked to their brain just as it was in women. He, more than most, was prepared to meet the issue head on and to suggest that since one cause of insanity in men was self-abuse, perhaps circumcision or other more radical surgery should be tried on men in order to cure their insanity.[107] However, there is no indication that he followed up on this idea.

Added to the criticism that the surgery in London focused only on women was concern about the repercussions of major abdominal procedures. Surgery was all well and good if the patient recovered her physical health and mental equilibrium, but since neither was assured, care had to be taken. Bucke himself believed that removal of a woman's ovaries would lessen or remove her sexual desires. Yet nowhere does he refer to this as a factor he took into consideration before giving permission for Hobbs to operate.[108] Neither did he seem to weigh in the balance the possibility of the patient's dying as a result of undergoing surgery. Yet patients did die. Ernest Hall, Bucke's most energetic supporter, described one of his own cases:

Although this patient presented sufficient pelvic disease to justify surgical measures under ordinary circumstances, the result shows that operation in this case was not indicated, and possibly detrimental, if, indeed, it did not hasten the fatal result. The mistake of undue haste need not be repeated. In future I shall abstain from operating until the possibility of acute cerebral cause is eliminated. It might be well to suggest that at least one year of expectant treatment be given following the appearance of mental trouble before operative measures be tried.[109]

Although death was a real possibility in any major surgery, Bucke and Hobbs seldom discuss whether, without surgery, their patients' lives were in danger or even unbearable. Surely the severity of the physical disease had to warrant the attempt to cure it.

Not only did critics question the frequency, morality, and consequences of the surgery, but some doubted whether it really had the result Bucke claimed for it. Bucke admitted at one time that any operation on an insane patient could very well lead to improvement, whether the organ operated on was diseased or not.[110] The very shock of the operation was enough to bring about recovery. Dr Russell suggested it was not the operation *per se* that resulted in what mental improvement was seen but the specialized nursing that came after it.[111] This made a good deal of sense. Asylums in the nineteenth century were incredibly large and impersonal institutions. In 1896 London had over 1000 patients. The kind of care provided was of necessity limited and cursory. When patients underwent surgery, however, they were placed in a special ward and given individualized nursing attention for the first time since their entry into the asylum. Such care might very well have created an environment in which the insanity would lessen on its own and eventually disappear. This care was the underpinning of moral treatment in which most superintendents, Bucke included, claimed to believe.[112]

As can be seen from the general criticism of the surgery being performed at London, one of Bucke's most vociferous critics was Dr Russell of the Hamilton Asylum. In an attempt to bolster his stance that resorting to surgery on the insane as a curative was too radical a departure from accepted treatment, he solicited opinions from 120 alienists both in Canada and the United States. In the *Canadian Practitioner* for 1898 he quoted liberally from them to suggest that opinions were almost unanimous in rejecting the surgery. Dr C.K. Clarke of the Rockwood Hospital for Insane in Kingston wrote: 'There is no room for such a fad ... These examinations, taken in conjunction with very extensive *post-mor-*

tem investigations, convince me that uterine disease is not any more common among the insane than among the sane, and as a factor in the production of mental disease may be considered as trivial and unimportant.' While not always quite as vehement, Workman and Ross of Toronto, T.W. Burgess, superintendent of the Protestant Hospital for Insane in Montreal, S. Vallee, medical superintendent of the Quebec Lunatic Asylum, and G.L. Sinclair, superintendent of the Hospital for Insane in Halifax, essentially agreed. Russell acknowledged that the laity and many medical men believed that pelvic disorders in women caused insanity. He could, consequently, understand the logic behind the operations. Nonetheless, he feared the predisposition to link pelvic disorders and insanity resulted in those operating finding what they were looking for. The surgical gynaecologist 'wages his most relentless fury on the ovaries, for in them he believes reside the chief demoniacal spirits that torment the unhappy lunatic.' Surgery on the insane in the hopes of curing their insanity he concluded was 'wholesale ... mutilation of helpless lunatics.' He described one woman patient who had come to the asylum after having had her ovaries as well as her clitoris removed, something he had great difficulty in accepting. Surgery had not helped this woman or others he had seen. Indeed, he worried that surgery on insane women could worsen their mental state. Had this possibility occurred to those who supported the surgery?[113] Anne Morrell, a patient in the Kingston Asylum was such a case. She was admitted on 3 April 1897 and the report on her indicated she had had her ovaries removed six months previously and as a result had become insane.[114] Despite the assurances of both Bucke and Hobbs that they operated to cure physical disease, Dr Russell and others were not convinced, and Bucke's and Hobbs's tendency to emphasize mental recoveries suggests they were not always clear in their own minds what their primary motivation for operating had been.

While the superintendent of the Hamilton Asylum was concerned about the nature and consequences of the surgery, the superintendent of the Toronto Asylum, Daniel Clark, was annoyed by the apparent grandstanding of Bucke. In his annual report for 1898, Clark referred to the co-operation he received from the Toronto General and St Michael's hospitals when his patients needed surgery; in an obvious reference to Bucke's penchant for providing detailed descriptions of the operations performed at the London Asylum, Clark made it clear that, in his opinion, 'it would be bad taste in us to go into details in an official report. Suffice it to say, that the various operations were successful.'[115] The next year, his report again suggested his irritation with and perhaps jealousy of Bucke: 'Our treatment has been cautious and conservative, and although we have not allowed novelties in treatment to control us, we can record a percentage of recoveries on the woman's side of the house of 40.4%.'[116] Such jealousy was understandable, since the approach taken by Bucke and Hobbs seemed to be a criticism of the non-interventionist methods followed by most asylum superintendents. It also brought notoriety to the asylum system which, as a government-funded enterprise, was not necessarily beneficial.[117]

It was not the operations themselves that seemed to perturb the superintendent of the Kingston Asylum, Dr Clarke. At Kingston in 1895 two women suffering from epilepsy had had a portion of their skull removed, a development to which Clarke attributed their mental improvement. However, he believed that any other operation could have had equal effect, especially when the shock of the operation was combined with special nursing afterwards.[118] Given this recognition, Clarke could hardly object to the surgery at London, but he could and did object to Bucke's efforts to lobby for support in the wider community. Clarke wrote to Inspector Christie on 1 February 1899 complaining that Hobbs and Bucke were appealing to the National Council of Women of Canada to endorse the gynaecological surgery they were performing. What was worse, the NCWC was apparently doing so. Christie was so in agreement with Clarke's concern that he sent a copy of Clarke's letter to Dr Russell of the Hamilton Asylum who, he probably correctly assumed, would be interested and sympathetic. To Clarke himself, Christie wrote in a way that left no doubt about his own deep reservations of what was occurring in London:

As you know, in discussing the matter with you, my judgment drew the line at the non-examination of females admitted to the asylums until conclusive evidence and the most thorough diagnosis of their condition made such examination a positive necessity for their welfare. The general and unlimited examination of females, either maids or matrons, would in my opinion, destroy all their finer sensibilities, and prostitute, even among the insane, all the elevating moral fibre of their being. Rather than have those nearest and dearest to me submitted to this indiscriminate examination, I would think it a mercy to consign ... [them] to the grave.[119]

Christie shared the conservative reluctance of many physicians to perform a pelvic examination on a woman. The problems of gaining informed consent for such an examination on the insane and the fact that in London the examinations often took place with the woman under anaesthesia simply compounded Christie's innate dislike of the procedure.

Bucke realized he could expect opposition to the surgery and that alone he would be unable to resist it. He needed support. To generate it, he sent out a circular letter to the physicians in the London district explaining the surgery and its results and seeking their approval of the work he and Hobbs were doing in London. He mailed at least 350 copies of the circular and received 249 replies. Of those doctors who responded, only one opposed the work, three were non-committal, eight moderately approved, thirty-four strongly approved, and 202 physicians not only strongly approved but also felt it was Bucke's duty to carry on the work. Two examples indicate how well Bucke had been able to elicit the support he wanted. Dr John Kingston from Aylmer wrote: 'Believing as we do that a large percentage of the cases of insanity in women proceeds from causes connected with the sexual organs, it would seem unjust and a neglect of duty to deprive those unfortunates of any treatment, surgical or medical.' Responding to the fear of some that the surgery was performed only for the cure of mental disorders, Dr Gray of Clinton wrote: 'Having been present at most of the Gynecological operations at the London Asylum during the years 1896–97, I am sure that the operations performed in each case was necessary for the physical welfare of the patient.' Bucke could not have drafted these replies better himself. Added to this, in December 1897 the London Medical Association resolved to endorse the surgery in no uncertain terms and urged the government to provide better facilities in London so the operations could continue.[120] Such an endorsation placed Bucke in a strong position to withstand any criticism of his work and gave him the backing to pressure the government to foster the surgery by improving the operating conditions in the asylum. This is something Bucke had been trying to do. In a letter dated 15 February 1897 he wrote to the inspector of asylums outlining the backing he had from the area's doctors. Not content to leave it at that, he suggested that all asylum superintendents follow his example or, better still, that all such surgical work for the Ontario asylum system be performed at London. In a rather extravagant use of statistics he assured the inspector that over 50 per cent of female inmates needed some kind of gynaecological surgery.[121] Bucke's ambition had never been more explicit.

Despite the support provided by the London area physicians, the controversy surrounding the operations did not go away. As already noted, Bucke appealed for backing from outside the medical fraternity, specifically from the local councils of women. Once again in his appeal to the councils, he stressed the mental improvement he believed was a result of the surgery. His willingness to solicit favour from a non-medical group for a medical procedure reveals how intense the debate had become and how defensive and threatened Bucke was feeling. In his annual report for 1898 he attempted to counter two major criticisms of his work. First, he reassured his readers that Hobbs never operated without the consent of the patient's friends or family. In addition, he always consulted the patient's personal physician and asked him to be present at the operation. For those physicians not in the area, of course, this latter would be a matter of form only. Second, he maintained that a doctor unconnected with the asylum always confirmed the diagnosis made on the patient. Bucke himself never made the original diagnosis but was present during surgery to ensure that the diagnosis was correct. In addition, a gynaecologist from outside the asylum system was present at the operation.[122]

Bucke's defence of the surgery and the procedures surrounding it was very convincing. Critics could raise questions about certain issues, but it was difficult for them to be adamant without knowing what actually was transpiring at the London Asylum. A closer examination of the operations themselves suggests that some of their concerns had validity and that Bucke and Hobbs were at times less than candid about what they were doling.

Between 1895 and 1901, 251 women underwent gynaecological surgery at the London Asylum. Unfortunately, the records kept were not always detailed. Of the sixty-one patients whose histories were reviewed, only forty-four actually mentioned the operation. The other seventeen contain no reference either to a pelvic examination or an operation taking place. Neither do the records suggest that the women undergoing the surgery needed it. Few references are made to any physical discomfort that would suggest gynaecological disorders. One of the exceptions was for Henrietta Cooper. Cooper had entered the asylum in 1877, aged twenty-six with one illegitimate child. The cause of her insanity was deemed to be 'seduction.' On 1 August her case notes refer to her having a prolapsed uterus. The attendant returned it to its proper position and Cooper remained in bed for several days. On 1 January 1885 the summary of her condition mentioned the recurrence of the prolapsed uterus but, after 1 May, no further mention is made to it until June 1895, when a vaginal hysterectomy was performed for the prolapse. Bctween May 1885 and June 1895 there is no indication she was receiving any treatment for it or that it was a continuing problem.[123]

Not only do the patient records lack detail, they do not always confirm what Bucke and Hobbs reported. The two men were very proud of the work they were doing at the asylum and especially insistent that the gynaecological surgery had led to mental recovery for some and mental improvement for others. Unfortunately, their enthusiasm often made them report the results or perceived results of the operations too quickly. Martha Carrington entered the asylum in September 1889. Aged forty-four, she was married with seven children. Her attack was her second one and characterized by 'abusive language' and violence. On 1 October, one of the physicians noted she had not been eating well and so Dr Bucke advised bed rest and an extra diet. In December she was on probation but in April 1890 returned to the asylum. Physicians examined her in October 1896 and discovered a hypertropied cervix and in November had it amputated. According to Bucke, after the operation she improved mentally and became much quieter. Yet her case file for 1 January 1899 indicates that her condition had deteriorated. Thus if she did improve it was only for a very short period. While Carrington's case might suggest some benefit, the fact that it did not last calls into question the accounts of Bucke and Hobbs. How long did they wait before they claimed recovery or improvement of patients?[124] More disturbing than the cases whose improvement was exaggerated were those for whom no evidence of improvement exists. Bucke claimed mental improvement for Agnes Clinton, yet no suggestion of this exists in the casebook. Similarly, improvement was reported for Marie Belliveau after her operation in February 1897, with no corroboration in her file. Caroline Hammond's case file indicates a somewhat different situation. She was forty years old and had been insane 'off and on' for six years before she came in 1898 to London, where her brother was also a patient. She was talkative, restless, sleepless, and incoherent. The notes on her life in the asylum reveal that, before the operation, she was already beginning to improve. Was the surgery given the credit for a recovery or improvement that would have occurred in any event? Several other cases suggest this to be a real possibility.[125] If the cases with these discrepancies are removed from the calculations, the cure rate for those operated on was actually less than for those not operated on.[126]

Operating on the insane was not as straightforward as operating on the sane. The latter could give informed consent, the former could not. To lessen concern about this problem, Bucke reassured his colleagues and the inspector that he received permission to operate from the friends of the patient before surgery. While Bucke sought permission before operating, he did so in such a way as to preclude refusal. On 14 December 1896 he wrote to the husband of Vancy Stuart seeking permission to perform surgery on her. Bucke stated that she had a tumour and that an operation was necessary and 'no doubt she will benefit by it in every way.' Such an appeal was going to be very difficult to resist. However, we will never know what Vancy's husband would have done. In January Hobbs operated on her but in March her husband wrote to Bucke claiming that he never received Bucke's letter explaining the operation. If true, how did Bucke receive permission for the surgery?[127] The chances are that Mr Stuart would not have refused permission. How could anyone deny treatment from which a loved one would 'benefit ... in every way.' Certainly the husband of Eliza Meecham could not. To Bucke's request he responded, 'I have full confidence in you and trust to your judgment, knowing that whatever you do will be done for the best.' After Meecham underwent the surgery, Bucke wrote to her brother expressing hope that the physical recovery would be followed by a mental recovery. Bucke was even more explicit about the chances of a mental improvement when he wrote to the father of Elizabeth Walker. He assured him that 'the operation is not a dangerous one' and that it would 'greatly relieve her condition physically and possibly help her mental condition.' He held out similar hope to the husband of Elizabeth Farriday in October 1898. Mr Farriday answered in the expected fashion, giving permission for surgery and saying the doctor knew better than he what would help his wife. After Bucke's death the letters sent out to families seeking permission to operate were more restrained about the possible consequences of the surgery. The new superintendent wrote to the husband of Gertie Timberlake informing him that his wife was suffering from uterine or ovarian irritation and advising surgery. He cautioned Mr Timberlake, however, 'that this step is only experimental and I do not guarantee that mental improvement will take place as a result.' Such a letter did not raise false hopes and, by referring to the experimental nature of the procedure, indicated that it was not accepted by all.[128]

The fact that Bucke sought permission to operate went some distance in reassuring his critics, although his method of doing so may not have. In a similar way, his efforts to obtain a second opinion on the physical diagnosis appeared comforting. There is

only limited evidence in the records that he did seek this corroboration and what there is raises questions of partiality. In May
1897 Dr Meek of London examined Susan Langstaff and discovered
a tumour. The next month she was operated on. In September
1897 Dr Meek again turns up in the records. This time, however,
he was not examining the patient but operating on Eliza Meecham.[129] The last reference to him was made in a 1901 letter from
Bucke to Christie to the effect that Dr Meek had come to the
asylum and was doing Hobbs's work while Hobbs was in New
York.[130] Dr Meek was clearly supportive of the work being done
at the asylum, had benefited from it, and consequently may not
have met the test of total disinterestedness that critics of the surgery would have demanded.

Although Bucke can be criticized for the way in which he sought
permission to operate and perhaps to a lesser extent from whom
he sought a second opinion, he does not seem to have concentrated his attention on any particular group of patients. Almost
all the patients examined were literate. Their religion reflected
that of the asylum population in general and that outside the
asylum. Similarly the ethnicity of the patients indicates no tendency to focus on groups who were disadvantaged in society. Most
of the women operated on were married rather than single or
widowed and so reflected the predominance of married women
in the asylum. The married status of these patients also indicates
they were not alone and friendless with no one to represent their
interests when the decision to operate was taken. While many
superintendents worried about insane women continuing to bear
children, little evidence suggests that this fear determined which
patients underwent surgery in the London Asylum. Ten of the
patients whose records were examined were in their twenties and
eighteen were in their thirties. These were the major childbearing
years. Twenty-one of the patients, however, were in their forties,
ten were in their fifties, and one in her sixties. Most of these
women were well beyond their most productive childbearing
years. In any case, not all the operations performed ended the
ability of women to bear children.

Any surgical procedure carries with it an element of risk. In reviewing the surgery in 1900, Bucke claimed that only four women had died as a direct result of the operations.[131] A review of the patients who died, whether as a direct result of the operations or not, raises some disturbing questions. Mary-Anne Radforth died on 18 February 1895 from double pneumonia during a flu epidemic and only eleven days after undergoing surgery. Did her weakened condition from the surgery lower her resistance and contribute to her death? Elsbeth Webster died one month after the operation from syphilitic ulcers which Bucke reported developed some time after the surgery. In truth her case file reveals she was already developing the syphilitic ulcers before the surgery. Should the operation have proceeded? Mary Quenton died five days after the operation from tuberculosis. As Bucke himself admits, her bodily health had been very weak. If that was so, why would she have even been considered as a candidate for surgery?[132] The case of Mary Quenton raises the question of the way Bucke and Hobbs chose which women would undergo surgery. According to them, they examined any woman who exhibited signs of gynaecological disease and made the decision to operate based on what they found. It did not matter whether the woman was chronically insane with little chance of recovery or acutely insane with an excellent chance of recovery. The purpose of the surgery was to cure physical disease, with mental recovery being an unexpected consequence.[133] But we have already seen that mental improvement was more than a consequence of the surgery; for Bucke and Hobbs it held primary interest. It may even have become the motivation for the surgery. Support for this conjecture can be found in an examination of the length of time the patients had actually been in the asylum before they underwent surgery. Almost 70 per cent of the women operated on had been in the asylum less than one year. These were the women who had the most chance to recover their sanity whether they underwent surgery or not.[134] In 1895, the first year of the operations, there were eighty-five new female admissions to London; eleven of these or just under 13 per cent underwent surgery. By the next year it had increased to one-third of all new admissions undergoing surgery. In 1900 three-quarters of the women admitted to the London Asy-

lum were chosen as candidates for surgery. There is no explanation for these figures in the records. Surely the women who
had been in the asylum for long periods were as susceptible to
gynaecological disorders as those just coming to the asylum? Were
they not as deserving of surgery to cure their physical ailments?
Bucke and Hobbs chose as candidates for surgery those women
whom all superintendents agreed had the best chance for mental
recovery – those who had spent the least amount of time in the
asylum. Certainly the mental improvement rate on the women
undergoing surgery was directly linked to the length of time they
had been in the asylum. Approximately 20 per cent of those who
had been in the asylum for more than ten years and were operated
on recovered. For women who had been in the asylum from five
to ten years and from one to five years it was 44 and 57 per cent,
respectively. For those who had spent less than a year in the
asylum the success rate was just over 71 per cent.

The idea that physical disease could cause insanity and that
insanity could be cured by treating the disease provided comfort
to the medical practitioners in charge of the insane. It integrated
them into the mainstream of the profession rather than leaving
them on the sidelines. Such an idea also provided solace to the
insane and their families. It was much less threatening to know
that insanity had a physical cause than to think that insanity was
the result of some form of moral deficiency, of God's judgment
on the individual, or the consequence of heredity.[135] What Bucke
did at the London Asylum had its own inner logic. Most physicians
recognized the influence of reflex action in disease causation.
Most acknowledged that through reflex action, gynaecological
disease could impair the functioning of the brain. It was only
reasonable to assume that if the gynaecological disease could be
eradicated, the mental instability would disappear. Until the 1890s,
however, many gynaecological disorders were not susceptible to
cure. Surgery which might have provided a solution to some problems was not safe, nor were there many individuals who felt com-
petent to undertake it. In the 1890s this situation had turned around
to the point that some physicians complained about how much
surgery was taking place. That Bucke and his medical colleague

Hobbs took advantage of this change in approach is not unusual. Performing the surgery gave them the opportunity to do something concrete for their patients and to be seen to be doing so. They examined them for physical disease and treated them for it. Certainly this was better than what Inspector Christie would have had them do. Except in obvious cases, he would have preferred the women to die than to undergo the experience of a pelvic examination. Conservatism in medicine could work against women just as it could work for them.

Conclusion

The operations performed at the London Asylum reveal how preconceived notions of women's bodies could affect treatment and how physicians working within a relatively closed ideological system were often unable to consider reasons other than those that fit that system to explain what they saw before them. Culture and medicine are interconnected. Physicians did not and do not divorce themselves from the society in which they live and work. It would be expecting the impossible to think they could. For this reason, the history of medicine offers insight into more than the science of medicine.

An examination of the medical treatment of women reveals how important the idea of nature was to Victorians. Doctors could use nature as an authoritative reference and know it would be accepted. They believed women were closer to nature than men because they assumed that women were more a reflection of their bodies. Yet Victorians were ambivalent about nature; they used it as a rationale for what was when they did not want to change, but considered it in need of improvement when this would increase their material wealth. Nature was God's creation and so women could bask in reflected glory; however, being close to nature suggested domination by body, not by mind. Women's bodies needed considerable energy at puberty in order to develop their reproductive capacities and, as a result, physicians and other Victorians believed their intellectual growth stopped. This in turn limited what women could and should do in society. No one was to blame for this; it was nature through women's bodies that dictated the limitation and, as Victorians were so fond of arguing, what was natural was what was right. Yet the interpretation of what was natural was fraught with value judgments. For one, doctors and others confused it with potential. Women had the potential for childbearing and, consequently, it was natural and, therefore, right that women should bear children. Sexual intercourse was necessary for the procreation of children, thus sex for this reason was natural. Sexuality for individual gratification was not.

Women were not alone in being seen as attuned to nature; physicians also viewed the past that way. They had a yearning for a world they thought had existed, a world where men and women knew their respective roles and where they could best perform them. They were uneasy with the modern woman. This woman, they thought, was unable to fulfil her childbearing responsibilities as well as her mother and grandmothers had. Even worse, she was rejecting the obligation to try. Doctors had a sense that women were healthier in the past, that they had dressed sensibly, had given birth easily, and had few gynaecological problems. It was a mythic golden age, one that may not have existed but that doctors wanted to exist. They comforted themselves with the conviction that if it had been that way before, it could be that way again. When pressed, however, few physicians wanted to return to that past or believed they could do so. Civilization had distorted nature's past. They regretted what women had lost but they also acknowledged what they felt women had gained. Women had become more refined, more spiritual than they had been. If the price they paid was a decline in health, then it was fortunate that medicine had developed to a stage where it could help them. Medicine through science had become nature's overseer.

Because of the close association physicians made between women and nature, they emphasized the link between body and every other aspect of personality for women more than they did for men. Physicians envisioned the individual as an organic whole in which every part was interconnected with every other. This went beyond the physical organs of the body being intercrelated through reflex action. Every aspect – physical, mental, emotional, and moral – was closely tied together. The physical, being the most basic and the most obvious, was given pride of place. Physiology could affect and indeed at times determine the mental, emotional, and moral make-up of the individual. Central to this understanding were the differences between men and women. Despite Victorian rhetoric to the contrary, the separate but equal ideology was not an accurate reflection of physicians' beliefs. Many were convinced that women's reproductive system made them not only different from men but also inferior to them both physically and intellectually. Because of this, physicians thought women required more medical care than men. This came partially from their inclination to use man as the norm by which to compare women. Doctors perceived the health problems of men (with few exceptions) as those of all humans; those of women were simply added to the list, which reinforced the notion of women's greater susceptibility to ill health. Once man was taken as the standard, then the differences between men and women became even more accentuated. Woman became the unknown. As physicians themselves admitted, they did not really understand how a normal female body worked.

Patterns of disease indicated that women certainly suffered or could suffer from a host of ailments to which men were not liable. Although seldom mentioned in the literature, the reverse was also true. But disease or illness was based on both gender and sex. In recent years, the literature on women has stressed the importance of gender as a variable of analysis. And the examination of women's health problems certainly reveals this to be the case. Women's susceptibility to tuberculosis was directly linked to the life style women led rather than to some inherent weakness of their bodies. Similarly, the symptoms of insanity in women were linked to gender as was some of the treatment they received in the asylum. So, too, was disease in men gender based. They, more than women, suffered from venereal disease and were more prone to accidents. One reflected their sexually active role in society and the other the kind of occupations they followed.

While gender is significant, sex cannot be ignored. Women's

and men's bodies are different and vulnerable to different ailments or problems, although how much this was a function of 'nature' rather than 'nurture' has yet to be determined. Any perusal of physician and hospital records reveals a wide variety of abnormalities and afflictions of men's genitalia that women's did not have, and vice versa. But for the nineteenth century, it was women's problems that were central. There were several reasons for this imbalance. Women's reproductive system is more complex than man's and more can go wrong with it. In addition, because the medical profession and others viewed the male as the norm, the problems of his body did not seem as deviant and thus as conspicuous as those of the female. And as we have seen, many of the problems of the female reproductive system may not have been problems at all but simply normal deviation within a healthy body which physicians interpreted as unhealthy. What is more, doctors viewed the reproductive system of women as the essence of womanhood, whereas they did not define manhood so narrowly. This would explain why ailments of the male reproductive system were not viewed as intrinsic to the nature of being male as women's were to being female. The childbearing ability of women only served to reinforce this perception.

Besides reflecting views and attitudes prevalent in the wider society, a study of medical treatment of women has revealed certain themes specific to the medical profession. One already mentioned is the influence of culture. The decisions physicians took were not always motivated by medical concerns alone. Their attitude towards birth control and their refusal to provide it to women is a case in point. It would appear that moral and social considerations determined their hostility to family limitation. But their moral and social stance was no more significant than anyone else's. The fact physicians were providing an aura of scientific legitimacy to their position made it influential. This was true of their statements on education for women, the benefits of marriage, their discussions of sexuality, and the appropriateness of certain types of exercise. By engaging in such topics and introducing them as legitimate concerns of medicine, they were expanding their influence in society.

This expansion was closely related to the professionalization of medicine. Throughout the latter half of the nineteenth century, regular practitioners were attempting to create a place for themselves in society as *the* professional medical care providers. At times, circumstances worked in their favour but, at others, they aggressively battled to secure pre-eminence. They used science to bolster their position and to give their arguments credibility. Looking back on the century, they had achieved much success. Many of their medical sect competitors had disappeared or had been absorbed by the regulars. Midwives had not strengthened their position and, by 1900, physicians had gained enough influence to ensure there would not be a resurgence in midwifery. Doctors had increasingly assumed care over many people who previously had not been considered patients, for example women in labour and the insane. Medical knowledge was becoming more specialized and those in society accepted that only 'experts' had access to it.

The expertise doctors had acquired changed their attitude towards women. From the middle to the end of the century there was a significant alteration in the way physicians regarded the female body and in the role they took in relation to their women patients. At mid-century they were reluctant to view the female body and to give an internal examination. By the end of the century this reticence had disappeared. As a result, they were able to learn more about the body, which was certainly of benefit to their patients. But it did alter the doctor/patient relationship since it made a doctor privy to much more information about a woman's anatomy than she was herself. He knew her more intimately in some respects than even her husband. Person and body became separate and the physician looked to the latter to provide the clues to disease instead of the patient who interpreted what her body was saying. While this would also be true with respect to male patients, the fact that their genitalia was external meant it did not happen to the same extent. Also, the commonality of gender as well as sex between male patients and their physicians would mean that male medical perusal did not appear quite as invasive for them as it was for women.

While there is no doubt that doctors were expanding their control over their patients and their influence in society, it is important to keep in mind that the medical profession was not a monolith. Doctors fought amongst themselves, specialists disagreed with general practitioners, and surgeons with non-surgeons. Neither were physicians as antagonistic to women as some studies have suggested. Doctors themselves were among the most vocal critics of the medical treatment of women. In fact, it would be difficult to criticize the medical profession in any way that some of its members had not already done. Many understood women's reluctance to go to male physicians and, while some tried to overcome that hesitancy, others accommodated women by writing health manuals for them so women could treat themselves medically. Many were very open about the management of birth, recognizing a woman's need for her husband or a friend to be present and not worrying about what birthing position the woman took. Nonetheless, the options women had during birth were narrowing as was their choice of medical therapeutics.

It is commonplace for historians to state that history is not linear, that it does not move from a golden age or towards one. The issue of intervention illustrates this point. It has been one of the strongest themes in the medical historiography, with historians arguing it increased dramatically over time as a result of changes in medical technology and the rise of hospitals. It is certainly true that doctors at the end of the century were intervening in women's bodies in ways almost unthought of at the beginning. The introduction of anaesthesia was partially responsible, as was the confidence provided by antiseptic medicine. In the case of gynaecological surgery, hospitals definitely provided the venue for increased intervention, but in obstetrics the situation was not as clear. Modern studies indicate that intervention increases with the status of the hospital concerned – that teaching hospitals tend to provide more interventionist care than other institutions and certainly more than general practitioners. Medical historians have assumed that the rise of hospitals encouraged that intervention. In the nineteenth century this did not seem to be the case. With respect to obstetrics, many teaching hospitals were very conservative in the treatment they provided compared with general practitioners. More research is needed before the reasons for this are clear. But what the nineteenth-century pattern suggests is that the association between intervention and increased hospitalization may not be a necessarily close one. What is more, the concentration of the historiography on intervention and whether it increased or not, and the tendency to associate intervention with bad medicine, may be misleading. More important is the type of intervention and when it occurs. Bucke's treatment of insane women was certainly interventionist and was not justified by the mental recovery results attained. But those opposing his work and those arguing for a more conservative approach would have had him not examine insane women at all. More to the point, the decision of when to intervene and when not to intervene is only partially a medical decision. Much depends on the patient herself and what she wants and even demands.

Patients are an integral part of medical history but, as this study has illustrated, it is not always easy to integrate them. They, more often than not, remain voiceless. But in their own time they were anything but silent. As consumers of medicine they were instrumental in the regular doctors' gaining the kind of monopoly they did. Women raised money for the building of hospitals and their expansion and sat on committees that oversaw the day-to-day running of them. They were the ones who encouraged the building of female wards. They took their children to doctors and they went to doctors themselves. They often were the ones who insisted on the use of forceps and anaesthesia. They were also the ones who looked to doctors for help in providing birth control and, while doctors did not respond in a positive way (at least publicly), that did not stop women from limiting the size of their families. Women did have a certain amount of power and they used it when they were able. But they were not always able. Many women did become ill and, when they did, they were vulnerable. Yet even that vulnerability was tinged with strength.

Women who were ill were not without choice. They could try to treat themselves with the aid of popular health manuals and patent medicines. They could rely on the help of neighbours, friends, and family. They could turn to those who had a reputation for healing but who were not physicians. For most of the century they could even choose among types of physicians. Perhaps when they did finally seek medical help they were at their most vulnerable, yet even then the strength of these women is visible. Perhaps more than anything, this examination of medical treatment of women has illuminated the discrepancy between image and reality in late nineteenth-century Canada. All the pundits described how physically weak and fragile women were because of their bodies. This is certainly what the medical profession stressed. But the medical records tell a somewhat different tale. They reveal a selected sample of women whose bodies were at risk but who, despite severe ailments, carried on with their daily responsibilities because they simply had no alternative. It is the strength of these women that is manifest, not weakness. That physicians and other Victorians could not recognize this strength says more about their value system than it does about the nature of women's bodies.

Note on Sources and Methodology

The major sources for this study are the textbooks used in Canadian medical schools, the medical journals published in this country, and the popular health manuals that were either published in this country or read by Canadians. In addition, patient records from both private and hospital practice have been examined. Each of these sources has its own strengths and limitations and, because such sources may be unfamiliar to most readers, I would like to describe some of them. The textbooks used in the medical schools in this country for the period under discussion are primarily non-Canadian in origin. The reason they are examined, however, is that being textbooks they were authoritative in that they represented the accepted wisdom of the profession. Also there is little reason to assume that students who learned from these books did not practise the kind of medicine described in them. The fact their teachers chose them to teach from also indicates their significance. The journals published in this country certainly represent Canadian content. Nevertheless, many of the articles published in these journals had their origins outside Canada, although the decision to republish does suggest approval of the contents, at least on the part of the editors. These journals also published much Canadian material, particularly in the form of case histories, which made it possible to confirm that what was being taught from the non-Canadian textbooks was being reflected in the practice of Canadian medicine. The journals represented one of the few forums in which physicians could discuss their concerns. And discuss they did through the various issues of numerous publications. In the nineteenth century alone, there were at least seventeen different medical journals published in Canada, although admittedly many did not survive for long.[1] How influential or representative these journals were is difficult to gauge, especially when their circulation is unknown. They were so numerous and edited by so many different individuals with differing perspectives, however, that it is unlikely any major approach to medicine (within the orthodox stream) was ignored. The variety also provides the historian with opportunity to have a sense of what the issues were, even if it is sometimes difficult to know how the medical profession divided on them.

One problem both the textbooks and journals share is the tendency for both these sources to publish the unusual rather than the normal case. A textbook on obstetrics would describe what an uncomplicated pregnancy and birth were like, but then in great detail would recount what could go wrong and how to cope with it. The same was true for the journals. A description of a normal pregnancy was not going to interest many readers but a description of one endangered by already existing pelvic disease would. It is understandable why more space was allotted to the unusual but it may create a false picture of actual medical practice; the fact that a majority of patients delivered normally without complications would not be reflected in the published record.

The examination of patient records helps to overcome the potential distortion of published records. In the actual case histories, the historian can determine what the physician did as opposed to what he said he did and determine how often the treatment corresponded to the unusual and interventionist approach that published sources emphasized. I chose records that represented both hospital and private physician practices as well as those in urban and rural areas. The use of patient records, however, raises important issues about the issue of confidentiality.[2] In my efforts to research this book I met with a variety of responses across the country and the openness of the records was clearly linked to whether they were held by an archives or a hospital. I was fortunate in that for the purposes of my work the records I needed were of Canadians who were no longer living and, consequently, authorities seemed predisposed to allow me access. Also for my needs, the specific identity of patients was not important and this made gaining access to their case histories easier. But for those writing about the twentieth century and/or for whom identities are important, access to records will be difficult. In this book I have changed the names of the patients to maintain their anonymity, although the initials do correspond to the real names. The statistical runs on the patients were all done using SPSSX (Statistical Package for the Social Sciences).

The last type of source material examined was the popular health manuals of the time. They were particularly important, for they reflected the opinions read by the wider lay community. The significance of popular literature is that 'it does not have to persuade – it does not innovate – it addresses readers who are ready for it.'[3] This readiness is perhaps best reflected in the circulation such manuals enjoyed. By 1895 R.V. Pierce's *People's Common Sense Medical Adviser* had gone into its tenth edition with a circulation figure in Canada and beyond of more than 2,3000,000.[4]

Notes

PREFACE

1 Alison Prentice et al., *Canadian Women: A History* (Toronto: Harcourt, Brace, Jovanovich 1988)

INTRODUCTION

1 Ivan Illich, *Medical Nemesis* (London: Calder & Boyars 1975), 125; Margarete Sandelowski, *Women, Health and Choice* (Englewood, NJ: Prentice-Hall 1981), 6; Pauline Bart, 'Social Structure and Vocabularies of Discomfort: What Happened to Female Hysteria,' in Dennis Brissett and Charles Edgley, eds., *Life as Theatre* (Chicago: Aldine 1975), 192; Janice Raymond, 'Medicine as Patriarchal Religion,' *Journal of Medicine & Philosophy* 7, 2 (May 1982): 208
2 Andrew Weil, *Health and Healing: A New Look at Medical Practice – From Folk Remedies to Chemotherapy – and What They Tell Us About* (Boston: Houghton Mifflin 1983), 221
3 Garfield Tourney, 'A History of Therapeutic Fashions in Psychiatry 1800–1966,' *American Journal of Psychiatry* 124, 6 (1967): 785
4 Michel Foucault, *The Birth of the Clinic: An Archaeology of Medical Perception* (New York: Pantheon Books 1973), 34
5 Sandelowski, *Women, Health and Choice*, 9
6 Vincente Navarro, *Medicine under Capitalism* (New York: Neal Watson Academic Publications 1976), 110–11

7 For example, see Barbara Ehrenreich and Deidre English, *For Her Own Good: 150 Years of the Experts' Advice to Women* (New York: Anchor Book/Doubleday 1978); Elizabeth Fee, ed., *Women and Health: The Politics of Sex in Medicine* (Farmingdale, NY: Baywood Publishing 1983); Linda Gordon, *Woman's Body, Woman's Right* (New York: Viking Press 1976); Sandelowski, *Women, Health and Choice*; Edward Shorter, *A History of Women's Bodies* (Don Mills: Fitzhenry and Whiteside 1982); Catherine Leslie Biggs, 'The Response to Maternal Mortality in Ontario, 1920–1940,' (MSc thesis, University of Toronto, 1983); Jane Donegan, *Women and Men Midwives: Medicine, Morality and Misogyny in Early America* (Westport, Conn.: Greenwood Press 1978); Rhona Kenneally, 'The Montreal Maternity, 1843–1926: Evolution of a Hospital,' (MA thesis, McGill University, 1983); Kathy Kuusisto, 'Midwives, Medical Men and Obstetrical Care in Nineteenth-Century Nova Scotia,' (MA thesis, University of Essex, 1980); Judith Walzer Leavitt, *Brought to Bed: Child-Bearing in America, 1750–1950* (New York: Oxford University Press 1986); Barabara Katz Rothman, *In Labour: Women and Power in the Birthplace* (London: Junction Books 1982); Margarete Sandelowski, *Pain, Pleasure, and American Childbirth: From the Twilight Sleep to the Read Method, 1914–1960* (Westport, Conn.: Greenwood Press 1984); Richard Wertz and Dorothy C. Wertz, *Lying-In: A History of Childbirth in America* (New York: Schocken Books 1979); G.J. Barker-Benfield, *The Horrors of the Half-Known Life: Male Attitudes Toward Women and Sexuality in Nineteenth-Century America* (New York: Harper and Row 1977); John Haller and Robin Haller, *The Physician and Sexuality in Victorian America* (Urbana: University of Illinois Press 1974); and Carroll Smith-Rosenberg, *Disorderly Conduct: Visions of Gender in Victorian America* (New York: Oxford University Press 1986).

8 The recent work by Gerda Lerner illustrates the strength of the notion of social control. In summarizing the development of society as we know it she claims: 'One must ... note that in all hunting/gathering societies, no matter what women's economic and social status is, women are always subordinate to men in some respects. There is not a single society known where women-as-a-group have decision-making power *over* men or where they define the rules of sexual conduct or control marriage exchanges.' Gerda Lerner, *The Creation of Patriarchy*

(New York: Oxford University Press 1986), 30. For an excellent summary of the social control perspective and its weakness see Thomas E. Brown, 'Foucault Plus Twenty: On Writing the History of Canadian Psychiatry in the 1980s,' *Canadian Bulletin of Medical History* 2, 1 (summer 1985): 33–8.

9 Historians of medicine generally were influenced by the increased involvement of the state in medicine and the competition represented by chiropractors and naturopaths. In addition, as historians and other Canadians came to appreciate environmentally induced health problems, many questioned medicine's efficacy in maintaining health. The physical fitness boom revealed a concern about physical well-being that had not existed for years and, as a result, more people became knowledgeable about their own bodies and dissatisfied with the medical care they received. There were accusations that medicine had lost sight of the humanness of the patient, that medicine had objectified not only the disease but also the patient. Richard Shryock, *The Development of Modern Medicine* (Madison: University of Wisconsin 1979), 15. For discussions on the way in which women are treated as patients in the present day see Phyllis Chesler, *Women and Madness* (New York: Avon 1972); Gena Corea, *The Hidden Malpractice: How American Medicine Treats Women as Patients and Professionals* (New York: Harper and Row 1977); Claudia Dreifus, *Seizing Our Bodies: The Politics of Women's Health* (New York: Vintage Books 1977); Robert Mendelsohn, *Male Practice: How Doctors Manipulate Women* (Chicago: Contemporary Books 1981); Gena Corea, *The Mother Machine: Reproductive Technologies from Artificial Insemination to Artificial Wombs* (New York: Harper and Row 1986); Shelley Romalis, ed., *Childbirth: Alternatives to Medical Control* (Austin: University of Texas Press 1982); and Diana Scully, *Men Who Control Women's Health: The Miseducation of Obstetrician-Gynecologists* (Boston: Houghton Mifflin 1980).

10 Eliot Freidson, 'The Social Meanings of Illness,' in his *The Profession of Medicine: A Study of the Sociology of Applied Knowledge* (New York: Dodd 1970), 317; Carroll Smith-Rosenberg, 'The Hysterical Woman: Sex Roles and Role Conflict in Nineteenth-Century America,' *Social Research* 39, 4 (winter 1972): 652–78; Ann Douglas Wood, '"The Fashionable Diseases": Women's Complaints and Their Treatment in

Nineteenth-Century America,' in Mary Hartman and Lois W. Banner, eds., *Clio's Consciousness Raised: New Perspectives on the History of Women* (New York: Harper Torchbooks 1974), 1–22

11 Shorter, *A History of Women's Bodies*, xi–xii; Edward Shorter, 'Women's Diseases before 1900,' paper presented to the American Historical Association, 1978, 9

12 Gail Parsons, 'Equal Treatment for All: American Medical Remedies for Male Sexual Problems, 1850–1900,' *Journal of the History of Medicine* 32 (Jan. 1977): 55–71; and Regina Morantz, 'The Lady and Her Physician,' in Hartman and Banner, eds., *Clio's Consciousness Raised*, 38–53. This latter is a response to an article in the same collection, Wood, 'Fashionable Diseases.'

13 For a discussion of such a view see Regina Markell Morantz-Sanchez, *Sympathy and Science: Women Physicians in American Medicine* (New York: Oxford University Press 1985), 204. Morantz-Sanchez claims that earlier historians viewed male doctors as deliberately hostile to women and even those who did not argued that the patriarchal views of American society could not help but influence doctors' treatment of women and make them insensitive to their needs. She does not really give references to historians supporting the first view but for those supporting the second she notes the following: Ann Douglas [Wood], '"The Fashionable Diseases": Women's Complaints and Their Treatment in Nineteenth-Century America,' *Journal of Interdisciplinary History* 4 (summer 1973): 25–52; Charles Rosenberg and Carroll Smith-Rosenberg, 'The Female Animal: Medical and Biological Views of Woman and Her Role in Nineteenth-Century America,' *Journal of American History* 60 (Sept. 1973): 332–56; Carroll Smith-Rosenberg, 'The Cycle of Femininity: Puberty and Menopause in 19th-Century America,' *Feminist Studies* 1 (winter 1973): 58–72; Smith-Rosenberg, 'The Hysterical Woman,' 652–78; Barker-Benfield, *The Horrors of the Half-Known Life.*

14 For example, see Leslie Biggs, 'The Case of the Missing Midwives: A History of Midwifery in Ontario from 1795–1900,' *Ontario History* 75, 1 (March 1983): 21–36; Donegan, *Women and Men Midwives*; Jean Donnison, 'Medical Women and Lady Midwives: A Case Study in Medical and Feminist Politics,' *Women's Studies: An Interdisciplinary Journal* 3, 3 (1976): 229–50; Margot Edwards and Mary Waldorf, *Reclaiming Birth: History and Heroines of American Childbirth Reform* (New

York: Crossing Press 1984); Frances Kobrin, 'The American Midwife Controversy: A Crisis of Professionalization,' *Bulletin of the History of Medicine* 40 (1966): 350–63; Judith Litoff, *American Midwives 1860 to the Present* (Westport, Conn.: Greenwood Press 1978).

15 Morantz-Sanchez, *Sympathy and Science*, 210, 215, 227–30

16 Margaret Conrad, '"Sundays Always Make Me Think of Home": Time and Place in Canadian Women's History,' in Veronica Strong-Boag and Anita Clair Fellman, eds., *Rethinking Canada: The Promise of Women's History* (Toronto: Copp Clark Pitman 1986), 73–4

17 Barbara Ehrenreich, *Complaints and Disorders: The Sexual Politics of Sickness* (New York: Old Westbury 1973), 5; Fee, *Women and Health*, 12

18 Sources for the prairies were relatively limited for this period because of its later development compared to the rest of the country. Western medical journals, however, were examined.

19 Archives of Ontario (AO), Lydia Christie Diary, microfilm MS-112, 1 Jan. 1886

20 A.A. Travill, 'Early Medical Co-education and Women's Medical College, Kingston, Ontario, 1880–1894,' *Historic Kingston* 30 (Jan. 1982), 80. Hospitals founded by women include the Maternity Home of Mercy (1840, Quebec City); the local hospital in Belleville (1886); the Home for Incurables (1892, London); Women's Hospital (1894, New Westminster); the Samaritan Free Hospital for Women (1895, Montreal); and the Home for Incurables (1898, Montreal). National Council of Women of Canada, *Women of Canada, Their Life and Work* (Ottawa 1900, reprinted NCWC 1975), 342–59

21 For the first major survey of minority medicine in Ontario see James Connor, 'Minority Medicine in Ontario, 1795 to 1903: A Study of Medical Pluralism and Its Decline' (PHD thesis, University of Waterloo, 1989).

22 AO, Dr Hugh Mackay Papers, Mss Misc. Coll. 1873 no. 6, MU 2118, Obstetrical Notebook

23 Marion Royce, *Eunice Dyke: Health Care Pioneer* (Toronto: Dundurn Press 1983), 18

24 Because the vast majority of physicians in nineteenth-century Canada were men, references to physicians will be in the masculine.

25 S.F. Wise, 'Sermon Literature and Canadian Intellectual History,' in Michael S. Cross and Gregory S. Kealey, eds., *Pre-Industrial Canada*

1760–1849: Readings in Canadian Social History, vol. 2 (Toronto: McClelland and Stewart 1982), 80

CHAPTER 1 The Victorian World: Doctors, Science, and 'Woman'

1 Jan Cochrane, Abby Hoffman, and Pat Kincaid, *Women in Canadian Life: Sports* (Toronto: Fitzhenry & Whiteside 1977), 26
2 'Woman's Sphere,' *The Harp*, Dec. 1874, 251
3 John Lanceley, *The Domestic Sanctuary* (Hamilton 1878), 13
4 Terry Chapman, 'Women, Sex and Marriage in Western Canada, 1890–1920,' *Alberta History* 33, 4 (autumn 1985): 2
5 Catherine Cleverdon, *The Woman Suffrage Movement in Canada* (Toronto: University of Toronto Press 1950), 6
6 Annual Report of the Maritime Woman's Christian Temperance Union, 1890, 43
7 B.F. Austin, 'What Christ Has Done for Woman,' in his *Woman: Her Characer, Culture and Calling* (Brantford, Ont. 1890), 203–4; Annual Report of the Woman's Auxiliary, Anglican Church, Toronto, 1896, 15
8 Joy Parr, 'Nature and Hierarchy: Reflections on Writing the History of Women and Children,' *Atlantis* 11, 1 (fall 1985): 40; Celia Davies, 'The Health Visitor as Mother's Friend: A Woman's Place in Public Health,' *Social History of Medicine* 1, 1 (April 1988): 40; Alice Kessler-Harris, 'Gender Ideology in Historical Reconstruction: A Case Study from the 1930s,' *Gender and History* 1, 1 (spring 1989), 31–45
9 Linda Kerber, 'Separate Spheres, Female Worlds, Woman's Place: The Rhetoric of Women's History,' *Journal of American History* 75, 1 (June 1988): 17
10 H.E. MacDermot, *History of the Canadian Medical Association, 1867–1921* (Toronto: Murray Printing 1935), 1; Ronald Hamowy, *Canadian Medicine: A Study in Restricted Entry* (Vancouver: Fraser Institute 1984), 14, 34; William Perkins Bull, *From Medicine Man to Medical Man: A Record of a Century and a Half of Progress in Health and Sanitation as Exemplified by Development in Peel* (Toronto: Perkins Bull Foundation, George J. McLeod 1934), 44; Mary Jane Price, 'The Professionalization of Medicine in Ontario during the 19th Century' (MA thesis, McMaster University, 1977), 36; James Connor, 'Minority Medicine in Ontario, 1795 to 1903: A Study of Medical Pluralism and Its Decline' (PHD thesis, University of Waterloo, 1989), 206–7

11 MacDermot, *History of the Canadian Medical Association*, 6, 8–9

12 Perkins Bull, *From Medicine Man*, 74; MacDermot, *History of the Canadian Medical Association*, 3–4; see Connor, 'Minority Medicine in Ontario,' chap. 4, for an excellent description of the rise and fall of Thomsonianism.

13 James Peter Warbasse, *The Doctor and the Public* (College Park, Maryland: McGrath Publishing 1970), 281

14 H.E. MacDermot, 'Early Medical Journalism in Canada,' *Canadian Medical Association Journal* 72 (1955): 537

15 Linda Lee, 'The Myth of Female Equality in Pioneer Society: The Red River Colony as a Test Case' (MA thesis, University of Manitoba, 1978), 109

16 Archives of Ontario (AO), Silverthorn Family Papers, Mss MU 2781, *Farmers' Directory and Housekeepers' Assistant*, 1851

17 Perkins Bull, *From Medicine Man*, 34

18 Elizabeth Gibbs, 'Professionalization of Canadian Medicine, 1850–1970,' paper presented to Annual Meeting, Canadian Historical Association, London, Ontario, 1978, 48

19 Alison Prentice et al., *Canadian Women: A History* (Toronto: Harcourt, Brace, Jovanovich 1988), 122

20 Price, 'The Professionalization of Medicine in Ontario,' 17–18, 23, 77

21 Not all regular or allopathic physicians resorted to bleeding on a regular basis. James Connor, for instance, has suggested that because many physicians practising in Canada were trained in Scotland where bleeding was in low repute, the degree to which they resorted to it was minimal. Very early records of some physicians reinforce this view. Connor, 'Minority Medicine in Ontario,' 251

22 Geoffrey Bilson, *A Darkened House: Cholera in Nineteenth-Century Canada* (Toronto: University of Toronto Press 1980), 161

23 James Connor, 'Of Irregulars and Regulars: Issues in the History of Sectarian Medicine in Nineteenth and Early Twentieth Century America,' unpublished paper, 1984, 32

24 Public Archives of Nova Scotia (PANS), Dr Alexander Forrest Papers, MG 3, Day Book 1830–55, 267–8

25 Kenneth G. Pryke, 'Poor Relief and Health Care in Halifax, 1827–1849,' in Wendy Mitchinson and Janice Dickin McGinnis, eds., *Essays in the*

History of Canadian Medicine (Toronto: McClelland and Stewart 1988), 42

26 In 1867 Quebec granted legal recognition to homeopaths but the educational requirements for them were identical to those for regular trained physicians, as set down in the 1847 act. In 1876 the province introduced a new act recreating the college and giving it additional powers to penalize unlicensed practitioners. Hamowy, *Canadian Medicine*, 49–50, 67, 135

27 MacDermot, *History of the Canadian Medical Association*, 11

28 In 1879 the representation of the Eclectics ceased because of their agreement to merge with the allopaths. Connor, 'Minority Medicine in Ontario,' 386

29 Price, 'The Professionalization of Medicine in Ontario,' 38; Colin D. Howell, 'Elite Doctors and the Development of Scientific Medicine: The Halifax Medical Establishment and 19th Century Medical Professionalism,' in Charles G. Roland, ed., *Health, Disease and Medicine: Essays in Canadian History* (Toronto: Hannah Institute for the History of Medicine 1984), 108–9

30 PANS, Halifax Medical Society Papers, MG 20, no. 181, Minutes of the Nova Scotia Medical Society, 3 June 1861

31 Price, 'The Professionalization of Medicine in Ontario,' 98

32 Charles M. Godfrey, 'The Evolution of Medical Education in Ontario' (MA thesis, University of Toronto, 1975), 38–9; Gibbs, 'Professionalization of Canadian Medicine,' 32

33 McGill University Archives, *Bylaws*, Montreal General Hospital, 1851, 19

34 The creation of medical examining boards or their equivalents in Prince Edward Island (1871), Manitoba (1871), Nova Scotia (1872), New Brunswick (1881), British Columbia (1886), and the North-West Territories (1888) followed the pattern set by Quebec and Ontario. With the exception of PEI, the boards required at the minimum a three- to four-year period of study at an approved medical school, giving preferential treatment to those accredited by a university-connected medical faculty or licence-granting body in the British Empire. Prince Edward Island, perhaps because of the limited number of physicians practising in the province, failed to stipulate a required time of study. It did, however, provide for a medical examination for those not licensed to practise from a recognized British college. Its act also

allowed for homeopathic practice if the physician could show proof of his ability and acquire five signatures of householders supporting his application. Hamowy, *Canadian Medicine*, 148–59. For a study of standardized training in Quebec see Jacques Bernier, 'La standardisation des études médicales et la consolidation de la professions dans la deuxième moitié du xixe siècle,' *Revue d'histoire de l'Amérique française* 37, 1 (juin 1983): 51–65.

35 Connor, 'Minority Medicine in Ontario,' 383. In turn many allopathic doctors proclaimed themselves homeopaths and practised as such.

36 David Coburn, George Torrance, and Joseph Raufert, 'Medical Dominance in Canada in Historical Perspective: The Rise and Fall of Medicine?' *International Journal of Health Services* 13, 3 (1983): 412; C. David Naylor, 'Rural Protest and Medical Professionalism in Turn-of-the-Century Ontario,' *Journal of Canadian Studies* 17, 4 (winter 1982–3): 5–20

37 *Canada Medical Record* 16, 10 (July 1888): 238–9

38 AO, William Canniff Papers, MU 490 package 1, *Historical Sketches of Canadian Medicine and Surgery* 15

39 Theodore Thomas, *A Practical Treatise on the Diseases of Women* (Philadelphia 1868), 50

40 *Canada Lancet* 3, 6 (Feb. 1871): 213

41 For a description of women's struggle to enter medical school see Prentice et al., *Canadian Women*, 160–1, and Carlotta Hacker, *The Indomitable Lady Doctors* (Toronto: Clarke, Irwin 1974).

42 University of Waterloo, Doris Lewis Rare Book Room, Elizabeth Smith Shortt Papers, Maud Service to Elizabeth Smith, Sept. 1877

43 Prentice et al., *Canadian Women*, 161

44 Revised Statutes of Ontario, 1897, c. 318, s. 30

45 Veronica Strong-Boag, 'Canada's Women Doctors: Feminism Constrained,' in Linda Kealey, ed., *A Not Unreasonable Claim: Women and Reform in Canada, 1880s–1920s* (Toronto: Women's Press 1979), 109–29

46 Elizabeth Smith Shortt Papers, letter to E. Shortt from Dr I.D. Macdonald, 18 Dec. 1886

47 *Canada Medical Record* 16, 12 (July 1888): 239; 18, 9 (June 1890): 215, 18, 5 (Feb. 1890): 118–19

48 M.L. Holbrook, 'Parturition without Pain,' in George Napheys, *The Physical Life of Woman: Advice to the Maiden, Wife and Mother* (Toronto 1890), 369–70

49 *Census of Canada*, 1891, vol. 2, 189. This small number meant that women had little impact as physicians in the care and treatment of women. As nurses, however, they were important and while this is a study focusing on physicians' treatment of women, it is necessary to remind ourselves of the existence of those women who often spent more time with patients than physicians.

50 John S. Haller, Jr, *American Medicine in Transition, 1840–1910* (Champaign, Ill.: University of Illinois Press, 1981), 202. Canadian statistics were calculated from figures in *Canada Year Book*, 1915, 90, and *Census of Canada*, 1921, vol. 4, 6.

51 Margaret Andrews, 'Medical Attendance in Vancouver, 1886–1920,' in S.E.D. Shortt, ed., *Medicine in Canadian Society: Historical Perspectives* (Montreal: McGill-Queen's University Press 1981), 417–46

52 McGill University Archives, Dr D.C. MacCallum Papers, MG 2031, 'Women's Medical Problems,' 1901, 1, 31

53 Thomas Laquer, 'Orgasm, Generation, and the Politics of Reproductive Biology,' in Catherine Gallagher and Thomas Laquer, eds., *The Making of the Modern Body* (Berkeley: University of California Press 1987), 4

54 William Buchan, *Domestic Medicine* (London 1813), 410. This book went through numerous editions in the nineteenth century.

55 Carl Berger, *Science, God and Nature in Victorian Canada* (Toronto: University of Toronto Press 1983), 32

56 Alexander Skene, *Medical Gynecology: A Treatise on the Diseases of Women from the Standpoint of the Physician* (New York 1895), 82

57 Gerda Lerner, *The Creation of Patriarchy* (New York: Oxford University Press 1986), 25

58 Holbrook, 'Parturition without Pain,' 312

59 Margarete Sandelowski, *Women, Health and Choice* (Englewood, NJ: Prentice-Hall 1981), 34

60 Elizabeth Spelman, 'Book Review,' *Journal of Medicine and Philosophy* 7, 2 (May 1982): 222

61 R. Pierce, *The People's Common Sense Medical Adviser in Plain English* (Buffalo 1882), 714

62 *Dr Williams Medical Handbook*, nd, np

63 Joy Parr, 'Nature and Hierarchy,' 40

64 Napheys, *The Physical Life of Woman*, 21

65 Hamilton Ayers, *Everyman His Own Doctor* ... (Montreal 1881), 449, suggests that old age for women began at the age of fifty-three and for men at the age of sixty.

66 Jesse Bernard, *The Future of Motherhood* (New York: Penguin 1975), 23

67 *Canadian Magazine* 5 (1895): 189

68 Eugene Becklard, *Physiological Mysteries and Revelations in Love, Courtship and Marriage* (New York 1842), 20, 112

69 Thomas, *A Practical Treatise on the Diseases of Women*, 497

70 Benjamin Grant Jefferis, *Searchlights on Health: Light on Dark Corners* (Fredericton 1894), 194; Pye Henry Chavasse, *Advice to a Wife on the Management of Her Own Health and on the Treatment of Some of the Complaints Incidental to Pregnancy, Labour, and Suckling* (Toronto 1882), 8, 89

71 Pierce, *The People's Common Sense Medical Adviser*, 736; Holbrook, 'Parturition without Pain,' 307; William Goodell, *Lessons in Gynaecology* (Philadelphia 1890), 570

72 Holbrook, 'Parturition without Pain,' 311

73 Napheys, *The Physical Life of Woman*, 24

74 Ibid., 269

75 Goodell, *Lessons in Gynaecology*, 550; Skene, *Medical Gynecology*, 78–91

76 Laquer, 'Orgasm, Generation, and the Politics of Reproductive Biology,' 4–5

77 Buchan, *Domestic Medicine*, 410

78 Becklard, *Physiological Mysteries*, 105

79 William Carpenter, *Principles of Human Physiology* (London 1869), 728–9

80 University of Western Ontario, Richard Maurice Bucke Papers, B 8, 'The Moral Nature and the Great Sympathetic' (New York 1878), 25; see also Skene, *Medical Gynecology*, 72, for a similar sentiment.

81 Henry Lyman, *The Practical Home Physician and Enclopedia of Medicine* (Guelph 1884), 842

82 Skene, *Medical Gynecology*, 66, 80, 70

83 Berger, *Science, God and Nature*, 32

84 Jefferis, *Searchlights*, 126, 60

85 Carpenter, *Principles of Human Physiology*, 911–12

86 Skene, *Medical Gynecology*, 80, 82
87 Bucke Papers, B 5, 'The Functions of the Great Sympathetic Nervous System,' 34
88 Pierce, *The People's Common Sense Medical Adviser*, 710
89 Jefferis, *Searchlights*, 25, 30
90 Berger, *Science, God and Nature*, xii
91 Carpenter, *Human Physiology*, 729
92 Skene, *Medical Gynecology*, 82 (emphasis mine)
93 *Manual of Hygiene for Schools and Colleges* (Toronto 1886), 240–5
94 *Dominion Medical Monthly* 3, 4 (Oct. 1894): 112
95 Dr D.C. MacCallum Papers, MG 2031, box 3, 'Inaugural Address,' 9
96 James Connor, 'To Be Rendered Unconscious of Torture: Anaesthesia in Canada, 1847–1920' (M. Phil. thesis, University of Waterloo, 1983), iv; James Connor, 'Joseph Lister's System of Wound Management and the Canadian Medical Practitioner, 1867–1900' (MA thesis, University of Western Ontario, 1981), 85; Charles G. Roland, 'The Early Years of Antiseptic Surgery in Canada,' *Journal of the History of Medicine and Allied Sciences* 22 (1967): 381–8. Not everyone agreed with the procedures set down by Lister. Those opposed based their objections not on 'experimental evidence but rather on emotion or on "common sense."' William Canniff, a Toronto surgeon and author of the first Canadian textbook in pathology, was a great believer in the healing power of nature and did not support the interference advocated by Lister. However, by the 1880s few practitioners were really challenging antiseptics or germ theory. S.E.D. Shortt, '"Before the Age of Miracles": The Rise, Fall and Rebirth of General Practice in Canada, 1890–1940,' in Roland, ed., *Health, Disease and Medicine*, 248
97 Howell, 'Elite Doctors,' 106
98 S.E.D. Shortt, 'Physicians, Science and Status: Historiographic Issues in the Professionalization of Nineteenth-Century Medicine,' paper presented for the Workshop on Professionals and Professionalization in the Nineteenth and Twentieth Centuries, University of Western Ontario, March 1981, 26. A reworked version of the paper was published as 'Physicians, Science, and Status: Issues in the Professionalization of Anglo-American Medicine in the Nineteenth Century,' *Medical History* 27 (1983): 51–68.

99 Henry B. Shafer, 'The American Medical Profession 1783 to 1850' (PHD thesis, Columbia University, 1937), 11

100 Berger, *Science, God and Nature,* 47

101 Silverthorn Papers, *Farmers' Directory and Housekeepers' Assistant* (1851)

102 Ruth Howes, 'Adelaide Hunter Hoodless,' in Mary Quayle Innis, ed., *The Clear Spirit: Twenty Canadian Women and Their Times* (Toronto: University of Toronto Press 1966), 112

103 In the early 1880s there was a significant expansion in the discovery of 'causal' agents of specific diseases – gonorrhoea, cholera, typhoid, tuberculosis, and diptheria. Shortt, 'Before the Age of Miracles,' 139

104 Regina Markell Morantz-Sanchez, *Sympathy and Science: Women Physicians in American Medicine* (New York: Oxford University Press 1985), 229

105 S.E.D. Shortt, 'The Canadian Hospital in the Nineteenth Century: An Historical Lament,' *Journal of Canadian Studies* 18, 4 (winter 1983–4), 8

106 PANS, Victoria General Hospital Papers, RG 25, series B, Patient Records, patient KM, no. 3532

107 Pryke, 'Poor Relief and Health Care in Halifax,' 39–61; Shortt, 'The Canadian Hospital in the Nineteenth Century,' 9

108 Queen's University Archives, Kingston General Hospital Papers, Admission Register, 1853, 1856, 1861, 1866

109 Margaret Angus, *Kingston General Hospital: A Social and Institutional History* (Montreal: McGill-Queen's University Press 1973), 22; based on the 1723 patients who entered in 1853, 1856, 1861, 1866; Queen's University Archives, Kingston General Hospital Papers, Annual Report, Kingston General Hospital 1860

110 City Archives of Vancouver, Royal Columbian Hospital Papers, Rules for Patients, 1861; Queen Elizabeth Hospital Archives, Annual Report, Toronto Home for Incurables, 1887, 11–12

111 *By-laws and Regulations,* Victoria General Hospital 1896, 28–9

112 Francis Shepherd, *Origin and History of the Montreal General Hospital,* nd, np, 14; Angus, *Kingston General Hospital,* 57, 63

113 British Columbia Archives and Record Service, Annual Report, Directors, Provincial Royal Jubilee Hospital, 1876, 42

114 Shortt, 'The Canadian Hospital in the Nineteenth Century,' 9

115 McGill University Archives, Annual Report, Montreal General Hospital, 1858, 13; 1878, 31–4

116 Sandelowski, *Women, Health and Choice*, vii

117 Spelman, 'Book Review,' 224

118 Skene, *Medical Gynecology*, 64, 76–7

119 Thomas, *A Practical Treatise on the Diseases of Women*, 511

CHAPTER 2 The Frailty of Women

1 Mary Carus-Wilson, *Medical Education of Women* (Montreal 1895), 22

2 Alexander Skene, *Medical Gynecology: A Treatise on the Diseases of Women from the Standpoint of the Physician* (New York 1895), 64

3 William Perkins Bull, *From Medicine Man to Medical Man: A Record of a Century and a Half of Progress in Health and Sanitation as Exemplified by Developments in Peel* (Toronto: Perkins Bull Foundation, George J. McLeod 1934), 33

4 Philanthropos, *A Medical Essay; or the Nurse and Family Physician* (np, 1834), 30

5 John Wright, 'Hysteria and Mechanical Man,' *Journal of the History of Ideas* 41, 2 (April 1980): 234

6 *Jayne's Medical Almanac and Guide to Health for British North America* (Philadelphia 1863), 7

7 *Canada Health Journal* 1, 5 (May 1870): 69

8 *Sanitary Journal* 2, 2 (Feb. 1876): 172–3

9 Pye Henry Chavasse, *Advice to a Wife on the Management of Her Own Health and on the Treatment of Some of the Complaints Incidental to Pregnancy, Labour and Suckling* (Toronto 1882), 2

10 Hamilton Ayers, *Ayers' Everyman His Own Doctor* (Montreal 1881), 295

11 Edward Playter, 'The Physical Culture of Women,' in B.F. Austin, ed., *Woman: Her Character, Culture and Calling* (Brantford 1890), 225

12 Chavasse, *Advice to Wife*, 3

13 *Canadian Practitioner* 8, 1 (Jan. 1886): 43

14 Alvin Wood Chase, *Dr Chase's Third, Last and Complete Recipe Book and Household Physician* (Detroit and Windsor 1892), 210

15 See Stephen Jay Gould, 'Hutton's Purpose,' in his *Hen's Teeth and Horse's Toes* (New York: W.W. Norton 1983), 79–83.

16 Chavasse, *Advice to Wife*, 22

17 Arthur Edis, *Diseases of Women: A Manual for Students and Practitioners* (Philadelphia 1882), 20

18 *Canada Medical and Surgical Journal* 10 (Jan. 1882): 343; *Canadian Practitioner* 21 (May 1896): 330

19 Playter, 'The Physical Culture of Women,' 214

20 Michael B. Katz, *The People of Hamilton, Canada West* (Cambridge Mass.: Harvard University Press 1975), 189–90

21 See Patricia Branca, *Silent Sisterhood: Middle Class Women in the Victorian Home* (Pittsburgh: Carnegie-Mellon University Press 1975).

22 Roderick P. Beaujot and Kevin McQuillan, 'Social Effects of Demographic Change: Canada 1851–1981,' *Journal of Canadian Studies* 21 (spring 1986): 59

23 F.H. Leacy, ed., *Historical Statistics of Canada* 2nd ed. (Ottawa: Statistics Canada 1983), B 59–74; Beth Light and Joy Parr, eds., *Canadian Women on the Move* (Toronto: New Hogtown and OISE Press 1983), 255

24 Statistics are based on the *Fourth Census of Canada*, 1901, 56–75.

25 Public Archives of Nova Scotia (PANS), Reports of the City of Halifax, RG 25, series B, vol. 1, Report for the Provincial and City Hospital, 1867, 6–7

26 Annual Report, Directors, Provincial Royal Jubilee Hospital, 1896, 25

27 Based on the annual reports of the Montreal General Hospital

28 Judith Fingard, *Jack in Port: Sailortowns of Eastern Canada* (Toronto: University of Toronto Press 1982), 125

29 *Sixth Census of Canada*, 1921, vol. 4, xii

30 Jacalyn Duffin, 'A Rural Practice in Nineteenth-Century Ontario: The Continuing Medical Education of James Miles Langstaff,' *Canadian Bulletin of Medical History* 5, 1 (summer 1988): 8

31 Margaret W. Andrews, 'Medical Attendance in Vancouver, 1886–1920,' in S.E.D. Shortt, ed., *Medicine in Canadian Society: Historical Perspectives* (Montreal: McGill-Queen's University Press 1981), 429

32 Academy of Medicine Library, Dr Alexander Primrose Papers, based on a survey of 1038 patients between 1888–1899

33 *Canada Lancet* 3, 3 (Nov. 1870): 91

34 *Canada Medical Record* 7, 12 (Sept. 1879): 319; Queen's University Archives, C.N. Mallory Papers, Notebook 1885; *Canada Medical Record* 16, 3 (Dec. 1888): 70; 19, 4 (Jan. 1891): 74; Henry Jacques Garrigues, *A Text-book of the Diseases of Women* (Philadelphia 1894), 125–9; Paul

Mundé, *A Practical Treatise on the Diseases of Women* (Philadelphia 1891), 35

35 William Goodell, *Lessons in Gynaecology* (Philadelphia 1890), 553

36 Garrigues, *A Text-book*, 125–9; Goodell, *Lessons in Gynaecology*, 552; Mundé, *Diseases of Women*, 34–5; Playter, 'The Physical Culture of Woman,' 226

37 Jane Lewis, ed., 'Introduction: Reconstructing Women's Experience of Home and Family,' in her *Labour and Love: Women's Experience of Home and Family 1850–1940* (Oxford: Basil Blackwell 1986), 15

38 George Napheys, *The Physical Life of Woman: Advice to Maiden, Wife and Mother* (Toronto 1890), 269

39 Garrigues, *A Text-book*, 125–9; Mundé, *Diseases of Women*, 35, 43–4

40 *Canadian Medical Times* 1, 10 (Aug. 1873): 78

41 Garrigues, *A Text-book*, 129; *Canada Medical Record*, 17, 5 (Feb. 1889): 98

42 *Dominion Medical Monthly and Ontario Medical Journal* 8, 2 (Feb. 1897): 146–7

43 McGill University Archives, Montreal General Hospital Papers, RG 96, Gynecological Casebook, vol. 273, Diseases of Women Casebook, patient EB, admitted 25 May 1882, 87

44 Ibid., patient Madam B, admitted 8 April 1882

45 Henry Lyman, *The Practical Home Physician and Encyclopedia of Medicine* (Guelph 1884), 1012

46 Napheys, *The Physical Life of Women*, 269

47 Garrigues, *A Text-book*, 125–8

48 Charles Penrose, *A Text-book of Diseases of Women* (Philadelphia 1905), 20

49 In 1881 11.3 per cent of women between the ages of 45 and 49 had never married and, in 1891, 9.4 per cent. Ellen Gee, 'Marriage in Nineteenth-Century Canada,' *Canadian Review of Sociology and Anthropology* 19, 3 (1982): 315

50 Alison Prentice et al., *Canadian Women: A History* (Toronto: Harcourt, Brace, Jovanovich 1988), 152–3

51 Dr Elizabeth Mitchell, 'The Rise of Athleticism among Women and Girls,' in National Council of Women of Canada Yearbook, 1895, 107, cited in Helen Lenskyj, *Out of Bounds: Women, Sport and Sexuality* (Toronto: Women's Press 1986), 23

52 Ira Warren, *The Household Physician* (Boston 1865), 91; *Sanitary Journal* 2, 2 (Feb. 1876): 172–3

53 Theodore Thomas, *A Practical Treatise on the Diseases of Women* (Philadelphia 1868), 53–4, 61; *Public Health Magazine and Literary Review* 1 (May 1876): 342–3

54 *Sanitary Journal* 2, 12 (Dec. 1876): 335

55 Garrigues, *A Text-book*, 126; Mundé, *Diseases of Women*, 36

56 *Canada Lancet* 12 (Feb. 1880): 187

57 *Canadian Practitioner* 9 (Dec. 1884): 363; *Canada Medical Record* 18, 2 (Nov. 1889): 25–7; Penrose, *A Text-book*, 20; *Canada Medical Record* 19, 4 (Jan. 1891): 74; Garrigues, *A Text-book*, 125–9; Mundé, *Diseases of Women*, 36

58 Mundé, *Diseases of Women*, 35; *Canada Medical Record* 18, 2 (Nov. 1889): 25–7; Penrose, *A Text-book*, 20; Goodell, *Lessons in Gynaecology*, 548–52

59 Skene, *Medical Gynecology*, 23

60 Playter, 'Physical Culture,' 216

61 Skene, *Medical Gynecology*, 20–3

62 Chavasse, *Advice to a Wife*, 270–2; Playter, 'Physical Culture,' 225

63 *Dominion Medical Monthly and Ontario Medical Journal* 7, 3 (Sept. 1896): 255–6; 8, 2 (Feb. 1897): 134–5

64 *Canada Medical Record* 24 (Aug. 1896): 555

65 See reference to this in *Canadian Practitioner* 21 (Nov. 1896): 848.

66 Ibid. (May 1896): 329–32; 21 (Nov. 1896): 848–9

67 *Dominion Medical Monthly and Ontario Medical Journal* 11, 1 (July 1898): 27–30

68 *Unfettered Canadian* (May 1894): 105

69 Thomas, *A Practical Treatise on the Diseases of Women*, 55–7

70 *Canada Health Journal* 1, 2 (Feb. 1870): 26–7

71 *Public Health Magazine and Literary Review* 1 (Dec. 1875): 172; 2 (April 1877): 308

72 *Sanitary Journal* 2, 12 (Dec. 1876): 335

73 *Canada Health Journal* 1, 2 (Feb. 1870): 26–7; *Public Health Magazine* 1 (Dec. 1876): 172–3

74 *Sanitary Journal* 2, 2 (Feb. 1876): 169–70

75 *Public Health Magazine* 2 (May 1877): 310–11

76 *Canada Medical Record* 7, 7 (April 1879): 188; Playter, 'Physical Culture,' 228

77 *Sanitary Journal* 2, 2 (Feb. 1876): 171

78 *Canada Medical Record* 8, 8 (May 1880): 216; Chavasse, *Advice to a Wife*, 63, 262; *Canadian Practitioner* 9 (Dec. 1884): 363; Lyman, *Practical Home Physician*, 885; *Manual of Hygiene for Schools and Colleges* (Toronto 1886), 140–1; *Canada Medical Record* 17, 3 (Dec. 1888): 60–70; 18, 2 (Nov. 1889): 25–7; 17, 5 (Feb. 1889): 98; Benjamin Grant Jefferis, *Searchlights on Health* (Fredericton 1894), 101–3; *Canada Medical Record* 19, 4 (Jan. 1891): 74; Garrigues, *A Text-book*, 125–9; Goodell, *Lessons in Gynaecology*, 548; Skene, *Medical Gynecology*, 11–15

79 Garrigues, *A Text-book*, 126–7

80 Mundé, *Diseases of Women*, 40

81 Goodell, *Lessons in Gynaecology*, 548

82 *Canadian Practitioner* 9 (Dec. 1884): 363; Garrigues, *A Text-book*, 125–9; Mundé, *Diseases of Women*, 35; *Canada Medical Record* 19, 4 (Jan. 1891): 74; Penrose, *A Text-book* 18–19; Goodell, *Lessons in Gynaecology*, 548

83 *Canada Lancet* 15 (May 1883): 264; *Manual of Hygiene*, 139

84 Chase, *Dr Chase's*, 210

85 Annual Report, Woman's Christian Temperance Union, Ontario, 1894, 110

86 Stephen Kern, *Anatomy and Destiny: A Cultural History of the Human Body* (Indianapolis: Bobbs-Merrill 1975), 15

87 *Canada Lancet* 15 (May 1883): 265

88 *Canada Medical Record* 8, 8 (May 1880): 216

89 Skene, *Medical Gynecology*, 12

90 Kern, *Anatomy and Destiny*, 10

91 *Canada Medical Record*, 17, 5 (Feb. 1889): 97; 17, 3 (Dec. 1888): 70; 19, 4 (Jan. 1891): 74

92 Chavasse, *Advice to a Wife*, 106

93 E.A. Hardy and Honora M. Cochrane, *Centennial Story: The Board of Education for the City of Toronto 1850–1950* (Toronto: Thomas Nelson 1950), 173

94 Edward Shorter has argued that the medical focus on corsets was without substance since most women did not wear them. Doctors, however, were responding to the class of women who did – largely

middle class. Edward Shorter, *A History of Women's Bodies* (New York: Basic Books 1982), 29–30

95 Doctors did not really know much about malnutrition. Vitamins had not been discovered and calories were unknown.

96 Sheila Ryan Johannson, 'Sex and Death in Victorian England: An Examination of Age and Sex Specific Death Rates, 1840–1910,' in Martha Vicinus, ed., *A Widening Sphere: Changing Roles of Victorian Women* (Bloomington: Indiana University Press 1972), 170–1

97 *Canada Lancet* 27 (Nov. 1894): 97

98 Annual Report of the National Council of Women of Canada, 1894, 230

99 Thomas, *Diseases of Women*, 52–8

100 *Canada Medical Record* 18, 2 (Nov. 1889): 25–30; Mundé, *Diseases of Women*, 34–5

101 Mundé, *Diseases of Women*, 34, 46; *Montreal Medical Journal* 25, 9 (March 1897); 682; Skene, *Medical Gynecology*, 70; Penrose, *A Text-book*, 18

102 Thomas, *Diseases of Women*, 53; Lyman, *The Practical Home Physician*, 981; Mundé, *Diseases of Women*, 34–5; *Canada Medical Record* 17, 2 (Nov. 1889): 27

103 Goodell, *Lessons in Gynaecology*, 548

104 *Canada Medical and Surgical Journal* 6 (Feb. 1878): 337–50; the version I used was in his papers, McGill University Archives, D.C. MacCallum Papers, MG 2031 'Report of the University Lying-in Hospital, Montreal for Eight Years, 1867–1875,' 5–6.

105 *Canada Medical Record* 17, 2 (Nov. 1889): 27; Joseph Cook, *A Nurse's Handbook of Obstetrics for Use in Training-Schools* (Philadelphia: J.B. Lippincott 1903), 21

106 Chase, *Dr Chase's*, 210

107 Chavasse, *Advice to a Wife*, 22; Pye Henry Chavasse, *Advice to a Mother on the Management of Her Children and on the Treatment on the Moment of Some of Their More Pressing Illnesses and Accidents* (Toronto 1879), 8; R. Pierce, *The People's Common Sense Medical Adviser in Plain English* (Buffalo 1882), 716–18

108 *Montreal Medical Journal* 25, 9 (March 1897): 682; Goodell, *Lessons in Gynaecology*, 548; Penrose, *A Text-book*, 20; Garrigues, *A Text-book*, 125–9

109 Goodell, *Lessons in Gynaecology*, 551, 561; *Montreal Medical Journal* 25, 9 (March 1897): 751–2; Penrose, *A Text-book*, 20
110 Skene, *Medical Gynecology*, 27–8
111 Robert Craig Brown and Ramsay Cook, *Canada 1896–1921: A Nation Transformed* (Toronto: McClelland and Stewart 1974), xiii
112 Skene, *Medical Gynecology*, 65
113 Michel Foucault, *The Birth of the Clinic: An Archaeology of Medical Perception* (New York: Pantheon Books 1973), 32

CHAPTER 3   Three Mysteries: Puberty, Menstruation, and Menopause

1 McGill University Archives, D.C. MacCallum Papers, MG 2031, 'Diseases Peculiar to Women,' 142
2 Carl Berger, *Science, God and Nature* (Toronto: University of Toronto Press 1983), 15
3 Henry Garrigues, *A Text-book of the Diseases of Women* (Philadelphia 1894), 114; William Carpenter, *Principles of Human Physiology* (London 1869), 832–3; William Tyler Smith, *The Modern Practice of Midwifery: A Course of Lectures on Obstetrics* (New York 1858), 86
4 Tyler Smith, *The Modern Practice of Midwifery: A Course of Lectures on Obstetrics*, 86
5 Carpenter, *Principles of Human Physiology*, 832–3
6 Arthur W. Edis, *Diseases of Women: A Manual for Students and Practitioners* (Philadelphia 1882), 133; Alfred Lewis Galabin, *A Manual of Midwifery* (Philadelphia 1886), 53
7 Ira Warren, *The Household Physician* (Boston 1865), 341–2
8 Archives of Ontario, William Canniff Papers, MU 491 package 5, taken from *The Leader*, 11 Oct. 1870
9 Austin Flint, *Physiology of Man* (New York 1874), 459
10 University of Western Ontario Archives, Richard Maurice Bucke Papers, B5, 'The Functions of the Great Sympathetic Nervous System,' 25
11 J. Price, *Indians of Canada: Cultural Dynamics* (Scarborough, Ont.: Prentice-Hall 1979), 194
12 Beth Light and Joy Parr, eds., *Canadian Women on the Move 1867–1926* (Toronto: New Hogtown Press and OISE 1983), 55
13 Henry Lyman, *The Practical Home Physician* (Guelph 1884), 872

14 R. Pierce, *The People's Common Sense Medical Adviser in Plain English* (Buffalo 1882), 710–11

15 Theophilus Parvin, *The Science and Art of Obstetrics* (Philadelphia 1886), 90; William Tyler Smith, *Parturition and the Principles and Practice of Obstetrics* (Philadelphia 1849), 89; see also P. Cazeaux, *Theoretical and Practical Treatise on Midwifery* (Philadelphia 1837), 103; Kenneth Neader Fenwick, *Manual of Obstetrics, Gynaecology and Pediatrics* (Kingston, Ont. 1889), 8; Galabin, *A Manual of Midwifery*, 53.

16 Alexander Skene, *Medical Gynecology: A Treatise on the Diseases of Women from the Standpoint of the Physician* (New York 1895), 80

17 George Grant, 'Education and Co-education,' *Canada Educational Monthly* (Oct. 1879), 514

18 George H. Napheys, *The Physical Life of Woman: Advice to the Maiden, Wife and Mother* (Toronto 1890), 24

19 William Buchan, *Domestic Medicine* (London 1813), 413

20 Warren, *The Household Physician*, 340; *Hostetter's United States Almanac for 1867*

21 Joseph Brown Cooke, *A Nurse's Handbook of Obstetrics for Use in Training-Schools* (Philadelphia 1903), 35; Buchan, *Domestic Medicine*, 411–12

22 *Manual of Hygiene for Schools and Colleges* (Toronto 1886), 240–5; John Baldy, *An American Text-book of Gynaecology* (Philadelphia 1894), 97; Skene, *Medical Gynecology*, 18–19

23 Parvin, *Science and Art of Obstetrics*, 91

24 Theodore Thomas, *A Practical Treatise on the Diseases of Women* (Philadelphia 1868), 54

25 Lyman, *Practical Home Physician*, 531

26 Vern Bullough and Martha Voight, 'Women, and Menstruation, and Nineteenth Century Medicine,' *Bulletin of the History of Medicine* 47, 1 (Jan.–Feb. 1973): 69–71

27 *Sanitary Journal* 1 (1874): 56

28 *Canada Lancet* 6, 7 (March 1874): 233–4

29 Garrigues, *A Text-book*, 125

30 *Canada Lancet* 6, 7 (March 1874): 233, *Canada Medical Record* 18, 2 (Nov. 1889): 25–7; Garrigues, *A Text-book*, 125–9; Paul Mundé, *A Practical Treatise on the Diseases of Women* (Philadelphia 1868), 34–5;

Canada Medical Record 19, 4 (Jan. 1891): 74; *Canadian Practitioner* 16, 6 (June 1891): 261; *Dominion Medical Monthly* 3, 4 (Oct. 1894): 112; William Goodell, *Lessons in Gynaecology* (Philadelphia 1890), 549; Charles Penrose, *A Text-book of Diseases of Women* (Philadelphia 1905), 20; Sir Thomas Watson, *Lectures on the Principles and Practice of Physic*, ed. David Francis Condie (Philadelphia 1858), 423

31 *Canada Medical Record* 7, 12 (Sept. 1879): 319

32 *Ibid.*, 18, 5 (Feb. 1890): 119

33 Judith Fingard, 'The New Woman Goes to College: Dalhousie Coeds 1881–1921,' unpublished paper, 1986, 15

34 Skene, *Medical Gynecology*, 32–4. Such an attitude was quite in keeping with notions in the wider society. An article in the *Queen's College Journal* of 1876 made it clear that it was fine for a woman to learn modern languages, but not the ancient ones; poetry, music, and painting, too, were safe, but not mathematics or metaphysics. Ramsay Cook and Wendy Mitchinson, eds., *The Proper Sphere: Woman's Place in Canadian Society* (Toronto: Oxford University Press 1976), 123–4

35 *Canada Medical and Surgical Journal* (Oct. 1887): 185

36 Goodell, *Lessons in Gynaecology*, 549

37 *Christian Guardian*, 16 Oct. 1872, 332; Mary Carus-Wilson, *Medical Education for Women* (Montreal 1895), 22; *Canadian Monthly and National Review* 1, 3 (March 1872): 249–64, cited in Cook and Mitchinson, eds., *The Proper Sphere*, 39

38 John William Dawson, *Thoughts on the Higher Education of Women* (Montreal 1871), 11–12; Principal Grant, 'Education and Co-Education,' *Rose Belford's Canadian Monthly* 2 (1879): 514; M, 'The Human Question,' *Rose Belford's Canadian Monthly* 2 (1879): 574

39 Fidelis, 'Higher Education for Women,' *Canadian Monthly* 7, 2 (Feb. 1875): 152, 148; Donna Ronish, 'The Development of Higher Education for Women at McGill University from 1857 to 1899 with Special Reference to the Role of Sir John William Dawson,' MA thesis, McGill University, 1972), 52

40 *Queen's College Journal*, 27 Jan. 1877

41 Hugh E. MacDermot, *Maude Abbott: A Memoir* (Toronto: Macmillan 1941), 10

42 Janice Delaney, M.J. Lupton, and Emily Toth. *The Curse: A Cultural*

History of Menstruation (New York: Mentor 1976), 14, 39; quotes are from King James Version.

43 Tyler Smith, *The Modern Practice of Midwifery*, 89

44 Alvin Wood Chase, *Dr Chase's Third, Last and Complete Receipt Book and Household Physician* (Detroit and Windsor 1892), 208

45 Warren, *The Household Physician*, 355

46 Thomas, *A Practical Treatise*, 57; Light and Parr, eds., *Canadian Women on the Move*, 57

47 Public Archives of Nova Scotia (PANS), Victoria General Hospital Papers, RG 25, series B, Patient Records box 35 202/00, patient AF, admitted 12 Feb. 1900

48 Lyman, *The Practical Home Physician*, 515; John Thorburn, *A Practical Treatise of the Diseases of Women* (London 1885), 96–7

49 *Canadian Practitioner* 9, 12 (Dec. 1884): 361

50 *Canada Medical and Surgical Journal* 6 (July 1877): 22–4

51 McGill University Archives, Montreal General Hospital Papers, RG 95, vol. 275, Gynecology Casebook, patient AS, 11 May 1888, 111–12

52 James Ricci, *One Hundred Years of Gynecology* 1800–1900 (Philadelphia 1945), 14

53 Harvey Graham, *Eternal Eve* (Altrincham, Eng.: William Heinemann 1950), 497–9

54 Carpenter, *Principles of Human Physiology*, 834

55 Delaney et al., *The Curse*, 60

56 *Canadian Practitioner* 9, 4 (April 1884): 115; Pierce, *The People's Common Sense Medical Advisor*, 221

57 MacCallum Papers, MG 2031, 'On Women's Medical Problems,' 130

58 Mundé, *A Practical Treatise on the Diseases of Women*, 35; Penrose, *A Text-book of Diseases of Women*, 20; Chase, *Dr Chase's*, 209

59 Garrigues, *A Text-book*, 127

60 Mundé, *Diseases of Women*, 40; *Montreal Medical Journal* 25, 9 (March 1897): 682; Garrigues, *A Text-book*, 127; Baldy, *An American Text-book of Gynaecology*, 97

61 John Hett, *The Sexual Organs: Their Use and Abuse* (Berlin, Ont. 1899), 33

62 PANS, Victoria General Hospital Papers, RG 25, series B 1892–3 (III-6)

63 Garrigues, *A Text-book*, 117

64 James Connor, 'Joseph Lister's System of Wound Management and the Canadian Medical Practitioner, 1867–1900' (MA thesis, University of Western Ontario, 1981), 132

65 MacCallum Papers, 'On Women's Medical Problems,' 133

66 Ibid., 111

67 *Montreal Medical Journal* 25, 9 (March 1897): 681

68 Caroline Whitbeck, 'Women and Medicine: An Introduction,' *Journal of Medicine and Philosophy* 7, 2 (May 1982): 121

69 PANS, Victoria General Hospital Papers, RG 25, series B, Patient Records box 35 452/00, patient Mrs H, admitted 24 Aug. 1900

70 William Buchan, *Domestic Medicine*, 416

71 Annual Report, Provincial and City Hospital, 1866–7, 70–1

72 Jayne's *Medical Almanac and Guide to Health for British North America* (Philadelphia 1863), 9

73 Light and Parr, eds., *Canadian Women on the Move*, 57

74 Pierce, *The People's Common Sense Medical Adviser*, 730–1; Light and Parr, eds., *Canadian Women on the Move*, 57

75 Montreal General Hospital Papers, RG 96, vol. 273, Diseases of Women Casebook (University Dispensary), patient Miss H, 17 June 1882, 107

76 Pye Henry Chavasse, *Advice to a Wife on the Management of Her Own Health and on the Treatment of Some of the Complaints Incidental to Pregnancy, Labour, and Suckling* (Toronto 1882), 111; Thornburn, *A Practical Treatise*, 192; Napheys, *The Physical Life of Woman*, 276–7

77 Napheys, *The Physical Life of Woman*, 274

78 Chavasse, *Advice to a Wife*, 105

79 Thornburn, *A Practical Treatise*, 192–3

80 Napheys, *The Physical Life of Woman*, 272, 275

81 Hamilton Ayers, *Ayers' Everyman His Own Doctor* (Montreal 1881), 451

82 William Playfair, *A Treatise on the Science and Practice of Midwifery* (London 1880), 85

83 Ayers, *Everyman*, 293

84 Baldy, *An American Textbook of Gynaecology*, 84–5

85 *Canadian Practitioner* 18, 11 (Nov. 1898): 847

86 MacCallum Papers, 'On Women's Medical Problems,' 153

87 Skene, *Medical Gynecology*, 80

88 *Canada Lancet* 26, 5 (Jan. 1894): 142; *Canadian Practitioner* 19, 7 (July 1894): 495

CHAPTER 4 Sexuality in Women

1 Mary Rubio and Elizabeth Waterston, eds., *Selected Journals of L.M. Montgomery*, vol. 1: *1889–1910* (Toronto: Oxford University Press 1986), 217

2 Patricia Branca, *Women in Europe since 1750* (London: Croom Helm 1978), 90

3 Arthur Imhof, 'From the Old Mortality Pattern to the New: Implications of a Radical Change from the Sixteenth to the Twentieth Century,' *Bulletin of the History of Medicine* 59, 1 (spring 1985): 12–13

4 Beth Light and Alison Prentice, eds., *Pioneer and Gentlewomen of British North America 1713–1867* (Toronto: New Hogtown Press 1980), 120

5 Peter Cominos, 'Late Victorian Sexual Respectability and the Social System,' *International Review of Social History* 8, 1 (1963): 37; Daniel Scott Smith and Michael Hindus, 'Premarital Pregnancy in America 1640–1971: An Overview and Interpretation,' in Vivian C. Fox and Martin H. Quitt, eds., *Loving, Parenting and Dying: The Family Cycle in England and America, Past and Present* (New York: Psychohistory Press 1980), 206; Mark Poster, *Foucault, Marxism and History: Mode of Production Versus Mode of Information* (Cambridge, Eng. Polity Press 1984), 122

6 Cominos, 'Late Victorian Sexual Respectability and the Social System,' 33; Edward Shorter has also seen the middle classes as exhibiting sexual control and the lower classes being much more open about their sexuality. See Elizabeth Fee, 'Psychology, Sexuality and Social Control in Victorian England,' *Social Science Quarterly* 58, 4 (March 1978): 632–3, for a critique of Shorter.

7 Stephen Kern, *Anatomy and Destiny: A Cultural History of the Human Body* (Indianapolis: Bobbs-Merrill 1975), 36–7

8 Daniel Scott Smith and Michael S. Hindus, 'Premarital Pregnancy in America 1640–1971: An Overview and Interpretation,' *Journal of Interdisciplinary History* 5, 4 (spring 1975): 549–51

9 Charles Rosenberg, 'Sexuality, Class and Role in 19th-Century America,' *American Quarterly* 25 (May 1975): 135

10 Marta Danylewycz, *Taking the Veil: An Alternative to Marriage, Motherhood, and Spinsterhood in Quebec, 1840–1920* (Toronto: McClelland and Stewart 1987), 39

11 Carol Bacchi, 'Race Regeneration and Social Purity: A Study of the Social Attitudes of Canada's English-Speaking Suffragists,' *Histoire Sociale* 9, 22 (Nov. 1978): 470

12 Carol Christ, 'Victorian Masculinity and the Angel in the House,' in Martha Vicinus, ed., *Suffer and Be Still: Women in the Victorian Age* (Bloomington: Indiana University Press 1977), 147

13 G.J. Barker-Benfield, *The Horrors of the Half-Known Life: Male Attitudes toward Women and Sexuality in Nineteenth-Century America* (New York: Harper and Row 1977), xiii

14 Peter Gay, *The Bourgeois Experience: Victoria to Freud* vol. 1: *The Education of the Sexes* (New York: Oxford University Press 1983), 197

15 Marion S. Goldman, *Goldiggers and Silver Miners: Prostitution and Social Life on the Comstock Lode* (Ann Arbor: University of Michigan Press 1981), 47

16 Kern, *Anatomy and Destiny*, 42; Regina Morantz, 'Making Women Modern: Middle Class Women and Health Reform in 19th Century America,' in Patricia Branca, ed., *The Medicine Show: Patients, Physicians and the Perplexities of the Health Revolution in Modern Society* (New York: Science History Publications 1977), 110; Goldman, *Goldiggers and Silver Miners*, 47; Christ, 'Victorian Masculinity,' 152

17 Bacchi, 'Race Regeneration,' 471–3. One of the problems with the historiographical discussion of sexuality is that most of the theories put forward to explain Victorian sexual norms remain in the realm of conjecture. They are difficult, if not impossible, to prove. They also treat the century as a monolith, which it was not. In *American Beauty*, Lois Banner discerned an openness around mid-century that gave rise to a new and different repressiveness by the 1870s, which for her was the 'real' Victorianism. But even this was in retreat by the 1890s. Lois W. Banner, *American Beauty* (Chicago: University of Chicago Press 1983), 8

18 Jennifer Stoddart, 'Feminism in Paris: A Review Article,' *Canadian Newsletter of Research on Women* 7, 1 (March 1978): 64; Michel Foucault, *The History of Sexuality* (New York: Vintage Books 1980), 17–49. One of the problems with Foucault's interpretation is that he does not see that discussion of sexuality and repression of it are not mutually exclusive. Poster also points out that Foucault's argument does not address the main issue: 'The bourgeois concern with the body

was not an erotic one; good diet and hygiene are not the same as sensuality.' Poster, *Foucault, Marxism and History*, 136

19 Carl Degler, '"What Ought to Be and What Was": Women's Sexuality in the Nineteenth Century,' *American Historical Review* 79, 5 (Dec. 1974): 1467–90; Gay, *The Bourgeois Experience*, 133–68. For an excellent critique of Degler's and Gay's emphasis on female sexual activity see Carol Z. Stearns and Peter N. Stearns, 'Victorian Sexuality: Can Historians Do It Better?' *Journal of Social History* 18, 4 (summer 1985): 625–34.

20 Poster, *Foucault, Marxism and History*, 133

21 Carl Degler, *At Odds: Women and the Family in America from the Revolution to the Present* (New York: Oxford University Press 1980), 269–72; Gay, *The Bourgeois Experience*, 133–68

22 Eugene Becklard, *Physiological Mysteries and Revelations in Love, Courtship and Marriage* (New York 1842), 69

23 *Canada Medical Journal and Monthly Record of Medical and Surgical Science* 3 (1867): 228

24 R. Pierce, *The People's Common Sense Medical Adviser in Plain English* (Buffalo 1882), 214

25 John Hett, *The Sexual Organs: Their Use and Abuse* (Berlin, Ont. 1899), 36

26 *Canada Medical Journal and Monthly Record of Medical and Surgical Science* 6 (1869): 294

27 William Carpenter, *Principles of Human Physiology* (London 1869), 826

28 *Canada Medical Record* 4 (Dec. 1875): 90; 9, 4 (Jan. 1880): 98

29 B.G. Jefferis, *Searchlights on Health: Light on Dark Corners* (Toronto 1900), 13–14

30 Liedewy Hawke, trans., *Hopes and Dreams: The Diary of Henriette Dessaulles 1874–1881* (Willowdale, Ont.: Hounslow Press 1986), 23

31 Jefferis, *Searchlights*, 393

32 *Canada Medical and Surgical Journal* 14 (Feb. 1886): 441

33 In her thesis Sibley notes that there was a difference between the British texts and the American texts used in Canada. The British tended to be very hostile to sexual excess whereas the American viewed sexuality as basically good. C.A. Sibley, 'The Early History and Development of Gynaecology in Canada, 1880–1910 (MA thesis, Queen's University, 1985), 83

34 Annual Report of the Dominion Woman's Christian Temperance Union, 1899, 81

35 John Buchanan, *The Eclectic Practice of Medicine and Surgery* (Philadelphia 1867), 714

36 John Haller and Robin Haller, *The Physician and Sexuality in Victorian America* (Urbana: University of Illinois Press 1974), 97

37 Gary Kinsman, *The Regulation of Desire: Sexuality in Canada* (Montreal: Black Rose Books 1987), 89

38 Carpenter, *Principles of Human Physiology*, 909

39 *Canada Medical and Surgical Journal* 5, 9 (March 1877): 415

40 *Canada Medical Record* 9, 3 (Dec. 1880): 53

41 Hamilton Ayers, *Ayers' Everyman His Own Doctor* (Montreal 1881), 461–2

42 Annual Report of the Maritime Woman's Christian Temperance Union, 1890, 42

43 *Canada Medical Record* 18, 2 (Nov. 1889): 29

44 Jefferis, *Searchlights* 127

45 William Acton, *The Functions and Disorders of the Reproductive Organs, in Childhood, Youth, Adult Age, and Advanced Life, Considered in Their Physiological, Social and Moral Relations* (Philadelphia 1894), 208–10

46 F. Barry Smith, 'Sexuality in Britain, 1800–1900: Some Suggested Revisions,' in Martha Vicinus, ed., *A Widening Sphere: Changing Roles of Victorian Women* (Bloomington: Indiana University Press 1977), 185

47 Carpenter, *Principles of Human Physiology*, 836; Matthew Mann, *A System of Gynecology by American Authors* (Philadelphia 1887), 442

48 *Canadian Practitioner* 15, 11 (Nov. 1890): 513

49 *Canada Medical Record* 18, 2 (Nov. 1889): 29

50 Alexander Skene, *Medical Gynecology: A Treatise on the Diseases of Women from the Standpoint of the Physician* (New York 1895), 83

51 Mann, *A System of Gynecology*, 106

52 Jill Conway, 'Stereotypes of Femininity in a Theory of Sexual Evolution,' *Victorian Studies* 14, 1 (Sept. 1970): 50

53 Pierce, *The People's Common Sense Medical Adviser*, 196

54 George Napheys, *The Physical Life of Woman: Advice to Maiden, Wife and Mother* (Toronto 1890), 51; Jefferis, *Searchlights*, 434

55 C.S. Clark, *Of Toronto the Good* (1898, Toronto: Coles 1970), 112

56 Hawke, *Hopes and Dreams*, 177, 243

57 *Canadian Practitioner* 19, 7 (July 1894): 495

58 *Canada Lancet* 26 (Jan. 1894): 142

59 Public Archives of Nova Scotia (PANS), Victoria General Hospital Papers, RG 25, series B, Patient Records box 33 62/99, patient HMcR, admitted 2 Nov. 1899

60 *Canada Medical Record* 11 (Aug. 1883): 255; Buchanan, *The Eclectic Practice of Medicine and Surgery*, 714; Pierce, *The People's Common Sense Medical Adviser*, 396; *Canada Lancet* 19 (Aug. 1887): 361; Annual Report of the Medical Superintendent of the Toronto Asylum (ARMS Toronto) 1862, *Sessional Papers* (*SP*) no. 66, Journal of the Legislative Assembly (JLA), 1863; ARMS Toronto 1863, *SP* no. 39, JLA, 1864; Victorians were worried about masturbation and referred to it as the secret vice. Rene A. Spitz has argued that it 'served as a convenient cover to express one's anti-sexuality while secretly practising it. That is adult males could rage ... about the widespread habit ... because it did not touch upon their own sexual activities with prostitutes, mistresses, and various forms of sadistic and masochistic behavior. Proof for this ... was in the fact that the harsh punishments for masturbation were directed primarily at children, women, and the insane, those least able to resist society, and also least able to express themselves.' Vern Bullough, *Sex, Society and History* (New York: Science History Publications 1976), 121–2

61 ARMS Saint John 1900, Journals of the House of Assembly 1901, 30

62 Gail Parsons, 'Equal Treatment for All: American Medical Remedies for Male Sexual Problems, 1850–1900,' *Journal of History of Medicine* 32 (Jan. 1977): 63–6

63 *British American Medical and Physical Journal* 6 (1851): 516–19, quoted in James Connor, 'Minority Medicine in Ontario, 1795 to 1903: A Study of Medical Pluralism and Its Decline' (PHD thesis, University of Waterloo, 1989), 307

64 Becklard, *Physiological Mysteries*, 100–1; *Canada Lancet* 19 (Aug. 1887): 362; Hett *Sexual Organs*, 95. That physicians were recognizing masturbation in the young suggests children were not viewed as particularly innocent. Smith, 'Sexuality in Britain 1800–1900,' 196. See also Jefferis, *Searchlights*, 436, 450; Pierce, *The People's Common Sense Medical Adviser*, 291; *Canada Lancet* 19 (Aug. 1887): 362; Henry Jacques

Garrigues, *A Text-book of the Diseases of Women* (Philadelphia, 1894), 290; Theodore Thomas, *A Practical Treatise on the Diseases of Women* (Philadelphia 1868), 89; Ayers, *Everyman*, 221; Henry Lyman, *The Practical Home Physician* (Guelph 1892), 541; McGill University Archives, D.C. MacCallum Papers, MG 2031, 'On Women's Medical Problems,' 11; Napheys, *The Physical Life of Woman*, 35; Henry MacNaughton-Jones, *Practical Manual of Diseases of Women and Uterine Therapeutics* (New York 1905), 9th ed., 4; *Canadian Practitioner* 21, 11 (Nov. 1896): 848; *Dominion Medical Monthly and Ontario Medical Journal* 7 (Sept. 1896): 256; 8 (Feb. 1897): 135

65 Garrigues, *A Text-book*, 290

66 Thomas, *A Practical Treatise*, 89; Ayers, *Everyman*, 221; Pierce, *The People's Common Sense Medical Adviser*, 749–50; *Canada Lancet* 19 (Aug. 1887): 362; Garrigues, *A Text-book*, 291; Napheys, *The Physical Life of Woman*, 35

67 Pierce, *The People's Common Sense Medical Adviser*, 748–9

68 Lyman, *Practical Home Physician*, 901; MacCallum Papers, 'On Women's Medical Problems,' 11

69 Lyman, *Practical Home Physician*, 541; Garrigues, *A Text-book*, 291

70 Napheys, *The Physical Life of Woman*, 35

71 MacNaughton-Jones, *Practical Manual of Diseases of Women*, 4

72 Academy of Medicine Library, Dr James Ross Papers, Ms Coll 99, Gynecology Record Book 1890–3, 289. Of course this was a two-way street; masturbation as a cause of disease allowed patients to explain their own symptoms and lessen their fear of the unknown. A.N. Gilbert, 'Doctor, Patient, and Onanist Diseases in the Nineteenth Century,' *Journal of the History of Medicine and Allied Sciences* 30, 3 (July 1975): 223–5

73 Garrigues, *A Text-book*, 289

74 *Canadian Practitioner* 21 (Nov. 1896): 848; an article in the *Dominion Medical Monthly and Ontario Medical Journal* 7 (Sept. 1896): 256, did the same thing.

75 *Canadian Practitioner* 21 (Nov. 1896): 849; *Dominion Medical Monthly and Ontario Medical Journal* 8 (Feb. 1897): 135

76 Christine Ball has argued that in the nineteenth century 'female sexuality was *never* viewed as existing separate from male sexuality.' The worry about masturbation indicates that this was not the case,

although the disapproval does suggest that women satisfying their sexual needs without men was perhaps what doctors feared. Christine Ball, 'Female Sexual Ideologies in Mid to Late Nineteenth-Century Canada,' *Resources for Feminist Research/Documentation sur la recherche féministe* 15, 3 (Nov. 1986): 26

77 Carl Degler argues that there was some recognition of female sexuality in the United States and that the mores of the period cannot be judged from the advice manuals. Certainly the manuals used in Canada, many of which were American, suggested that people realized that women had sexual desires. Degler, ' "What Ought to Be and What Was," ' 1467–90

78 P. Cazeaux, *Principles of Comparative Physiology* (Philadelphia 1854), 67

79 Austin Flint, *Physiology of Man* (New York 1874), 338

80 *Dominion Medical Monthly and Ontario Medical Journal* 8, 2 (Feb. 1897): 135; William Tyler Smith, *The Modern Practice of Midwifery: A Course of Lectures on Obstetrics* (New York 1858), 58; Alfred Lewis Galabin, *A Manual of Midwifery* (Philadelphia 1886), 54; William Goodell, *Lessons in Gynaecology* (Philadelphia 1890), 568

81 Becklard, *Physiological Mysteries*, 74

82 Pierce, *The People's Common Sense Medical Adviser*, 279

83 *Canadian Practitioner* 12, 6 (June 1887): 180

84 Garrigues, *A Text-book*, 39; Cazeaux, *Theoretical and Practical Treatise on Midwifery*, 60–1; Francis Ramsbotham, *The Principles and Practice of Obstetric Medicine and Surgery* (London 1841), 54; Fleetwood Churchill, *On the Theory and Practice of Midwifery* (Philadelphia 1843), 48; William Tyler Smith, *Parturition and the Principles and Practice of Obstetrics* (Philadelphia 1849), 74; Flint, *Physiology of Man*, 336; William Playfair, *A Treatise on the Science and Practice of Midwifery* (London 1880), 42–3. Even when the centrality of the clitoris was denied, which was rarely, physicians still acknowledged its importance. Theophilus Parvin, *The Science and Art of Obstetrics* (Philadelphia 1885), 49

85 Queen Elizabeth Hospital Archives, Toronto Home for Incurables Papers, Annual Report 1887, 11–12; *Bylaws*, Montreal General Hospital, 1875, 23

86 Nancy Thompson, 'The Controversy Over the Admission of Women to University College, University of Toronto' (MA thesis, University of Toronto, 1974), 81: 2

87 Goldwin Smith, 'The Woman's Rights Movement,' *Canadian Monthly* 6 (March 1872): 255, 260; 'Co-Education of the Sexes,' *Christian Guardian*, 16 Oct. 1872, 332

88 J. Millar, 'The Co-Education of the Sexes,' *Canada Educational Monthly* 6 (1879): 293; Smith, 'The Woman's Rights Movement,' 253–4

89 Mann, *A System of Gynecology by American Authors*, 444; Skene, *Medical Gynecology*, 120

90 *Medical Chronicle or, Montreal Monthly Journal of Medicine and Surgery* 6 (Oct. 1858): 230–9

91 James Connor, 'To Be Rendered Unconscious of Torture: Anaesthesia in Canada, 1847–1920' (MPhil. thesis, University of Waterloo, 1983), 60–6

92 *Canadian Practitioner* 8 (Feb. 1883), 49

93 Connor, 'To Be Rendered Unconscious,' 130

94 *Canada Lancet* 18 (March 1886): 213

95 Edward Shorter, *A History of Women's Bodies* (Don Mills: Fitzhenry and Whiteside 1982), 12. Historians have focused on a change from, in earlier centuries, recognizing female sexuality as a lesser version than the male's, just as women were lesser versions of men, to the belief in the nineteenth century of female sexuality being almost non-existent, as a reflection of a new way of viewing women as quite separate from men and driven by their reproductive instincts. While this may be true, both views seemed to hold sway in the Canadian context – that is, recognizing female sexuality but seeing women as predominantly reproductive beings. Catherine Gallagher and Thomas Laquer, eds., *The Making of the Modern Body* (Berkeley: University of California Press 1987), viii

96 Becklard, *Physiological Mysteries*, 44; Galabin, *A Manual of Midwifery*, 55; Skene, *Medical Gynecology*, 83; MacCallum Papers, 'On Women's Medical Problems,' 109

97 Goodell in the *Canadian Practitioner* 19 (July 1894): 495; Napheys, *The Physical Life of Woman*, 77; Alfred Galabin, *Diseases of Women* (London 1893), 498; *Canadian Practitioner* 12, 6 (June 1887): 181

98 Tyler Smith, *Parturition and the Principles and Practice of Obstetrics*, 128

99 *Canadian Practitioner*, 11, 1 (Jan. 1886): 43

100 Elizabeth Fee has suggested in 'Psychology, Sexuality, Social Control in Victorian England,' *Social Science Quarterly* 58, 4 (March 1978): 642–3, that in the nineteenth century sexuality was controlled for the purpose of production – that is, for procreation; by the early twentieth century sexuality was seen as necessary to satisfy the individual needs of both spouses – that is, it now served consumption.

101 Ira Warren, *The Household Physician* (Boston 1865), 351

102 Alvin Wood Chase, *Dr Chase's Third, Last and Complete Receipt Book and Household Physician* (Detroit and Windsor 1892), 210; Garrigues, *A Text-book*, 125; Goodell, *Lessons in Gynaecology*, 551

103 Napheys, *The Physical Life of Woman*, 78

104 Goodell, *Lessons in Gynaecology*, 560–2

105 Garrigues, *A Text-book*, 128

106 PANS, Victoria General Hospital Papers, RG 25, series B, Clinical Records III-40, case 53/00

107 *Canada Lancet* 26 (Jan. 1894): 143

108 Napheys, *The Physical Life of Woman*, 80

109 Pierce, *The People's Common Sense Medical Adviser*, 739–40, 223

110 Flint, *Physiology of Man* 333

111 Ayers, *Everyman*, 303; Lyman, *The Practical Home Physician*, 959; Napheys, *The Physical Life of Woman*, 83; Garrigues, *A Text-book*, 115; Hett, *Sexual Organs: Their Use and Abuse*, 28

112 Jefferis, *Searchlights on Health*, 206–11

113 F.B. Strong, 'Sex, Character and Reform in America, 1830–1920' (PHD thesis, Stanford University, 1972), 10–11. Foucault has described the tendency of the medical profession to create normative models: 'Medicine must no longer be confined to a body of techniques for curing ills and of the knowledge that they require; it will also embrace a knowledge of *healthy man*, that is, a study of *non-sick* man and a definition of the *model man*.' Michel Foucault, *The Birth of the Clinic: An Archaeology of Medical Perception* (New York: Pantheon Books 1973), 34

114 Toronto General Hospital, Obstetrics Register 1878–82 of the Burnside Lying-In Hospital patient no. 7, admitted 25 Oct. 1878

115 PANS, Victoria General Hospital Papers, RG 25, series III B.3, Patient Records, patient AF, 529, 539

CHAPTER 5 A Modern Issue Emerges: Birth Control

1 Liedewy Hawke, *Hopes and Dreams: The Diary of Henriette Dessaulles 1874–1881* (Willowdale: Hounslow Press 1986), 338
2 The literature on birth control is vast. See J.A. Banks and Olive Banks, *Feminism and Family Planning in Victorian England* (New York: Shocken Books 1977); Joseph Banks, *Prosperity and Parenthood: A Study of Family Planning among the Victorian Middle Classes* (London: Routledge, Kegan Paul 1954); S. Green, *The Curious History of Contraception* (London: Ebury 1971); N.E. Himes, *Medical History of Contraception* (New York: Gamut Press 1963); David Kennedy, *Birth Control in America: The Career of Margaret Sanger* (New Haven: Yale University Press 1970); Angus McLaren; *Reproductive Rituals: Perceptions of Fertility in Britain from the Sixteenth Century to the Nineteenth Century* (Toronto: Methuen 1984); Angus McLaren, *Birth Control in Nineteenth-Century England* (New York: Holmes and Meier 1978); James Mohr, *Abortion in America: The Origins and Evolution of National Policy, 1800–1900* (New York: Oxford University Press 1978); James Reed, *The Birth Control Movement and American Society: From Private Vice to Public Virtue* (Princeton, NJ: Princeton University Press 1978); Richard Allen Soloway, *Birth Control and the Population Question in England, 1877–1930* (Chapel Hill: University of North Carolina Press 1982); Linda Gordon, *Woman's Body, Woman's Right: A Social History of Birth Control in America* (New York: Grossman 1976).
3 Edward Shorter, 'Female Emancipation and Fertility in European History,' *American Historical Review* 78 (June 1973): 612–13
4 Gordon, *Woman's Body, Woman's Right*, 28, 41, 42, 45
5 Patricia Branca, *Women in Europe since 1750* (London: Croom Helm 1978), 129. Demographer Thomas McKeown has even suggested that contraception and the decline in birth rates led to the general decline of mortality from non-infective causes such as infanticide and starvation in the eighteenth and nineteenth centuries. Thomas McKeown, *The Modern Rise of Population* (London: Edward Arnold 1976), 154
6 Jacques Henripin, *Trends and Factors of Fertility in Canada* (Ottawa: Federal Census Bureau 1972), 19, 21, 38

7 In 1851 average age of marriage for men was 26.1 years and in 1891, 29.1. Ellen Gee, 'Marriage in Nineteenth Century Canada,' *Canadian Review of Sociology and Anthropology* 19, 3 (1982): 315

8 Henripin, *Trends and Factors of Fertility in Canada*, 81. In Halifax the legitimate fertility rate was 72 compared to the provincial index of 100 in 1871 and 97 in 1891; Winnipeg's was 84 in 1891.

9 For an explanation of the American situation see Stuart M. Blumin, 'Rip Van Winkle's Grandchildren: Family and Household in the Hudson Valley, 1800–1860,' in Tamara Hareven, ed., *Family and Kin in Urban Communities, 1700–1930* (New York: New Viewpoints 1977), 100–21; Laurence A. Glasco, 'The Life Cycles and Household Structure of American Ethnic Groups,' in Hareven, *Family and Kin*, 122–43

10 Joy Parr, 'Hired Men: Ontario Agricultural Wage Labour in Historical Perspective,' *Labour/le travail* 15 (spring 1985): 91–103; David Gagan, *Hopeful Travellers: Family, Land, and Social Change in Mid-Victorian Peel County, Canada West* (Toronto: University of Toronto Press 1981), 40–60; the discussion of urban and farm families was worked out in consultation with Alison Prentice, Beth Light, Paula Bourne, Gail Cuthbert Brandt, and Naomi Black.

11 *Canada Lancet* 27 (Nov. 1894): 98

12 *Canada Health Journal* 1, 5 May 1870): 66; Paul Mundé, *A Practical Treatise on the Diseases of Women* (Philadelphia 1891), 43

13 *Canada Lancet* 7 (June 1875): 291

14 Public Archives of Nova Scotia (PANS), Minutes of the Nova Scotia Medical Society, MG 20, no. 181, 15 Dec. 1863

15 *Canada Lancet* 7 (June 1875): 291

16 *Canada Health Journal* 1, 5 (May 1870): 66

17 *Canada Lancet* 4, 4 (Dec. 1871): 185–6

18 Mary Ellen Wright, 'The Desperate Alternative: Infanticide and Its Alternatives in Halifax, 1850–1875,' unpublished paper, 1983, 3

19 Constance Backhouse, 'Involuntary Motherhood: Abortion, Birth Control and the Law in Nineteenth Century Canada,' *Windsor Yearbook of Access to Justice* 3 (1983): 85–6; Clio Collective, *Quebec Women: A History* (Toronto: Women's Press 1987), 139–40; Gilbert Malcolm Sproat, *The Nootka: Scenes and Studies of Savage Life* (Victoria: Sono Nis Press 1987), 169; Peter Gossage, 'Absorbing Junior: The Use of Patent

Medicines as Abortifacients in Nineteenth-Century Montreal,' *The Register* 3, 1 (March 1982) 5

20 *Canada Health Journal* 1, 5 (May 1870): 66

21 *Canada Lancet* 4, 4 (Dec. 1871): 185; 7 (June 1875): 291

22 Gossage, 'Absorbing Junior,' 1–2

23 Angus Mclaren and Arlene Tigar Mclaren, *The Bedroom and the State: The Changing Practices and Politics of Contraception and Abortion in Canada, 1880–1980* (Toronto: McClelland and Stewart 1986), 16

24 *Canada Health Journal* 1, 5 (May 1870): 66–7

25 *Canada Lancet* 7 (June 1875): 291

26 Henry Lyman, *The Practical Home Physician and Encyclopedia of Medicine* (Guelph 1884), 988

27 George Napheys, *The Physical Life of Woman: Advice to Maiden, Wife and Mother* (Toronto 1890), 91–3

28 R. Pierce, *The People's Common Sense Medical Adviser in Plain English* (Buffalo 1882), 754; *Canada Lancet* 34, 12 (Aug. 1901): 663; Martin Holbrook, 'Parturition without Pain,' in Napheys, *The Physical Life of Woman*, 315

29 *Canada Health Journal* 1, 5 (May 1870): 66–7

30 *Canada Lancet* 4, 4 (Dec. 1871): 185–6

31 *Sanitary Journal* 2, 12 (Dec. 1876): 335

32 Holbrook, 'Parturition without Pain,' 315

33 Backhouse, 'Involuntary Motherhood,' 80–1

34 McGill University Archives, University Lying-in Hospital Papers, RG 95, vol. 97, Register, patient entered 19 May 1896 and discharged 24 May 1896

35 *Canada Lancet* 7 (June 1875): 291

36 Napheys, *The Physical Life of Woman*, 98; *Canada Medical Record* 18, 9 (June 1889): 194

37 Backhouse, 'Involuntary Motherhood,' 64–76

38 Terry Chapman, 'Women, Sex and Marriage in Western Canada, 1890–1920,' *Alberta History* 33, 4 (fall 1985): 6

39 Backhouse, 'Involuntary Motherhood,' 74–5

40 *Canada Lancet* 5 (June 1875): 291; 21, 7 (March 1889): 218

41 Gossage, 'Absorbing Junior,' 2

42 *Provincial Medical Journal* 1 (May 1868): 13–16

43 *Canada Medical and Surgical Journal* 12 (Nov. 1884): 252

44 Backhouse, 'Involuntary Motherhood,' 91–2

45 *Canada Health Journal* 1, 5 (May 1870): 67–8

46 Linda Lee, 'The Myth of Female Equality in Pioneer Society: The Red River Colony as a Test Case' (MA thesis, University of Manitoba, 1978), 103

47 Annual Report, Dominion Woman's Christian Temperance Union, 1891, 81–2

48 *Canada Lancet* 8, 1 (Sept. 1875): 24

49 Gossage, 'Absorbing Junior,' 7–9

50 *Canada Lancet* 21, 7 (March 1889): 217–18

51 Backhouse, 'Involuntary Motherhood,' 92–3, 96

52 *Canada Medical Journal and Monthly Record of Medical and Surgical Science* 3 (1867): 226–7; *Canada Health Journal* 1, 5 (May 1870): 68–9; Henry Jacques Garrigues, *A Text-book of the Diseases of Women* (Philadelphia 1894), 128–9; Napheys, *The Physical Life of Woman*, 98

53 *Canada Health Journal* 1, 5 (May 1870): 70

54 Pierce, *The People's Common Sense Medical Adviser*, 734; Holbrook, 'Parturition without Pain,' 315

55 PANS, Victoria General Hospital Papers, RG 25, series B, section 3, no. 6, Patient Records, LS admitted 29 Sept. 1891

56 Backhouse, 'Involuntary Motherhood.' 116

57 Kristin Luker, *Abortion and the Politics of Motherhood* (Berkeley: University of California Press 1984), 8, 32

58 *Canada Lancet* 7, 10 (June 1875): 291

59 Ibid., 289

60 Archives of Ontario (AO), Hugh Mackay Papers, Mss Misc. Coll. 1873 no. 6, MU 2118, Obstetrical Notebook, patient Mrs F, delivered 21 Sept. 1873, 244

61 McGill University Archives, Montreal General Hospital Papers, RG 96, vol. 275, Gynecology Casebook, Jane H, admitted 29 Jan. and discharged 15 Feb. 1886, 44

62 In 1892 the Criminal Code lessened the penalty for a woman aborting herself to seven years.

63 McGill University Archives, University Lying-in Hospital, RG 25, vol. 97, Register, preface

64 Wright, 'The Desperate Alternative,' 6

65 Mackay Papers, Mss Misc. Coll. 1873 no. 6, MU 2118, Obstetrical Notebook, patient M, 30 March 1876, 251

66 James Conner, 'Minority Medicine in Ontario, 1795 to 1903: A Study of Medical Pluralism and Its Decline' (PHD thesis, University of Waterloo, 1989), 172

67 Ibid., 171–2

68 Backhouse, 'Involuntary Motherhood,' 98–9, 109

69 Eugene Becklard, *Physiological Mysteries and Revelations in Love, Courtship and Marriage* (New York 1842), 40–2

70 Pierce, *The People's Common Sense Medical Adviser*, 224

71 *Queen's Medical Quarterly* 3, 1 (Oct. 1898): 164–5

72 See, for example, the article in *Canada Medical Record* 18, 9 (June 1889): 194, that advised avoiding intercourse for ten days prior to menstruation.

73 Napheys, *The Physical Life of Woman*, 95–6

74 Reuben Ludlam, *Lectures Clinical and Didactic on the Diseases of Women* (Chicago 1872), 32–3

75 William Goodell, *Lessons in Gynaecology* (Philadelphia 1890), 571–2

76 Norman E. Himes, *Medical History of Contraception* (London: George Allen and Unwin 1936), 213

77 *Canada Medical Journal and Monthly Record* 3 (1867): 226

78 *Canadian Practitioner* 18 (April 1883): 296; John Hett in *The Sexual Organs: Their Use and Abuse* (Berlin, Ont. 1899), 104, argued that coitus interruptus had the same serious side effects on men as masturbation.

79 *Canadian Practitioner* 18 (April 1883): 296; Garrigues, *A Text-book*, 127; Goodell, *Lessons in Gynaecology*, 568

80 B.F. Jefferis, *Searchlights on Health* (Toronto 1895), 247–8

81 Goodell, *Lessons in Gynaecology*, 566

82 McLaren and McLaren, *The Bedroom and the State*, 21–2

83 Clio Collective, *Quebec Women*, 138

84 Wright, 'The Desperate Alternative,' 2

85 Backhouse, 'Involuntary Motherhood,' 122–3

86 Clio Collective, *Quebec Women*, 138

87 Gordon, *Woman's Body, Woman's Right*, 25

88 Theodore Thomas, *A Practical Treatise on the Diseases of Women* (Philadelphia 1868), 58–9

89 Lyman, *The Practical Home Physician*, 990

90 *Canada Medical Journal and Monthly Record of Medical and Surgical Science* 3 (Oct. 1866): 226; 3 (1867): 228; Paul Mundé, *A Practical Treatise on the Diseases of Women* (Philadelphia 1891), 35; Napheys, *The Physical Life of Woman*, 96–7; Goodell, *Lessons in Gynaecology*, 571, 562

91 John Thorburn, *A Practical Treatise of the Diseases of Women* (London 1885), 525

92 *The Medical Chronicle or, Montreal Monthly Journal of Medicine and Surgery* 4 (June 1856): 35

93 Lyman, *The Practical Home Physician*, 990

94 Goodell, *Lessons in Gynaecology*, 562, 570

95 *Queen's Medical Quarterly* 3, 1 (Oct. 1898): 165

96 *Canada Lancet* 25 (July 1893): 372–3

97 Backhouse, 'Involuntary Motherhood,' 124

CHAPTER 6 The Emergence of Medical Obstetrics

1 Beth Light and Alison Prentice, eds., *Pioneer and Gentlewomen of British North America 1713–1867* (Toronto: New Hogtown Press 1980), 137–8

2 Beth Light and Joy Parr, eds., *Canadian Women on the Move 1867–1920* (Toronto: New Hogtown Press and the Ontario Institute for Studies in Education 1983), 133

3 Ramsay Cook and Wendy Mitchinson, eds., *The Proper Sphere: Woman's Place in Canadian Society* (Toronto: Oxford University Press 1976), 226

4 Catherine Gallagher and Thomas Laquer, eds., *The Making of the Modern Body* (Berkeley: University of California Press 1987), viii

5 Mary O'Brien, 'Politics of Reproduction,' *Resources for Feminist Research/Documentation sur la recherche féministe* 8, 2 (spring 1979): 29

6 William Tyler Smith, *Parturition and the Principles and Practice of Obstetrics* (Philadelphia 1849), 19

7 Richard A. Leonardo, *History of Gynecology* (New York: Froben Press 1944), 255

8 Reay Tannahill, *Sex in History* (London: Abacus 1981), 330

9 *Canada Lancet* 3, 2 (Oct. 1870): 46–7

10 R. Pierce, *The People's Common Sense Medical Adviser in Plain English* (Buffalo 1882), 208–9

11 Tyler Smith, *Parturition*, 95; Austin Flint, *Physiology of Man* (New York 1874), 293; Alfred Galabin, *Diseases of Women* (London 1893), 72; McGill University Archives, D.C. MacCallum Papers, MG 2031, 'On Women's Medical Problems,' 111; George Napheys, *The Physical Life of Woman: Advice to the Maiden, Wife and Mother* (Toronto 1890), 71; Pierce, *The People's Common Sense Medical Adviser*, 221

12 P. Cazeaux, *Theoretical and Practical Treatise on Midwifery* (Philadelphia 1837), 123; Benjamin Grant Jefferis, *Searchlights on Health: Light on Dark Corners* (Fredericton 1894), 236

13 Napheys, *The Physical Life of Woman*, 83, 90

14 *Canadian Practitioner* 11, 1 (Jan. 1886): 43

15 Cazeaux, *Theoretical and Practical Treatise*, 124

16 William Carpenter, *Principles of Human Physiology* (London 1869), 906

17 Flint, *Physiology of Man.*, 346

18 Jefferis, *Searchlights*, 256; Henry Lyman, *The Practical Home Physician and Encyclopedia of Medicine* (Guelph 1894), 938

19 Pierce, *The People's Common Sense Medical Adviser*, 212

20 Annual Report, Dominion Woman's Christian Temperance Union, 1899, 60. The belief that children carried maternal impressions all their lives was a long held belief, predating the understanding of women's role in conception and harkening back to age-old superstitions.

21 *Medical Chronicle or, Montreal Monthly Journal of Medicine & Surgery* 4 (July 1856): 72

22 *Canada Health Journal* 1, 2 (Feb. 1870): 17, 20

23 *Canada Medical Record* 17, 10 (July 1888): 240; 23, 6 (March 1894): 140

24 John Hett, *The Sexual Organs: Their Use and Abuse* (Berlin, Ont. 1899), 46–7

25 Flint, *Physiology of Man*, 347, 350–1

26 Napheys, *The Physical Life of Woman*, 115–16

27 Flint, *Physiology of Man*, 350–1; Archives of Ontario (AO), Hugh Mackay Papers, Mss Misc. Coll. 1873 no. 6, MU 2118, Obstetrical Notebook, 245

28 Toronto General Hospital, Burnside Lying-In Hospital, Obstetrical Register, patient admitted 4 May 1881

29 Lyman, *The Practical Home Physician*, 924–5

30 Roderick P. Beaujot and Kevin McQuillan, 'Social Effects of Demographic Change: Canada 1851–1981,' *Journal of Canadian Studies* 21 (spring 1986): 58–9

31 Public Archives of New Brunswick (PANB), Thomas Clowes Brown Papers, Obstetrical Cases, 1860–89. Every patient record was examined, representing just over 1100 patients.

32 Mackay Papers, Mss Misc. Coll. 1873 no. 6, MU 2118, based on 816 of his cases between 1873 and 1888. Each case was examined.

33 Academy of Medicine Library, Dr James Ross Papers, Ms Coll. 97, 98, Obstetrical Register, 1853–91, based on an analysis of every patient, every other year, or over 1400 patients.

34 Ira Warren, *The Household Physician* (Boston 1865), 59

35 *Canadian Practitioner* 11, 1 (Jan. 1886): 43

36 *Canada Medical Record* 18, 2 (Nov. 1889): 25–30 (my emphasis)

37 Pye Henry Chavasse, *Advice to a Wife on the Management of Her Own Health and on the Treatment of Some of the Complaints Incidental to Pregnancy, Labour and Suckling* (Toronto 1882), 22–3; Lyman, *The Practical Home Physician*, 981

38 Napheys, *The Physical Life of Woman*, 94, 253

39 Margaret W. Andrews, 'Medical Attendance in Vancouver, 1886–1920,' in S.E.D. Shortt, ed., *Medicine in Canadian Society: Historical Perspectives* (Montreal: McGill-Queen's University Press 1981), 432–3

40 Judith S. Lewis, 'Maternal Health in the English Aristocracy: Myths and Realities, 1790–1840,' *Journal of Social History* 17, 1 (fall 1983): 106

41 Jan Lewis and Kenneth A. Lockridge, '"Sally Has Been Sick": Pregnancy and Family Limitation among Victorian Gentry Women, 1780–1830,' *Journal of Social History* 22, 1 (fall 1988): 14

42 Ann Oakley, 'Wisewoman and Medicine Man: Changes in the Management of Childbirth,' in Juliet Mitchell and Ann Oakley, eds., *The Rights and Wrongs of Women* (Harmondsworth, Middlesex: Penguin 1976), 18

43 Gena Corea, *The Hidden Malpractice: How American Medicine Treats Women as Patients and Professionals* (New York: Harper Colophon Books 1977), 14

44 For an article indicating that midwifery practice in early twentieth-century America was safe see Eugene Declerq, 'The Nature and Style of

Practice of Immigrant Midwives in Early Twentieth-Century Massachusetts,' *Journal of Social History* 19, 1 (fall 1985): 113–30.

45 Judith Walzer Leavitt and Whitney Walton, ' "Down to Death's Door": Women's Perceptions of Childbirth in America,' in Judith Leavitt, ed., *Women and Health in America* (Madison: University of Wisconsin Press 1984), 156

46 Edward Shorter, *A History of Women's Bodies* (New York: Basic Books 1982), 58–62

47 Jane Donegan, 'Midwifery in America, 1760–1860: A Study in Medicine and Morality' (PHD thesis, Syracuse University, 1972), 55, 26, 96

48 James Connor argues that in Britain, midwives were able to align themselves with consultants and thus gain powerful supporters. James Connor, 'Minority Medicine in Ontario, 1795 to 1903: A Study of Medical Pluralism and Its Decline' (PHD thesis, University of Waterloo, 1989), 6

49 Judy Litoff, *American Midwives 1860 to the Present* (Westport, Conn.: Greenwood Press 1978), 139–41; John S. Haller, *American Medicine in Transition, 1840–1910* (Champaign, Ill.: University of Illinois Press 1981), 190

50 Connor, 'Minority Medicine in Ontario,' 166–8, 138

51 *Upper Canada Journal of Medical, Surgical and Physical Science* 1 (June 1851): 109; Dickson had been trained to practise midwifery in Glasgow and consequently had a positive view of midwives. I should thank Dr Tony Travill for communicating this information to me.

52 *Medical Chronicle or, Montreal Monthly Journal of Medicine & Surgery* 2 (Dec. 1854): 261–2

53 Connor, 'Minority Medicine in Ontario,' 146

54 Ibid., 132

55 AO, William Canniff Papers, MU 490 package 1, *An Historical Sketch of Canadian Medicine and Surgery*, 12

56 *Belcher's Farmer's Almanac for 1889* (Halifax: T.C. Allen 1889), 187

57 Colin Howell, 'Reform and the Monopolistic Impulse: The Professionalization of Medicine in the Maritimes,' *Acadiensis* 11, 1 (autumn 1981): 20–1

58 *Census of Canada*, 1850–1, vol. 1, 516–19, 542–5. An indication of how the census figures underestimate the number of midwives is that the *British American Journal of Medical & Physical Science*, in 1850 published the names of eleven midwives 'duly licensed' to attend

midwifery cases in Montreal Quebec and Chambly. Connor, 'Minority Medicine in Ontario,' 131; *Census of Canada*, 1860–1, vol. 1, 566–7, 544–5; *Census of Canada*, 1870–1, vol. 2, 340–1

59 Leslie Biggs, 'The Case of the Missing Midwives: A History of Midwifery in Ontario from 1795–1900,' *Ontario History* 75, 1 (March 1983): 25

60 Jo Oppenheimer, 'Childbirth in Ontario: The Transition from Home to Hospital in the Early Twentieth Century,' ibid., 41

61 Peter Ward, ed., *Charlotte Führer, The Mysteries of Montreal: Memoirs of a Midwife* (Vancouver: University of British Columbia Press 1984), 9

62 *By-laws, Rules and Regulations for the Management of the University Lying-in Hospital* (Montreal 1859), 15

63 Rhona Kenneally, 'The Montreal Maternity Hospital 1843–1926: Evolution of a Hospital' (MA thesis, McGill University, 1983), 25

64 Connor, 'Minority Medicine in Ontario,' 175

65 Marta Danylewycz, *Taking the Veil: An Alternative to Marriage, Motherhood, and Spinsterhood in Quebec, 1840–1920* (Toronto: McClelland and Stewart 1987), 20

66 Public Archives of Nova Scotia (PANS), Halifax Medical Society Papers, MG 20, no. 181, Minutes, 6 May 1861

67 For an excellent article on who midwives were and the kind of work they did in the Unite States see Charlotte G. Borst, 'The Training and Practice of Midwives: A Wisconsin Study,' *Bulletin of the History of Medicine* 62, 4 (winter 1988): 606–27.

68 Connor, 'Minority Medicine in Ontario,' 148

69 Charles Roland and Bohodar Rubashewsky, 'The Economic Status of the Practice of Dr Harmaunus Smith in Wentworth County, Ontario, 1826–67,' *Canadian Bulletin of Medical History* 5, 1 (summer 1988): 36–8

70 PANS, Dr Samuel Burns Papers, MG 1, vol. 1689, Ledger 1881–92; Dr J.R. Collie Papers, MG 1, vol. 1774, no. 5, Account Book

71 PANS, British Medical Association, Nova Scotia Branch, Papers, MG 20, no. 203, Minutes, 19 March 1902, 36

72 Jacalyn Duffin, 'A Rural Practice in Nineteenth-Century Ontario: The Continuing Medical Education of James Miles Langstaff,' *Canadian Bulletin of Medical History* 5, 1 (summer 1988): 19–20

73 Light and Prentice, eds., *Pioneer and Gentlewomen of British North America*, 139

74 Duffin, 'A Rural Practice in Nineteenth-Century Ontario,' 11

75 PANB, Brown Papers, Obstetrical Cases, 1860–93. Between 1860 and 1893 Brown attended 1096 cases or an average of thirty-three cases a year. In the same period Dr Hugh Mackay of Woodstock averaged forty-nine cases a year. AO, MacKay Papers, Mss Misc. Coll. 1873 no. 6, MU 2118, Obstetrical Notebook

76 Donegan, 'Midwifery in America,' 4

77 William Buchan, *Domestic Medicine* (London 1813), 419

78 *Upper Canada Journal of Medical, Surgical & Physical Science* 1 (June 1851): 107–9

79 *Medical Chronicle or, Montreal Monthly Journal of Medicine & Surgery* 2 (April 1855): 436

80 Tyler Smith, *Parturition*, 19, 28–9

81 *Canada Lancet* 7 (Oct. 1874), 57

82 Connor, 'Minority Medicine in Ontario,' chap. 2

83 N. Devitt, 'The Statistical Case for Elimination of the Midwife: Fact versus Prejudice 1890–1935,' *Women and Health* 4, 1 (spring 1979): pt 1, 91

84 Oppenheimer, 'Childbirth in Ontario,' 41

85 *British American Journal of Medical & Physical Science* 6 (Nov. 1850): 333

86 Kenneally, 'Montreal Maternity Hospital,' 19–20. The University Lying-in Hospital was renamed the Montreal Maternity Hospital in 1887.

87 Oppenheimer, 'Childbirth in Ontario,' 41

88 Halifax Medical College Calendar, 1900, 11

89 Veronica Strong-Boag and Kathryn McPherson, 'The Confinement of Women: Childbirth and Hospitalization in Vancouver, 1919–1939,' *BC Studies* 69–70 (spring–summer 1986): 147

90 Nurses also were antagonistic to the VON assuming midwife duties, for nurses saw VON activities as 'home helpers' as poor role models. Suzann Buckley, 'Ladies or Midwives? Efforts to Reduce Infant and Maternal Mortality,' in Linda Kealey, ed., *A Not Unreasonable Claim: Women and Reform in Canada 1880s–1920s* (Toronto: Women's Press 1979), 136–7

91 Connor, 'Minority Medicine in Ontario,' 128–78, 154

92 James Connor, 'To Be Rendered Unconscious of Torture: Anaesthesia in Canada, 1847–1920' (M. Phil. thesis, University of Waterloo, 1983), 8, 27

93 *The British American Journal of Medical & Physical Science* 4 (April 1848): 324; R.C. Fuller, *50 Years of Pharmacy in Nova Scotia* (Halifax: Nova Scotia Pharmaceutical Society 1925), 21–2; Connor, 'To Be Rendered Unconscious,' 35

94 Walter Radcliffe, *Milestones in Midwifery* (Bristol: Wright 1967), 81

95 Tyler Smith, *Parturition*, 129

96 Connor, 'To Rendered Unconscious,' 36–9

97 Ibid., 43, 68

98 Duffin, 'A Rural Practice in Nineteenth-Century Ontario,' 13

99 *Canada Medical Journal and Monthly Record of Medical and Surgical Science* 4 (1867–8): 443–5, cited in Connor, 'To Be Rendered Unconscious,' 95–6

100 William Tyler Smith, *The Modern Practice of Midwifery: A Course of Lectures on Obstetrics* (New York 1858), 732–3

101 *Canada Medical and Surgical Journal* 12 (Feb. 1884): 423

102 Napheys, *The Physical Life of Woman*, 189; Holbrook, 'Parturition without Pain,' in Napheys, *The Physical Life of Woman*, 317, 367. Just as doctors saw middle-class women as weaker than working-class women, so did judges perceive that middle-class women had a lower threshold than working-class women to take abuse from their husbands. James Snell, 'Marital Cruelty: Women and the Nova Scotia Divorce Court, 1900–1939,' *Acadiensis* 18, 1 (autumn 1988): 20

103 Connor, 'To Be Rendered Unconscious,' 145–6

104 Toronto General Hospital, Burnside Lying-In Hospital, Obstetric Register, 1878–82. Out of 517 cases, only nineteen indicated that anaesthesia had been used.

105 AO, Mackay Papers, Obstetrical Notebook, 1873–89; Casebook, Misc. Coll. 1873 no. 6, MU 2118, 253. In James Connor's thesis he notes Mackay used chloroform in only eighteen out of 935 cases. Connor, 'Minority Medicine in Ontario,' 158. The difference between my findings and Connor's may reflect my counting chloroform any time it was used, even in minimal dosage. In any event, thirty-five times out of 816 cases is not a high percentage. More difficult to explain is C.A. Sibley's claim that Mackay used chloroform in 18.2 per cent of his cases. C.A. Sibley,

'The Early History and Development of Gynaecology in Canada, 1880–1910' (MA thesis, Queen's University, 1985), 157

106 *Canada Lancet* 18 (Sept. 1885): 26

107 Academy of Medicine, Alexander McPhedran Papers, C 21, Ms Coll. 57, Casebook 1884–7

108 Kenneally, 'Montreal Maternity Hospital, 55

109 PANB, Brown Papers, Obstetrical Cases, 1860–93

110 Connor, 'To Be Rendered Unconscious,' 146

111 *British American Journal of Medical & Physical Science* 3, 12 (April 1848): 324

112 Connor, 'Minority Medicine in Ontario,' 159

113 Mary Poovey, '"Scenes of an Indelicate Character": The Medical "Treatment" of Victorian Women,' in Catherine Gallagher and Thomas Laquer, eds., *The Making of the Modern Body* (Berkeley: University of California Press 1987), 152

114 Connor, 'Minority Medicine in Ontario,' 162

115 Connor, 'To Be Rendered Unconcious,' 83

116 *Canadian Medical Review* 6 (1897): 157

117 Kenneally, 'Montreal Maternity Hospital,' 48

118 David Hamilton, 'The Nineteenth-Century Surgical Revolution – Antisepsis or Better Nutrition?' *Bulletin of the History of Medicine* 56, 1 (spring 1982): 30–40

119 *Canadian Medical Review* 6, 5 (Nov. 1897): 155, 157

120 *Canada Lancet* 18 (Sept. 1885): 26

121 PANS, *British Medical Association*, Nova Scotia Branch Papers, MG 20 no. 203, Minutes, 14 April 1892, 128

122 *Canada Medical Record* 14, 8 (May 1885): 171

123 Barbara Rothman, *In Labour: Women and Power in the Birthplace* (London: Junction Books 1982), 15–16

124 Kathleen Pickard, 'Choosing Hospitalised Childbirth: The Ottawa Maternity Hospital, 1895–1924' (MA thesis, Queen's University, 1986), 66–7

125 Annual Report, Halifax Visiting Dispensary, 1856, 6; 1868, 10–12; and 1875, 10–11

126 McGill University Archives, Montreal General Hospital Papers, RG 96, Diseases of Women, vol. 273 (University Dispensary), 1882–3, patient MC, first seen 18 March 1882

127 PANS, Victoria General Hospital Papers, RG 25, series B, Patient Records, patient LH, admitted 5 Nov. 1894

128 Pickard, 'Choosing Hospitalised Childbirth,' 5; McGill University Archives, University Lying-in Hospital Papers, RG 96, vol. 352–60, Archibald Hall, 'Statistics of the University Lying-in Hospital, Montreal,' reprint from *British American Journal of Medical & Physical Science* 1 (1860): 1–2 of reprint

129 S.E.D. Shortt, *Victorian Lunacy: Richard M. Bucke and the Practice of Late Nineteenth-Century Psychiatry* (London: Cambridge University Press 1986), 8; *By-laws, Rules and Regulations, for the Management of the University Lying-In Hospital* (Montreal 1859), 6–14

130 Pickard, 'Choosing Hospitalised Birth,' 5; Oppenheimer,' Childbirth in Ontario,' 41–2

131 Peter Ward, 'Unwed Motherhood in Nineteenth-Century English Canada,' Canadian Historical Association, *Historical Papers* 1981, 50

132 Pickard, 'Choosing Hospitalised Birth,' 23

133 Lydia Macpherson, *Historical Sketch of the Woman's Christian Temperance Union of British Columbia 1883–1953* (Vancouver: np 1953), 4–5

134 Pickard, 'Choosing Hospitalised Childbirth,' 5

135 Hall, 'Statistics of the University Lying-in Hospital,' 4 of reprint; Ward, 'Unwed Motherhood,' 50; for an excellent description of the University Lying-in Hospital see Peter Ward and Patricia Ward, 'Infant Weight and Nutrition in Industrializing Montreal,' *American Historical Review* 89, 2 (April 1984): 324–45.

136 Toronto General Hospital, Burnside Lying-In Hospital Obstetrical Register, 1878–82

137 Ward, 'Unwed Motherhood,' 50; McGill University Archives, University Lying-in Hospital Papers, RG 95, vol. 97, Register 1851–1900, based on calculations from every tenth patient record or 717 cases

138 Toronto General Hospital, Burnside Lying-In Hospital, Obstetrical Register, 1878–82. Every case or 517 patient records were examined. For only 499 were the age of the patient and period before entry known. For these patients, 54.9 per cent (n = 274) entered two weeks before delivery: 59.5 per cent (n = 22) of those in their thirties and 100 per cent (n = 4) of those in their forties.

139 Anual Report, Montreal Maternity Hospital 1888, 5–6; 1859, 13

140 The records of the Burnside Lying-In Hospital suggest that at least one of their patients went out to wet nurse. Toronto General Hospital, Burnside Lying-In Hospital, Obstetrical Register, 1878–82

141 Sibley, 'The Early History and Development of Gynaecology in Canada,' 100

142 *By-laws, University Lying-in Hospital*, 1859, 11. This was also true for the Ottawa Maternity Home (1895). Pickard, 'Choosing Hospitalised Birth,' 65

143 *By-Laws, University Lying-in Hospital*, 1859, 7–8, 13

144 Toronto General Hospital, Burnside Lying-In Hospital, Obstetrical Register, 1878–82 patient admitted 4 Feb. 1881

145 *Canadian Medical Review* 6, 5 (Nov. 1897), 155

146 Kenneally, 'Montreal Maternity Hospital,' 14, 23–5, 99–101

147 McGill University Archives, University Lying-in Hospital, RG 95, vol. 97, Register 1851–1904, patient admitted 11 June 1894 and discharged 29 June 1894

148 Pickard, 'Choosing Hospitalised Birth,' 6

149 Annual Report, Montreal Maternity Hospital 1892, 4; 1895, 3; 1894, 4

150 Kenneally, 'Montreal Maternity Hospital,' 41

151 Queen's University Archives, Dean J.C. Connell, *History of the Kingston General Hospital* (np: np 1925), np

152 British Columbia Archives and Record Service, Annual Report, Board of Directors, Royal Jubilee Hospital, 1896, 4

153 Pickard, 'Choosing Hospitalised Childbirth,' 31–61

154 Leavitt and Walton, 'Down to Death's Door,' 161

155 Buchan, *Domestic Medicine*, 420

156 *Upper Canada Journal of Medical, Surgical and Physical Science* 1 (July 1851): 152

157 Judith Walzer Leavitt, *Brought to Bed: Child-Bearing in America, 1750–1950* (New York: Oxford University Press 1986), 217

CHAPTER 7 Changing Obstetric Care

1 Public Archives of Nova Scotia (PANS), Victoria General Hospital Papers, RG 25, series B, Patient Records, patient Mrs M, admitted 24 March 1893

2 Ibid., patient LB, admitted 23 June 1893

3 Judith Leavitt, *Brought to Bed: Child-bearing in America, 1750–1950* (New York: Oxford University Press 1986), 73–4

4 Barbara Rothman, *In Labour: Women and Power in the Birthplace* (London: Junction Books 1982), 134. Emphasis is Rothman's.

5 Dalhousie University, Tupper Medical Library, J. Lowder manuscript, 99. From the manuscript it would appear that Lowder was trained overseas.

6 P. Cazeaux, *Theoretical and Practical Treatise on Midwifery* (Philadelphia 1837), 238; Pye Henry Chavasse, *Advice to a Wife on the Management of Her Own Health and on the Treatment of Some of the Complaints Incidental to Pregnancy, Labour, and Suckling* (Toronto 1882), 115

7 McGill University Archives, Montreal General Hospital Papers, RG 96, vol. 273, Diseases of Women Casebook, University Dispensary, patient AP 297

8 Archives of Ontario (AO), Hugh Mackay Obstetrical Notebook, Mss Misc. Coll. 1873 no. 6, MU 2118, patient JM, 4 March 1873, 240

9 Margaret Andrews, 'Medical Services in Vancouver, 1886–1920: A Study in the Interplay of Attitudes, Medical Knowledge, and Administrative Structures' (PHD thesis, University of British Columbia, 1979), 73

10 Annual Report, Montreal Maternity Hospital, 1898, 7; 1899, 7

11 Jacalyn Duffin, 'A Rural Practice in Nineteenth-Century Ontario: The Continuing Medical Education of James Miles Langstaff,' *Canadian Bulletin of Medical History* 5, 1 (summer 1988): 11, 6–7

12 Rothman, *In Labour*, 35

13 Kenneth Neader Fenwick, *Manual of Obstetrics, Gynaecology and Pediatrics* (Kingston 1889), 44–5

14 Gunning Bedford, *The Principles and Practice of Obstetrics* (New York 1861), 352

15 McGill University Archives, D.C. MacCallum Papers, MG 2031, 'On Women's Medical Problems,' 1092

16 Cazeaux, *Theoretical and Practical Treatise on Midwifery*, 392

17 William Playfair, *A Treatise on the Science and Practice of Midwifery* (London 1880), 276

18 Chavasse, *Advice to a Wife*, 211

19 Benjamin Grant Jefferis, *Searchlights on Health: Light on Dark Corners* (Toronto 1900), 302; William Tyler Smith, *The Modern Practice*

of Midwifery: A Course of Lectures on Obstetrics (New York 1858), 358–9

20 *Canada Lancet* 6, 8 (April 1874): 267

21 MacCallum Papers, 'On Women's Medical Problems,' 1093–5

22 *Canada Medical Record* 6 (Jan. 1878): 82

23 *Canada Lancet* 16, 1 (Aug. 1884): 371

24 MacCallum Papers, 'On Women's Medical Problems,' 1111

25 Reuben Ludlam, *Lectures Clinical and Didactic on the Diseases of Women* (Chicago 1872), 32–3; *Canada Medical Record* 24 (March 1896): 266–7; Alexander Skene, *Medical Gynecology: A Treatise on the Diseases of Women from the Standpoint of the Physician* (New York 1895), 4; George Napheys, *The Physical Life of Woman: Advice to the Maiden, Wife and Mother* (Toronto 1890), 186

26 *By-Laws, Rules and Regulations, for the Management of the University Lying-in Hospital* (Montreal 1859), 12

27 Ludlam, *Lectures*, 32–3; quote is by Skene, *Medical Gynecology*, 4. But if some refused to nurse, other women went to the opposite extreme and nursed their children too long – a practice which William Goodell, a leading American gynaecologist, warned could cause illness in women. Equally worrisome to opponents of birth control were women who extended their breast feeding in order to prevent conception. Clearly, women were to moderate their nursing as they were to moderate most other aspects of their lives. William Goodell, *Lessons in Gynaecology* (Philadelphia 1890), 571

28 Napheys, *The Physical Life of Woman*, 215

29 Ibid., 216–17; William Lusk, *The Science and Art of Midwifery* (New York 1889), 256. These references are made in the non-Canadian literature, so it is difficult to know how prevalent it was in this country. Certainly in the historiographical literature it is associated more with Britain and Europe than with North America. A recent article has focused on wet-nursing in the United States. Janet Golden, 'From Wet Nurse Directory to Milk Bank: The Delivery of Human Milk in Boston, 1909–1927,' *Bulletin of the History of Medicine* 62, 4 (winter 1988): 589–605

30 *Upper Canada Journal of Medical, Surgical and Physical Science* 2 (Oct. 1852): 180–1

31 Henry Lyman, *The Practical Home Physician and Encyclopedia of Medicine* (Guelph 1884), 954

32 *Canada Medical Record* 9, 12 (Sept. 1881): 301

33 Paul Mundé, *A Practical Treatise on the Diseases of Women* (Philadelphia 1891), 98, 35; *Canada Medical Record* 24 (March 1896): 268; 17, 5 (Feb. 1889): 98; MacCallum Papers, 'On Women's Medical Problems,' 1241; Napheys, *The Physical Life of Woman*, 187; Henry Garrigues, *A Text-book of the Diseases of Women* (Philadelphia 1894), 128

34 Kathleen Pickard, 'Choosing Hospitalised Childbirth: The Ottawa Maternity Hospital, 1895–1924' (MA thesis, Queen's University, 1986), 58, 33

35 McGill University Archives, University Lying-in Hospital Register, 1851–1900, RG 95, vol. 97. Figures are based on an analysis of every tenth patient, for each year, or 717 cases. The number of valid cases were 554. In the 1850s 13.5 per cent (n = 12) stayed longer than two weeks. This declined to 9.7 per cent (n = 12) in the 1860s but after that increased until 35.3 per cent (n = 48) in the 1890s stayed longer than two weeks. There is no indication that women were kept after their confinement in order to perform domestic duties to pay for their stay.

36 Toronto General Hospital, Burnside Lying-In Hospital Register, 1878–82, analysis of the 517 cases in the register

37 Annual Report, Montreal Maternity Hospital, 1896, 5

38 *Bylaws, University Lying-in Hospital*, 1859, 17

39 Toronto General Hospital, Burnside Lying-In Hospital Register, 1878–82, patient admitted 7 June 1879 and delivered 7 July 1879

40 It is intervention in childbirth that most critics focus on today. For example, Ann Oakley had pointed out that there is a direct correlation between the amount of depression a woman experiences after birth and the amount of intervention which occurred during childbirth. Ann Oakley, *Women Confined: Towards a Sociology of Childbirth* (Oxford: Martin Robertson 1980), 174

41 Tyler Smith, *The Modern Practice of Midwifery*, 29

42 McGill University Archives, University Lying-in Hospital Papers, RG 96, vol. 352–60. Dr Archibald Hall, 'Statistics of the University Lying-in Hospital, Montreal,' reprint from *British American Journal of Medical & Physical Science* 1 (1860): 20–1 of reprint.

43 *Canada Medical Record* 4 (Feb. 1876): 129

44 Chavasse, *Advice to a Wife*, 206; *Canada Lancet* 18 (Sept. 1885): 25; *Canada Medical Record* 18, 4 (Jan. 1890): 73–5 *Maritime Medical News* 10, 10 (Oct. 1898): 337

45 *Canada Medical Record* 18, 5 (Feb. 1889): 9

46 *Maritime Medical News* 4, 7 (July 1892): 125

47 *Canada Medical Record* 19, 4 (Jan. 1890): 94

48 *Canada Lancet* 7, 2 (Oct. 1874): 57

49 Rothman, *In Labour*, 145–6

50 In some respects, by making the pregnant woman a patient and deeming her ill or in need of assistance the physician '[robbed her] of autonomy and authority.' Ann Oakley, 'Wisewoman and Medicine Man: Changes in the Management of Childbirth,' in Juliet Mitchell and Ann Oakley, eds., *The Rights and Wrongs of Women* (Harmondsworth, Middlesex: Penguin Books 1976), 57

51 Mackay Papers, Obstetrical Notebook, patient Mrs ww, 248

52 Rhona Kenneally in her study of the Montreal Maternity Hospital indicated that intervention in childbirth increased considerably after the 1890s. Rhona Kenneally, 'The Montreal Maternity, 1843–1926: Evolution of a Hospital' (MA thesis, McGill University, 1983), 58

53 Walter Radcliffe, *Milestones in Midwifery* (Bristol: Wright 1967), 82–3

54 William Buchan, *Domestic Medicine* (London 1813), 419

55 McGill University Archives, University Lying-in Hospital Register, 1851–1900

56 Upper Canada Journal of Medical, Surgical and Physical Science 1 (Aug. 1851): 195–6

57 Ibid. (July 1851): 152

58 Hall, 'Statistics,' 19, 21

59 A.C. Siddall, 'Bloodletting in American Obstetric Practice, 1800–1945,' *Bulletin of the History of Medicine* 54, 1 (spring 1980): 107. In the United States bleeding continued until the late nineteenth century in cases of puerperal convulsions and into the twentieth century in gynaecological cases. John Haller, *American Medicine in Transition, 1840–1910* (Champaign Ill.: University of Illinois Press 1981), 64

60 Hall, 'Statistics,' 8–13. The general practice of James Langstaff from the 1850s to the 1870s indicates that the type of bleeding shifted from venesection to cupping and that the percentage of patients he bled and

the quantity of blood removed also decreased. Duffin, 'A Rural Practice,' 16–17

61 *Canadian Medical Review* 6, 5 (Nov. 1897): 161–2

62 Hall, 'Statistics,' 16–17

63 Public Archives of New Brunswick (PANB), Theodore Clowes Brown Papers, Obstetrical Cases 1860–93, analysis based on 1096 cases in the record

64 Mackay Papers, Obstetrical Notebook, 1873–88, based on an analysis of 816 patients in the notebook; Academy of Medicine Library, Dr James Ross Obstetric Record 1852–91, Ms Coll. 97, 98, based on an analysis of over 1400 patients, every patient record, for 1853, 1856, and every fifth year after that.

65 *Canada Lancet* 16 (Aug. 1884): 372

66 Ibid. 18 (Sept. 1885): 26

67 PANS, British Medical Association – Nova Scotia Branch, MG 20, no. 203, Minutes, 9 April 1891, 107; Dr Adam Wright of the Burnside Lying-In Hospital also advocated a 'Modified Credé' method in the third stage of labour. *Canadian Medical Review* 6, 5 (Nov. 1897): 158

68 Radcliffe, *Milestones in Midwifery*, 71; Mackay Papers, Obstetrical Notebook, 1873–88; Alvin Chase, *Dr Chase's Third, Last and Complete Receipt Book and Household Physician* (Detroit and Windsor 1892), 87

69 McGill University Archives, University Lying-in Hospital Register, 1851–1900

70 Toronto General Hospital, Burnside Lying-In Hospital Register

71 *Medical Chronicle or, Montreal Monthly Journal of Medicine & Surgery* 2 (Dec. 1854): 261

72 *Upper Canada Journal of Medical, Surgical and Physical Science* 1 (Aug. 1851): 198; *Provincial Medical Journal* 1 (May 1868): 14

73 PANS, Halifax Medical Society Minutes, MG 20, no. 181, Tuesday, 1 Oct. 1861

74 *Canadian Journal of Medical Science* 5 (Jan. 1880): 45

75 Ibid.; *Canada Lancet* 6, 7 (March 1874): 219; *Upper Canada Journal of Medical, Surgical and Physical Science* 2 (July 1852): 66–7

76 PANS, Halifax Medical Society Minutes, MG 20, no. 181, 1 Oct. 1861

77 Academy of Medicine Library, James Ross Obstetrical Record 1852–91, Ms Coll. 97, 98

78 Duffin, 'A Rural Practice,' 12

79 Toronto General Hospital, Burnside Lying-In Hospital Register, patient admitted 7 April 1881 and gave birth 10 April 1881

80 Harvey Graham, *Eternal Eve* (Altrincham: William Heinemann 1950), 188–205

81 Claudia Dreifus, *Seizing Our Bodies: The Politics of Women's Health* (New York: Random House 1978), xxii

82 There were 1344 valid cases, of which 7.3 per cent (n = 98) were forceps delivery. Of those women in labour for over twenty-four hours, 22 per cent (n = 46) experienced a forceps delivery.

83 Radcliffe, *Milestones in Midwifery*, 49; Jane Donegan, 'Midwifery in America, 1760–1860: A Study in Medicine and Morality' (PHD thesis, Syracuse University, 1972), 22

84 Tupper Medical Library, Dalhousie University, Lowder Manuscript, 142

85 McGill University Archives, University Lying-in Hospital Register, RG 95, vol. 97; Hall, 'Statistics,' 14; D.C. MacCallum, *Report of the University Lying-In Hospital for Eight Years* (Montreal 1878) 2, 5

86 Judith Schneid Lewis, 'Maternal Health in the English Aristocracy: Myths and Realities, 1790–1840,' *Journal of Social History* 17, 1 (fall 1983): 104

87 Tyler Smith, *The Modern Practice of Midwifery*, 30

88 Gunning Bedford, *The Principles and Practice of Obstetrics* (New York 1861), 569–75

89 *Maritime Medical News* 9, 5 (May 1897): 153

90 *Canadian Journal of Medical Science* 2 (Oct. 1877): 338–9

91 James Connor, 'Minority Medicine in Ontario, 1795 to 1903: A Study of Medical Pluralism and Its Decline' (PHD thesis, University of Waterloo, 1989), 155

92 *Canadian Medical Times* 1, 22 (Nov. 1873): 174

93 *Canada Medical Record* 7, 7 (April 1879): 184

94 AO, William Canniff Papers, MU 490 package 3, Canada Medical Association 1882 reports from newspapers

95 PANS, Victoria General Hospital Papers, RG 25, series B, Patient Records, patient RM, admitted 18 Dec. 1886; patient Mrs M, admitted 11 July 1893

96 *Canadian Medical Review* 6, 5 (Nov. 1897): 158

97 Toronto General Hospital, Burnside Lying-In Hospital Register, patient admitted 28 March 1881 and delivered the same day

98 Annual Report, Montreal Maternity Hospital, 1891, 5; Pickard, 'Choosing Hospitalised Birth,' 69

99 Support for this is suggested in British obstetric history. One observer
noted that physicians in England used forceps frequently, but their use
decreased substantially with no ill effects when midwives attended.
Canada Medical Record 26 (Jan. 1898): 14–15

100 The list consisted of 1 pair of obstetrical forceps (Barnes-Simpson
modified), 1 pair of obstetrical forceps (for use on phantom), 1 uterine
dressing forceps, 1 needle forceps – Russian, 1 Bullet forceps, 1 artery
forceps, 1 polypus forceps, 1 pair of scissors (curved on flat), 1
hypodermic syringe, 1 stethoscope, 1 speculum (Sims), 1 pair of needles
and silk. McGill University Archives, University Lying-in Hospital
Register, preface

101 Duffin, 'A Rural Practice,' 12–13

102 *Canadian Medical Association Journal* 40 (1939): 184

103 C.A. Sibley in her 'The Early History and Development of Gynaecology
in Canada, 1880–1910' (MA thesis, Queen's University, 1985) estimated a
17 per cent rate.

104 Mackay Papers, Obstetrical Notebook, patient Mrs WM, delivered 14
Feb. 1882, 351, and patient Mrs M, delivered 23 Feb. 1882, 327

105 *Canada Lancet* 18 (Sept. 1885): 73

106 *Canada Medical Record* 26 (Jan. 1898): 20

107 In the United States, Leavitt has argued that the increased use of
anaesthesia in home births did not result in increased use of forceps
but that in early twentieth-century hospital births it did. Leavitt,
Brought to Bed, 182

108 Alfred King, *A Manual of Obstetrics* (Philadelphia 1884), 204

109 Radcliffe, *Milestones in Midwifery*, 94

110 Connor, 'Minority Medicine in Ontario, 1795 to 1903,' 146

111 *Canadian Journal of Medical Science* 2 (Oct. 1877): 338

112 PANB, Theodore Brown Obstetrical Register, 1860–93

113 Mackay Papers, Obstetrical Notebook, patient AO 257

114 Toronto General Hospital, Burnside Lying-In Hospital Register, patient
admitted 3 Nov. 1879 and delivered 19 Nov. 1879

115 McGill University Archives, Montreal General Hospital Papers, RG 96
Gynaecology Casebook, vol. 275, 173; PANS, Halifax Medical Society,
Minutes, 3 Nov. 1862

116 McGill University Archives, University Lying-in Hospital Register,
1851–1900

117 *Canadian Practitioner* 11, 10 (Oct. 1886): 321–2

118 King, *Manual of Obstetrics*, 210

119 Ibid., 198

120 Graham, *Eternal Eve*, 160; King, *Manual of Obstetrics*, 198

121 *Dominion Medical Monthly* 1, 1 (July 1893): 26

122 *Canadian Practitioner* 20, 2 (Feb. 1895): 92; Annual Report of Montreal Maternity Hospital, 1898, 7; McGill University Archives, University Lying-in Hospital, Register, patient admitted 16 Oct. 1904 and discharged 24 Nov. 1904

123 Radcliffe, *Milestones in Midwifery*, 94

124 A. Charpentier, *Encyclopedia of Obstetrics and Gynecology*, vol. IV (New York 1887), 207

125 King, *Manual of Obstetrics*, 199

126 Canniff Papers, package 1, 'An Historial Sketch of Canadian Medicine and Surgery,' 15

127 King, *Manual of Obstetrics*, 198–9

128 Radcliffe, *Milestones in Midwifery*, 69

129 *Canada Medical and Surgical Journal* 12, 1 (Aug. 1884): 15

130 Kenneally, 'Montreal Maternity Hospital,' 68

131 It is interesting to note that in the present day many critics of the increase in Caesarian sections performed having pointed to a change in attitude by the medical profession. Whereas as we have seen in the past that priority was given to the mother, now it is given to the child. As Barbara Rothman has argued, 'In other situations in which taking a chance with the health of one person [mother] might possibly, though not certainly, benefit another person [infant], the question would almost surely be phrased as a moral/ethical problem.' However, in the present day it is defined as a medical problem. Here she is not arguing against Caesarian sections, but against the decision to perform one being a medical decision only. Rothman, *In Labour*, 278

132 PANS, Victoria General Hospital Papers, Patient Records, patient Mrs MS, admitted 17 Nov. 1893

133 Kenneally, 'Montreal Maternity Hospital,' 69

134 McGill University Archives, University Lying-in Hospital Register, 1851–1900. In a cross-tabulation of interference by length of labour, 2.8 per cent (n = 16) of the cases experienced interference, although 4.7 per cent (n = 6) of medium labour cases (twelve hours to under

twenty-four hours) and 8.8 per cent (n = 5) of long labours (twenty-four hours or more) did.

135 Toronto General Hospital, Burnside Lying-In Hospital Register 1872–82. Of 512 valid cases, 5.3 per cent (n = 27) were interfered with and of those with non-head presentation, 22.2 per cent (n = 14) were. Of 517 valid cases, 5.2 per cent (n = 27) were interfered with and of those with birth complications, 48.1 per cent (n = 13) were.

136 Mackay Papers, Obstetrical Notebook. In a cross-tabulation of interference with number of labours, 29.9 per cent (n = 218) were interfered with but 39.7 per cent (n = 81) of first labours were. When interference is cross-tabulated with length of labour, 32 per cent (n = 188) experienced some form of interference. Of those undergoing protracted labour (n = 74, 12.6 per cent), 45.9 per cent (n = 34) experienced some form of interference.

137 In New Jersey in 1974 almost one-third of all births were induced and 95 per cent were performed under anaesthesia. In 1982 18.5 per cent of all babies were delivered through Caesarian section in the United States. In Canada the 1980 figure was 14.9 per cent. Gena Corea, *The Hidden Malpractice: How American Medicine Mistreats Women* (New York: Harper and Row 1986), 224, 227, 243. Statistics Canada, *Women in Canada: A Statistical Report* (Ottawa: Statistics Canada 1985), 93

138 PANB, Brown Obstetrical Register. Of the 1096 cases, for only 424 was the date of the previous pregnancy known.

139 Andrews, 'Medical Services in Vancouver,' 75

140 Toronto General Hospital, Burnside Lying-In Hospital Register. Altogether, 9.6 per cent of the babies died, but 58.8 per cent of those with a non-head presentation died and 38.5 per cent of births with complications died.

141 Of those experiencing protracted labours (n = 209), 33.7 per cent (n = 29) had birth complications whereas the general rate for Ross's practice was only 6.4 per cent (n = 86).

142 Mackay Papers, Obstetrical Notebook. Of cases recorded (816), 1.3 per cent (n = 92) did not have a living child. For those having a non-head presentation compared to a head presentation, the figures were 64 per cent (n = 16) and 5.5 per cent (n = 37), respectively. For those experiencing protracted labour compared to normal, the figures were 16.9 per cent (n = 12) and 4.7 per cent (n = 23)

143 Ibid. For primipara women compared to multipara, the figures on complications were 39.7 per cent (n = 81) and 19.2 per cent (n = 101). For farm women (n = 197), 18.3 per cent (n = 36) experienced complications whereas for the general practice it was over 23 per cent.

144 Ibid., 333

145 PANS, Victoria General Hospital Papers, RG 25, series B III.3, Patient Records, patient Mrs M admitted 14 June 1882, 578; patient Mrs C admitted 14 July 1882, 603

146 McGill University Archives, Montreal General Hospital Papers, Diseases of Women Casebook, RG 96, vol. 273, Mrs ML, admitted 17 Aug. 1882, 157; Mrs HL, seen 18 July 1882, 139–40

147 PANS, Victoria General Hospital Papers, RG 25, series B III.3, Patient Records, Mrs O, admitted 7 Nov. 1900

148 Academy of Medicine Library, Dr Alexander McPhedran Casebook, 132

149 Theodore Thomas, *A Practical Treatise on the Diseases of Women* (Philadelphia 1868), 59; *Canada Medical Record* 17, 5 (Feb. 1889): 98; Garrigues, *A Text-book*, 128–9

150 Lyman, *Practical Home Physician*, 980

151 Charles Penrose, *A Text-book of Diseases of Women* (Philadelphia 1905), 18–19; *Canada Medical Record* 26 (Jan. 1898)): 4; Joseph Cooke, *A Nurse's Handbook of Obstetrics for the Use in Training Schools* (Philadelphia 1903), 13

152 *Canada Medical Record* 26, 1 (Jan. 1898): 4

153 *Canadian Practitioner* 23 (Oct. 1898): 581

154 Stephen Kern, *Anatomy and Destiny: A Cultural History of the Human Body* (Indianapolis: Bobbs-Merrill 1975), 37. For a different view of puerperal fever see Margaret Delacy, 'Puerperal Fever in Eighteenth-Century Britain,' *Bulletin of the History of Medicine* 63, 4 (winter 1989): 521–56

155 For an excellent study of the introduction of antiseptic techniques in Canada see James Connor, 'Joseph Lister's System of Wound Management and the Canadian Medical Practitioner, 1867–1900' (MA thesis, University of Western Ontario, 1981).

156 Fleetwood Churchill, *Essays on Puerperal Fever and Other Diseases Peculiar to Women* (Philadelphia 1850), 9

157 Kenneally, 'Montreal Maternity Hospital,' 51, 53

158 Between 1895 and 1925 fourteen out of fifty-seven maternal deaths at the Ottawa Civic Hospital were from puerperal fever. Suzann Buckley, 'The Search for the Decline of Maternal Mortality: The Place of Hospital Records,' in Wendy Mitchinson and Janice Dickin McGinnis, eds., *Essays in the History of Canadian Medicine* (Toronto: McClelland and Stewart 1988), 151

159 Sheila Ryan Johannson, 'Sex and Death in Victorian England: An Examination of Age – and Sex Specific Death Rates, 1840–1910,' in Martha Vicinus, ed., *A Widening Sphere: Changing Roles of Victorian Women* (Bloomington and London: Indiana University Press 1977), 167

160 It must be recognized that men were more prone to die from accidents compared to women.

161 William Carpenter, *Principles of Human Physiology* (London 1869), 909

162 *Canadian Journal of Medical Science* 2, 10 (Oct. 1877): 338

163 Napheys, *The Physical Life of Woman*, 190

164 Peter Ward and Patricia Ward, 'Infant Birth Weight and Nutrition in Industrializing Montreal,' *American Historical Review* 89, 2 (April 1984): 325, 327

165 In a recent study of slum areas in nineteenth- and twentieth-century England it was discerned that poverty was not linked to maternal mortality except as poverty resulted in poor obstetric practice. If women attended outdoor charities run by trained individuals, the maternal mortality rates, even in slum areas, declined. Irvine Loudon, 'Maternal Mortality: 1880–1950. Some Regional and International Comparisons,' *Social History of Medicine* 1, 2 (Aug. 1988). 220

166 McGill University Archives, University Lying-in Hospital Register, 1851–1900, preface

167 Peter Ward, ed., *The Mysteries of Montreal: Memoirs of a Midwife* by Charlotte Führer (Vancouver: University of British Columbia Press 1984), 8

168 Ward, ed., *Mysteries of Montreal*, 16

169 Duffin, 'A Rural Practice,' 11

170 *Census of Canada*, 1851–2, vol. 2, 34, 5

171 Ibid. 1870–1, vol. 2, tables VII and XVIII; ibid., 1880–1, vol. 2, tables VII and XIX

172 Duffin, 'A Rural Practice,' 11, 14

173 *Canadian Journal of Medical Science* 2 (Oct. 1877): 338

174 *Canada Medical Record* 6 (Jan. 1878): 81

175 MacCallum, 'Report,' 1, 7

716 Annual Report, Montreal Maternity Hospital 1891, 5

177 Connor, 'Minority Medicine in Ontario,' 164

178 Pickard, 'Choosing Hospitalised Birth,' 72; this included years up to 1924.

179 *Census of Canada*, 1850–1, vol. 1, 310–12, 558–68

180 Ibid., 1860–1, vol. 1, 528–9, 524–5, 592–3. A total of 990 women died between the ages of fifteen and forty, and of these 188 died owing to childbirth complications.

181 Ibid., 356–9, 582–3. A total of 991 women died during potential childbearing years and 185 died of childbirth complications.

182 For Ontario the rate was 10.8 per cent; for Quebec, 9.5 per cent; for New Brunswick, 8.1 per cent and for Nova Scotia, 7.5 per cent. Ibid., 1870–1, vol. 2, 398–9, 412–18, 522–4

183 Ibid., 1890–1, vol. 2, 70–1, 106–36

184 Roderick P. Beaujot and Kevin McQuillan, 'Social Effects of Demographic Change: Canada 1851–1981,' *Journal of Canadian Studies* 21 (spring 1986): 61

185 David Gagan, *Hopeful Travellers: Families, Land, and Social Change in Mid-Victorian Peel County, Canada West* (Toronto: University of Toronto Press 1981), 89

186 George Graham-Cummings, 'Health of the Original Canadians, 1867–1967,' *Medical Services Journal, Canada* 23 (Feb. 1967): 120

187 Nancy Schrom Dye, 'Modern Obstetrics and Working-Class Women: The New York Midwifery Dispensary, 1890–1920,' *Journal of Social History* 20, 3 (spring 1978): 559

CHAPTER 8 The Rise of Gynaecology

1 *Canada Medical Record* 16, 2 (Nov. 1887): 25–6

2 George Napheys, *The Physical Life of Woman: Advice to the Maiden, Wife and Mother* (Toronto 1890), 253; *Canada Medical Record* 19, 4 (Jan. 1891): 73

3 British Columbia Archives and Record Service (BCARS), John Helmcken Casebook, Add. Mss 505, A-810, vol. 3. The casebooks also indicate a high degree of syphilitic problems. While syphilis was not confined to men,

the medical literature of the day certainly seemed to feel that men more than women contracted it. The patient records of the Victoria General Hospital in Halifax also suggest that some of the treatment meted out to men could be extremely painful. One young boy was treated for a wound to the urethra. Part of the treatment consisted of inserting a bougie into it. Public Archives of Nova Scotia (PANS), Victoria General Hospital, RG 25, series B.III.4, Patient Records, 539

4 Academy of Medicine Library, Alexander Primrose Papers, Patient Records 1888–99

5 James Fraser, *The Emigrants Medical Guide* (Glasgow 1853), 129

6 Alvin Wood Chase, *Dr Chase's Third, Last and Complete Receipt Book and Household Physician* (Detroit and Windsor 1892), 210

7 Henry Lyman, *The Practical Home Physician* (Guelph 1892), 1018

8 Alexander Skene, *Medical Gynecology: A Treatise on the Diseases of Women from the Standpoint of the Physician* (New York 1895), 64

9 PANS, City and Provincial Hospital Annual Report 1867, 11. There was one case of hysteria which nineteenth-century physicians associated only with women. In addition, there were midwifery cases. The City and Provincial Hospital later became the Victoria General Hospital.

10 Ira Warren, *The Household Physician* (Boston 1865), 348

11 *Sanitary Journal* 2, 2 (Feb. 1876): 171

12 C.A. Sibley, 'The Early History and Development of Gynaecology in Canada, 1880–1910' (MA thesis, Queen's University, 1985), 54, 78, ii. G.M. White, 'The History of Obstetrical and Gynaecological Teaching in Canada,' *American Journal of Obstetrics and Gynecology* 77 (1959): 468

13 BCARS. *Pioneer Days* (Victoria, B.C.: Provincial Royal Jubilee Hospital 1924), 14–20

14 Annual Report, Halifax Visiting Dispensary, 1874, 17–18; 1876, 12

15 Queen's University Archives, Kingston General Hospital Papers, H 101, Dean J.C. Connell, *History of the Kingston General Hospital* (np 1925), np

16 Annual Report of the Victoria General Hospital 1895, Journals of the House of Assembly, Nova Scotia 1896, appendix 3B, 23

17 Queen's University Archives, Register for Kingston General Hospital, 1853, 1856, 1861, 1866. An analysis of over 1700 patients revealed a variety of health problems which I collapsed into the following categories:

general poor health, digestive, accident, mental, ear-eye-nose-throat, genito-urinary, respiratory, fever, contagious, heart-liver-kidney, skin, moral, motor, brain-nervous, pregnancy, and other. Accidents represent 11.8 per cent (n = 193) of the cases and men represented 81.9 per cent (n = 158) of the total. Genito-urinary ailments represented 10 per cent (n = 162) of the cases and women represented 51.9 per cent (n = 84) of this category, despite the fact that they only represented 38.6 per cent (n = 627) of the patients.

18 *Canada Medical Record* 7 (April 1879): 184
19 Calculated from the annual reports of the Halifax Visiting Dispensary
20 Annual Report, Royal Victoria Hospital, 1895, 9, 13; 1901, 24
21 Sibley, 'The Early History and Development of Gynaecology,' 157–60
22 Primrose Papers, based on an analysis of over 1000 patients between 1888 and 1899, examining every patient, every other year
23 Harvey Graham, *Eternal Eve* (Altrincham: William Heinemann 1950), 442–5
24 PANS, Halifax Medical Society Minutes, MG 20, no. 181, 8 July 1862, 5 Nov. 1866
25 McGill University Archives, Montreal General Hospital, University Dispensary, Diseases of Women Casebook, 18 March 1882–23 October 1883, RG 96, vol. 273
26 *Canadian Practitioner* 23, 10 (Oct. 1898): 579
27 PANS, Victoria General Hospital Papers, RG 25, series B, 4C, H.L. Scammell, *A History of the Victoria General Hospital*, 23
28 Theodore Thomas, *A Practical Treatise on the Diseases of Women* (Philadelphia 1868), 47
29 *Canada Lancet* 19, 2 (Nov. 1886): 71; see also McGill University Archives, D.C. MacCallum Papers, MG 2031, 'On Diseases Peculiar to Women,' 1–2
30 *Canada Lancet* 16, 12 (Aug. 1884): 384
31 Ibid., 16, 12 (Aug. 1884): 384
32 *Maritime Medical News* 10 (Oct. 1898): 337
33 *Canadian Journal of Medicine and Surgery* 4, 5 (Nov. 1898): 294
34 Archives of Ontario (AO), Rev. William Cochrane Papers, MS 409, reel 2, series B-6, Diary, 1 Jan. 1871
35 *Radway's Almanac for 1872 and Guide to Health* (Montreal 1872), 26; *Radway's Almanac and Guide to Health 1886* (Montreal 1886), 25–6

36 Warren, *The Household Physician*, 339, 352, 348

37 Chase, *Dr Chase's*, 212–14

38 Jefferis's prescription for amenorrhoea was quite complex and included bichloride of mercury, arsenite of sodium, sulphite of strychnine, carbonate of potassium, and sulphate of iron. Once mixed, the woman was to divide it into sixty pills and to take one after every meal. Benjamin Grant Jefferis, *Searchlights on Health: Light on Dark Corners* (Fredericton 1894), 360

39 R. Pierce, *The People's Common Sense Medical Adviser in Plain English* (Buffalo 1882), 762

40 Dalhousie University, Tupper Library, John Lowder Manuscript, 99–100, 30

41 *British American Journal of Medical & Physical Science* 6, 4 (Aug. 1850): 161–2. Even today criticism has been made against the unwillingness of many physicians to realize how difficult it is for women to be examined by a male physician. Joan Emerson, 'Behaviour in Private Places: Sustaining Definitions of Reality in Gynecological Examinations,' in H. Dreitzel, *Recent Sociology* 2 (New York: Macmillan 1970), 333

42 *Medical Chronicle or, Montreal Monthly Journal of Medicine & Surgery* 1 (March 1854): 300

43 Henry MacNaughton-Jones, *Points of Practical Interest in Gynaecology* (London 1901), 4

44 MacCallum Papers, 'On Diseases Peculiar to Women,' 2–4

45 *Medical Chronicle or, Montreal Monthly Journal of Medicine & Surgery* 4 (Sept. 1856): 147

46 Ibid., 1 (Jan. 1854): 219–20

47 *Canada Medical and Surgical Journal* 2, 1 (July 1873): 1–2

48 Friederich Scanzoni von Lichtenfels, *A Practical Treatise on the Diseases of Women* (New York 1861), 38

49 PANS, Victoria General Hospital Papers, RG 25, series III.4, patient MC, admitted 25 Oct. 1885

50 Thomas, *Practical Treatise on the Diseases of Women*, 66; *Canada Medical Record* 5 (Nov. 1876): 56

51 PANS, Victoria General Hospital Papers, RG 25, series B, Patient Records, patient CM, admitted 22 Dec. 1894

52 *Canada Medical Record* 20, 4 (Jan. 1891): 74; Alban Doran, *Handbook of Gynaecological Operations* (London 1887), 45

53 Arthur Edis, *Diseases of Women: A Manual for Students and Practitioners* (Philadelphia 1882), 20–3; *Canada Medical and Surgical Journal* 2, 1 (July 1873): 2

54 MacCallum Papers, 'On Diseases Peculiar to Women,' 6–7

55 McGill University Archives, Montreal General Hospital Papers, RG 96, Diseases of Women Casebook, University Dispensary, vol. 273, 403, 73

56 Ibid., Gynecology Casebook, University Dispensary, patient Mrs S, admitted 1 April 1882

57 PANS, Victoria General Hospital Papers, Patient Records, patient MD, admitted 22 July 1894

58 Ibid., RG 25, series III.4, 1875–82, patient RN, admitted 31 Aug. 1881

59 *Medical Chronicle or, Montreal Monthly Journal of Medicine & Surgery* 4 (Sept. 1856): 145, 149; PANS, Halifax Medical Society Minutes, MG 20, no. 181, 2 Aug. 1864; *Canada Medical and Surgical Journal* 2, 1 (July 1873): 1; *Canada Lancet* 17, 11 (July 1885): 320

60 AO, Hugh Mackay Papers, Misc. Coll. 1873 no. 6, MU 2118, Obstetrical Notebook, 191–2

61 McGill University Archives, Montreal General Hospital Papers, RG 96, Diseases of Women Casebook, University Dispensary, vol. 273, patient Mrs B, admitted 1 April 1882

62 *Canada Lancet* 4 (June 1863), 25; Henry Garrigues, *A Text-book of the Diseases of Women* (Philadelphia 1894), 182

63 *British American Journal of Medical & Physical Science* 2, 3 (July 1846): 61–2

64 *Canada Medical and Surgical Journal* 14 (Feb. 1886): 411

65 *Medical Chronicle or, Montreal Monthly Journal of Medicine & Surgery* 1, 10 (March 1854): 302

66 Von Lichtenfels, *A Practical Treatise on the Diseases of Women,* 61

67 Thomas, *A Practical Treatise on the Diseases of Women,* 73–86

68 Patricia Branca, *Women in Europe since 1750* (London: Croom Helm 1978), 115

69 *Canada Lancet* 19, 3 (Nov. 1886): 72

70 Sibley, 'The Early History and Development of Gynaecology in Canada,' 36

71 *Canada Medical and Surgical Journal* 16, 1 (July 1888): 19

72 McGill University Archives, Montreal General Hospital Papers, RG 96, Diseases of Women Casebook, University Dispensary, vol. 273

73 *Canada Lancet* 24, 3 (Nov. 1891): 92

74 PANS, Victoria General Hospital Papers, Patient Records, RG 25, series B.III.3, patient BR, admitted 8 May 1882, 538

75 Ibid., patient AD, admitted 29 July 1893

76 *Canada Medical Record* 22 (Oct. 1893): 18, published a piece in which the author complained about unskilled people getting involved in gynaecology.

77 Garrigues, *A Text-book of the Diseases of Women*, 129

78 MacCallum Papers, 'On Diseases Peculiar to Women,' 55

79 Academy of Medicine Library, Dr J. Ross Papers, Ms Coll. 99, Gynecological Record Book 1890–3, 105

80 Pierce, *The People's Common Sense Medical Adviser*, 764–5; MacCallum Papers, 'On Diseases Peculiar to Women,' 168

81 Sibley, 'The Early History and Development of Gynaecology in Canada,' 32

82 Ibid., 109–15

83 BCARS, Royal Jubilee Hospital, Discharge Register, based on analysis of 1517 patients from 1891, 1896, and 1901. Altogether, 36 per cent of patients stayed in the hospital for under ten days, but of those undergoing gynaecological surgery only 14 per cent did.

84 The above information comes from Sibley, 'The Early History and Development of Gynaecology in Canada,' 109–21.

85 McGill University Archives, Montreal General Hospital Papers, Gynecology Casebook, vol. 275, patient MM, 110

86 Ibid., Disease of Women Casebook, University Dispensary, patient MS, 587

87 PANS, Victoria General Hospital Papers, Patient Records, patient RM, admitted 18 Dec. 1888

88 Ross Papers, Ms Coll. 99, Gynecological Record Book 1890–3, patient MM, 16 June 1890, 5–6

89 See James Connor, 'Joseph Lister's System of Wound Management and the Canadian Medical Practitioner, 1867–1900' (MA thesis, University of Western Ontario, 1981).

CHAPTER 9 Gynaecological Surgery

1 Public Archives of Nova Scotia (PANS), Halifax Medical Society Minutes, MG 20, no. 181, 8 July 1862

2 Annual Report, Royal Victoria Hospital, 1895, 36–44

3 Abraham Groves, *All in the Day's Work: Leaves from a Doctor's Casebook* (Toronto: Macmillan 1934), 3–4

4 Report of the Commissioners of Public Charities, 1899, Medical Board, Victoria General Hospital, Journals of the House of Assembly, Nova Scotia 1900, app. 3B, 80

5 Francis Shepherd, *Origin and History of the Montreal General Hospital* (np, nd), 19

6 McGill University Archives, Annual reports of the Montreal General Hospital, 1891–2, 1900–1

7 S.E.D. Shortt, 'The Canadian Hospital in the Nineteenth Century: An Historical Lament,' *Journal of Canadian Studies* 18, 4 (winter 1983–4): 10

8 James Ricci, *The Development of Gynaecological Surgery and Instruments* (Philadelphia: Blakiston 1949), 279; Harvey Graham, *Eternal Eve* (New York: Doubleday 1951), 492; see also James Ricci, *One Hundred Years of Gynaecology 1800–1900* (Philadelphia: Blakiston 1945), 35.

9 Annual Report, Montreal General Hospital, 1861, 16

10 Bernard Stern, *Social Factors in Medical Progress* (New York: AMS Press 1968), 23–4

11 G. Barker-Benfield, 'Sexual Surgery in Late-Nineteenth-Century America,' in Claudia Dreifus, ed., *Seizing Our Bodies: The Politics of Women's Health* (New York: Vintage Books 1977), 21–3

12 *Canada Medical Journal and Monthly Record* 2 (Jan. 1866): 347

13 *Canada Medical and Surgical Journal* 14, 1 (July 1886): 108

14 *Canada Medical Record* 16, 4 (Jan. 1888): 80

15 Report of the Commissioners of Public Charities, 1898, Medical Board, Victoria General Hospital, Journals of the House of Assembly, Nova Scotia 1899, app. 3B, 50

16 C.A. Sibley, 'The Early History and Development of Gynaecology in Canada, 1880–1910' (MA thesis, Queen's University, 1985), 123–5

17 Ricci, *One Hundred Years of Gynaecology*, 166–71

18 *Canada Medical Record* 28, 5 (Feb. 1890): 97–9

19 Archives of Ontario, Hugh Mackay Papers, Misc. Col. 1873 no. 6, MU 2118, Notebook, 204

20 Margaret Angus, *Kingston General Hospital: A Social and Institutional History* (Montreal: McGill-Queen's University Press 1973), 67, 72, 39, 45

21 Directors Report, Provincial Royal Jubilee Hospital, 1895–6, 31–3

22 McGill University Archives, Royal Victoria Hospital Papers, RG 95, Annual Report, Royal Victoria Hospital, Montreal, 1895

23 *Canada Medical Record* 26, 4 (Jan. 1898): 4

24 McGill University Archives, Montreal General Hospital Papers, University Dispensary, RG 96, Gynaecology Casebook, vol. 275, patient Mme B, admitted 8 April 1882

25 *Canadian Practitioner* 9, 9 (Sept. 1884): 274

26 *Canadian Medical Record* 16, 2 (Nov. 1887): 25

27 *Canadian Practitioner and Review* 19 (July 1894): 500

28 Ricci, *One Hundred Years of Gynaecology*, 432

29 *Canada Medical Journal and Monthly Record of Medical and Surgical Science* 4, 5 (Nov. 1867): 207–9

30 Henry MacNaughton-Jones, *Points of Practical Interest in Gynecology* (London 1901), 88–90

31 Henry Garrigues, *A Text-book of the Diseases of Women* (Philadelphia 1894), 292

32 G.J. Barker-Benfield, *The Horrors of a Half-Known Life: Male Attitudes toward Women and Sexuality in Nineteenth-Century America* (New York: Harper Colophon Books 1976), 120

33 Annual Report of the Royal Victoria Hospital 1895, 59

34 Theodore Thomas, *A Practical Treatise on the Diseases of Women* (Philadelphia 1868), 49, 561

35 *Canadian Practitioner* 12 (Oct. 1887): 307

36 Lawrence D. Longo, 'The Rise and Fall of Battey's Operation: A Fashion in Surgery,' *Bulletin of History of Medicine* 53, 2 (summer 1979): 252

37 J.A. Price, 'The Early Ovariotomists – Pioneers in Abdominal Surgery,' *Ulster Medical Journal* 36 (winter 1967): 5, 8

38 *Canada Medical and Surgical Journal* 14, 22 (Sept. 1885): 108

39 Thomas, *A Practical Treatise on the Diseases of Women*, 566

40 *Medical Chronicle or, Montreal Monthly Journal of Medicine & Surgery* 4 (Dec. 1856): 260

41 Thomas, *A Practical Treatise on the Diseases of Women*, 563–5

42 *Canada Medical Journal and Monthly Record of Medical and Surgical Science* 8, 3 (Sept. 1871): 98

43 *Canada Medical and Surgical Journal* 10 (Jan. 1882): 341

44 *Canadian Practitioner* 10, 12 (Dec. 1885): 361

45 *Canada Medical and Surgical Journal* 4 (Feb. 1876): 13

46 *Canadian Practitioner* 12 (Oct. 1887): 312

47 Annual Report, Montreal General Hospital, 1864, 16

48 James Connor, 'Joseph Lister's System of Wound Management and the Canadian Medical Practitioner, 1867–1900' (MA thesis, University of Western Ontario, 1981), 6

49 *Canada Medical Journal and Monthly Record of Medical and Surgical Science* 8, 3 (Sept. 1871): 97–9

50 Charles G. Roland, 'The Early Years of Antiseptic Surgery in Canada,' *Journal of the History of Medicine* 22 (1967): 388

51 *Obstetric Journal of Great Britain and Ireland* 43 (Oct. 1876): 429, 432

52 Longo, 'The Rise and Fall,' 255; *Canada Medical Record* 4 (June 1876): 217, 220

53 *Canada Medical Record* 6, 5 (Feb. 1878): 159; 13, 2 (Nov. 1884): 25–8

54 Ibid., 13, 2 (Nov. 1884): 25; *Canadian Practitioner* 9 (Sept. 1884): 272

55 *Canada Medical and Surgical Journal* 15 (Oct. 1887): 141

56 *Canadian Practitioner* 12 (Oct. 1887): 312

57 Annual Report of the Montreal General Hospital, 1884–5 and 1900–1

58 Annual Report of the Royal Victoria Hospital, Montreal, 1895, 47, 59

59 PANS, Victoria General Hospital Papers, RG 25, series B, Patient Records, patient RG, admitted 2 July 1887

60 Report of the Commissioners of Public Charities, 1894, 1899, Medical Board, Victoria General Hospital, Journals of the House of Assembly, Nova Scotia 1895, 1900, app. 3B

61 Annual Directors Report 1896, Provincial Royal Jubilee Hospital, 31–2

62 Thomas, *A Practical Treatise on the Diseases of Women*, 563

63 *Canada Lancet* 9 (March 1877): 210

64 *Canada Medical and Surgical Journal* 8 (Oct. 1879): 128

65 *Obstetric Journal of Great Britain and Ireland* 43 (Oct. 1876): 426

66 *Canada Medical Record* 4 (June 1876): 217–19

67 Arthur Edis, *Diseases of Women: A Manual for Students and Practitioners* (Philadelphia 1882), 273

68 *Canada Medical and Surgical Journal* 10 (Jan. 1882): 340

69 *Canada Medical Record* 13, 2 (Nov. 1884): 25; *Canadian Practitioner* 12 (Oct. 1887): 310

70 Longo, 'The Rise and Fall,' 256

71 *Canadian Practitioner* 9 (Sept. 1884): 273; 12 (Oct. 1887): 309

72 *Canada Medical Record* 13, 2 (Nov. 1884): 27

73 *Canadian Practitioner* 12 (Oct. 1887): 309

74 Garrigues, *A Text-book*, 130

75 MacNaughton-Jones, *Points of Practical Interest in Gynaecology*, 69–70

76 Barker-Benfield, in *The Horrors of a Half-Known Life*, 122, wrote: 'Doctors claimed success for castration when it returned woman to her normal role, subservient to her husband, her family and household duties.'

77 *Canada Lancet* 8, 6 (Feb. 1876): 176–7; 26 (Jan. 1894): 143

78 William Goodell, *Lessons in Gynaecology* (Philadelphia 1890), 413

79 *Canadian Practitioner* 9 (Sept. 1884): 273

80 Trenholme was apparently the first to remove the ovary of a patient for a myoma in 1876. Ricci, *One Hundred Years of Gynecology*, 102

81 *Canada Medical Record* 13, 2 (Nov. 1884): 26

82 *Canada Medical and Surgical Journal* 13 (Oct. 1884): 173–5

83 Longo, 'The Rise and Fall,' 263

84 *Canada Medical and Surgical Journal* 13, 3 (Oct. 1884): 227

85 *Canadian Practitioner* 12 (Oct. 1887): 309; 15 (Nov. 1890): 513

86 *Manitoba and West Canada Lancet* 6, 4 (Aug. 1898): 34

87 *Canada Medical and Surgical Journal* 10 (Jan. 1882): 342

88 *Canadian Practitioner* 9 (Dec. 1884): 364–5

89 Ibid. 19 (July 1894): 496; *Canada Lancet* 26 (Jan. 1894): 143

90 Longo, 'The Rise and Fall,' 266

91 *Dominion Medical Monthly and Ontario Medical Journal* 11, 5 (Nov. 1898): 225 (my emphasis)

92 *Canadian Practitioner* 11 (Oct. 1886): 322

93 *Canada Medical and Surgical Journal* 10 (Jan. 1882): 342

94 *Canadian Practitioner* 15 (Nov. 1890): 513; 9 (Sept. 1884): 272

95 *Canada Medical and Surgical Journal* 14 (July 1886): 716

96 *Canada Practitioner* 12 (Oct. 1887): 308

97 *Canada Medical and Surgical Journal* 12 (Aug. 1884): 26; 15 (Oct. 1887): 143–4; 14 (Nov. 1886): 214

98 *Canada Practitioner* 19 (July 1894): 499

99 *Canada Medical Journal and Monthly Record of Medical and Surgical Science* 8 (Sept. 1871): 97

100 *Canadian Practitioner* 10 (Dec. 1885): 360; 15 (Nov. 1890): 514; 23 (Oct. 1898): 581; 19 (July 1894): 499–500; *Dominion Medical Monthly* 12, 6 (June 1899): 280

101 *Canadian Practitioner* 10 (Dec. 1885): 361

102 Ibid. 12 (Oct. 1887): 311; *Canada Medical Record* 16, 2 (Nov. 1887): 26; *Canada Medical Record* 16, 4 (Jan. 1888): 80; Dr J. Campbell of Seaforth, Ontario, expressed similar views in the *Dominion Medical Monthly and Ontario Medical Journal* 5, 6 (Dec. 1895): 674; even the eminent gynaecologist William Goodell expressed caution, though he had earned much of his reputation through such surgery. *Canadian Practitioner* 19 (July 1894): 497

103 *Dominion Medical Monthly and Ontario Medical Journal* 12, 6 (June 1899): 280–1

104 Ibid. 11 (Nov. 1898): 225

105 *Canadian Practitioner* 23 (Oct. 1898): 580. Sibley in her thesis has also suggested that class as well as gender played a part. We have noted the tendency to operate more on working-class women because of their need to get back to work as quickly as possible. Sibley, however, suggests that the class bias goes beyond practical reasons. She maintains that some of the medical texts in the 1890s linked diseases with class, vice, and poverty: 'The tendency for a general practitioner in Canada, too busy or ill-equipped for pathological tests, and laden with the aforementioned class-based biases, to misdiagnose and perform a hysterectomy unnecessarily in an indigent patient, may have been a regrettable and all too frequent occurrence.' Sibley, 'The Early History and Development of Gynaecology in Canada,' 82

106 *Obstetrical Journal of Great Britain and Ireland* 43 (Oct. 1876): 425

107 *Canadian Practitioner* 12 (Oct. 1877): 308

108 McGill University Archives, D.C. MacCallum Papers, MG 2031, 'On Women's Medical Problems,' 87

109 *Canadian Practitioner* 9 (Sept. 1884): 272; 10 (Dec. 1885): 361, quoted from *Medical News*

110 *Canada Medical and Surgical Journal* 15 (Oct. 1886): 143

111 *Canadian Practitioner* 10 (Dec. 1885): 360

112 Ibid. 19 (July 1894): 495–6

113 PANS, Victoria General Hospital Papers, RG 25, series B, Patient Records, patient SMI, admitted 6 June 1896, box 42, no. 839, 1900; patient Mrs M, admitted 11 Sept. 1900

114 PANS, Victoria General Hospital Patient Records, 1900, patient BC, no. 869

115 *Canada Medical and Surgical Journal* 19 (Jan. 1882): 341

116 Goodell, *Lessons in Gynaecology*, 410–13

117 *Canadian Practitioner* 19 (July 1894): 493–4; Charles Penrose, *A Text-book of Diseases of Women* (Philadelphia 1905), 52

118 *Canada Lancet* 26 (Jan. 1894): 143

119 Thomas, *A Practical Treatment on the Diseases of Women*, 509

120 *Canada Lancet* 3, 5 (Jan. 1871): 182 (my emphasis)

121 *Canadian Practitioner* 19 (July 1894): 497

122 Alexander Skene, *Medical Gynecology: A Treatise on the Diseases of Women from the Standpoint of the Physician* (New York 1895), 18

123 *Canadian Practitioner* 15 (Nov. 1890): 513

124 Penrose, *A Text-book*, 52

125 *Canada Medical and Surgical Journal* 10 (Jan. 1882): 341

126 Goodell, *Lessons in Gynaecology*, 410–11

127 *Canadian Practitioner* 19 (July 1894): 494–5

128 Ibid. 10 (Dec. 1885): 360

129 Ibid. 15 (Nov. 1890): 513

130 Penrose, *A Text-book*, 535

131 *Canada Medical and Surgical Journal* 15, 9 (April 1887): 572

132 *Canada Medical Record* 22 (Oct. 1893): 18

133 *Canadian Practitioner* 23 (Oct. 1898): 579

134 *Dominion Medical Monthly* 12, 6 (June 1899): 278–9

135 When the ovariotomy 'craze' was declining in general practice it was picked up by a few asylums. See Andrew Scull and Diane Favreau, '''A Chance to Cut is a Chance to Cure'': Sexual Surgery for Psychosis in Three Nineteenth Century Societies,' *Research in Law, Deviance and Social Control* 8 (1986): 3–39.

CHAPTER 10 Women and Mental Health

1 *Maritime Medical News* 6 (Jan. 1894): 211

2 *Canada Lancet* 33, 1 (Sept. 1899): 56

3 *Canada Medical Record* 22 (April 1894): 168

4 John Haller, Jr, 'Neurasthenia: The Medical Profession and the "New Woman" of the Late Nineteenth Century,' *New York State Journal of Medicine* 71 (Feb. 1971): 474

5 *Canada Medical Record* 4 (Aug. 1875): 92; *Canada Medical and Surgical Journal* 13 (Oct. 1884): 165; Annual Report, Montreal General Hospital, 1891–2; Public Archives of Nova Scotia (PANS), Victoria General Hospital Papers, RG 25, series B, Patient Records, patient CF, admitted 19 Feb. 1894 and discharged 21 Aug. 1894

6 *Sanitary Journal* 2 (Feb. 1876): 172; *Canada Medical Record* 8 (Sept. 1879): 319; *Montreal Medical Journal* 25, 9 (March 1897): 751–2. See also Alexander Skene, *Medical Gynecology: A Treatise on the Diseases of Women from the Standpoint of the Physician* (New York 1895), 30.

7 Benjamin Miller and Elaine Keane, *Encyclopedia and Dictionary of Medicine, Nursing and Allied Health* (Philadelphia: W.B. Saunders 1978), 500–1

8 Carroll Smith-Rosenberg, 'The Hysterical Woman: Sex Roles and Role Conflict in Nineteenth-Century America,' in her *Disorderly Conduct: Visions of Gender in Victorian America* (New York: Oxford University Press 1985), 200. Elaine Showalter has an extensive discussion of the relationship between feminism and hysteria in her *The Female Malady: Women, Madness, and English Culture, 1830–1980* (New York: Pantheon Books 1985), 145–64.

9 Showalter, *The Female Malady*, 5

10 Hannah Decker, 'Freud and Dora: Constraints on Medical Progress,' *Journal of Social History* 14, 3 (spring 1981): 449

11 Edward Shorter, 'Women's Diseases before 1900,' paper presented to the American Historical Association, 1978, 30. Shorter also maintains that feminist historians have made doctors the villains of the piece by insisting that they tried to convince women they were sick when they were not. However, this is a misreading of the literature. The emphasis that feminist historians have made was on the role of the woman and what she was responding to, not the role of the physician, which seems to be central in Shorter's hypothesis.

12 Yet we have to use them warily; for most of the century non-paying patients predominated in such institutions and the hysterics among

them were not necessarily representative of the hysterical population as
a whole.

13 Dalhousie University, Annual Report, Halifax Visiting Dispensary, 1857,
1868, 1874, and 1878; PANS, Annual Report of the Provincial and City
Hospital, Halifax, 1882–8, 1889–98. Of the 1770 patients examined at the
Kingston General Hospital at mid-century, only seven were hysterical.
The low number may reflect the few women who entered the hospital.
Annual Report, Montreal General Hospital, 1865, 16. The annual reports
of the Montreal General Hospital indicate that in 1871 there were
fourteen cases. This fluctuated from no cases in 1874 to twenty-five
cases in 1891–2.

14 *Canada Medical and Surgical Journal* 15 (Aug. 1887): 2

15 *Canada Medical Record* 4 (Feb. 1876): 140

16 *Canada Lancet* 12 (Jan. 1880): 146. The association of women with
hysteria was a long-standing one. Galen devoted one of his studies to
the 'affections of the female genitalia,' most of which concerned
hysteria. Haly Abbas (d. 994), a Persian physician, argued that hysteria
varied depending on whether menstrual products or semen was
retained in the uterus and became putrid. Harvey Graham, *Eternal Eve*
(Altrincham: William Heinemann 1950), 83, 103. In 1682 Thomas
Sydenham wrote that next to fever, hysteria was the most common
disease among women. John Wright, 'Hysteria and Mechanical Man,'
Journal of the History of Ideas 41, 2 (April 1980): 233. In the eighteenth
century physicians connected hysteria in women to disease of the
spleen. Veida Skultans, *English Madness: Ideas on Insanity 1580–1890*
(London: Routledge and Kegan Paul 1979), 28–9. Nineteenth-century
physicians simply adopted what by then was conventional wisdom –
hysteria was a woman's complaint. William Buchan, *Domestic Medicine*
(London 1813), 377; Thomas Watson, *Lectures on the Principles and
Practice of Physic* (Philadelphia 1848), 414; James Fraser, *The
Emigrant's Medical Guide* (Glasgow 1853), 129–37; Henry Guernsey,
*The Application of the Principles and Practice of Homoeopathy to
Obstetrics and the Disorders Peculiar to Women and Young Children*
(Philadelphia 1867), 150; Arthur Edis, *Diseases of Women: A Manual
for Students and Practitioners* (Philadelphia 1882), 523; Ernst
Strumpell, *Textbook of Medicine* (New York 1886), 757; *Canada*

Medical and Surgical Journal 15 (Aug. 1887): 2; Hamilton Ayers, *Ayers' Everyman His Own Doctor* (Montreal 1881), 317

17 *Canada Medical Record* 8 (June 1880): 237

18 Edis, *Diseases of Women*, 524

19 Guernsey, *The Application of the Principles and Practice of Homeopathy*, 155; *Canada Medical Record* 7, 2 (Sept. 1879): 319; Edis, *Diseases of Women*, 523–4; *Canada Lancet* 24 (Sept. 1891) 11; *Dominion Medical Monthly* 10, 3 (March 1898): 89

20 Guernsey, *The Application of the Principles and Practice of Homoeopathy*, 155; *Canada Medical Journal and Monthly Record of Medical and Surgical Science* 7 (Sept. 1870): 185–6; Edis, *Diseases of Women*, 524; *Maritime Medical News* 6, 3 (Jan. 1894): 211; *Canada Lancet* 25 (Jan. 1892): 164; *Dominion Medical Monthly* 1, 3 (Sept. 1893): 68

21 University of Western Ontario, Richard Maurice Bucke Collection, B5, 'The Functions of the Great Nervous System,' 24

22 Watson, *Lectures on the Principles and Practice of Physic*, 416

23 Guernsey, *The Application of the Principles and Practice of Homoeopathy*, 148, 155; *Canada Medical Journal and Monthly Record of Medical and Surgical Science* 7 (Sept. 1870): 185–6; Reuben Ludlam, *Lectures Clinical and Didactic on the Diseases of Women* (Chicago 1872), 87–8

24 R. Pierce, *The People's Common Sense Medical Adviser in Plain English* (Buffalo 1882), 710–11

25 *Canada Medical Journal and Monthly Record of Medical and Surgical Science* 7 (Sept. 1870): 185–6; *Canada Medical and Surgical Journal* 7, 11 (May 1879): 439; Pye Henry Chavasse, *Advice to a Wife on the Management of Her Own Health and on the Treatment of Some of the Complaints Incidental to Pregnancy, Labour, and Suckling* (Toronto 1882), 105

26 Edis, *Diseases of Women*, 524

27 Henry Lyman, *The Practical Home Physician and Encyclopedia of Medicine* (Guelph 1884), 906; Chavasse, *Advice to a Wife*, 102; Ayers, *Ayers' Everyman His Own Doctor*, 316

28 Beth Light and Joy Parr, eds., *Canadian Women on the Move 1867–1920* (Toronto: New Hogtown Press and OISE 1983), 57

29 Guernsey, *The Application of the Principles and Practice of Homoeopathy*, 152; see also Michael J. Clark, 'Rejection of Psychological Approaches to Mental Disorder in Late Nineteenth-Century British Psychiatry,' in Andrew Scull, ed., *Madness, Mad-Doctors, and Madmen: The Social History of Psychiatry in the Victorian Era* (Philadelphia: University of Pennsylvania Press 1981), 295.

30 Ira Warren, *The Household Physician* (Boston 1865), 364; *Canada Lancet* 24 (Sept. 1891), 8–9

31 McGill University Archives, Montreal General Hospital Papers, RG 96, Medical Casebook 1882, vol. 132, patient ML, 196, and patient MH, 181

32 PANS, Victoria General Hospital Papers, RG 25, series B, Patient Records, patient BM, admitted 31 May 1894

33 Lyman, *Practical Home Physician*, 199, 905; Chavasse, *Advice to a Wife*, 317

34 PANS, Victoria General Hospital Papers, RG 25, series B.III.5, 1882–7, patient SE, admitted 16 May 1885

35 Laurence Humphry, *A Manual of Nursing: Medical and Surgical* (London 1898) 47. In the nineteenth century this belief focused on women. However, in the First World War, shell-shock victims with symptoms of hysteria had difficulty persuading many physicians of the reality of their problem. These men were often accused of malingering. See T.E. Brown, 'Shell Shock in the Canadian Expeditionary Force, 1914–1918: Canadian Psychiatry in the Great War,' in Charles G. Roland, ed., *Health, Disease and Medicine: Essays in Canadian History* (Toronto: Hannah Institute of Medicine 1984), 310.

36 *Canada Lancet* 12 (April 1880): 244; *Canada Medical and Surgical Journal* 15 (Aug. 1886): 15

37 Buchan, *Domestic Medicine*, 378–80

38 William Perkins Bull, *From Medicine Man to Medical Man: A Record of a Century and a Half of Progress in Health and Sanitation as Exemplified by Development in Peel* (Toronto: Perkins Bull Foundation, George J. McLeod 1934), 38

39 John Eyre, *A European Stranger in America: With the Family Physician and the Farmer's Companion* (New York 1839), 3

40 Fraser, *The Emigrant's Medical Guide*, 135. Archy McCurdy's lecture notes in 1873 from Trinity College Medical School also suggest that a

dash of cold water on the face was effective treatment. Light and Parr, eds., *Canadian Women on the Move*, 58

41 Eugene Becklard, *Physiological Mysteries and Revelations in Love, Courtship and Marriage* (New York 1842), 75–6

42 Archives of Ontario (AO), Hugh Mackay Papers, Mis. Coll. 1873 no. 6, MU 2118, Medical Notebook, 193

43 *Canada Lancet* 12 (April 1880): 244

44 McGill University Archives, Montreal General Hospital Papers, Medical Casebook, vol. 132, patient AD, admitted 21 Aug. 1882, 217

45 *Canada Medical Journal and Monthly Record of Medical and Surgical Science* 4, 5 (Nov. 1867): 207

46 *Canada Lancet* 15, 9 (May 1883): 310

47 *Canada Medical and Surgical Journal* 9 (Jan. 1881): 372–3

48 It was suggested within the American context that women may have actually encouraged operations for nervous disorders because the operation was a recognition of the validity of their symptoms. F.G. Gosling and Joyce M. Ray, 'The Right to Be Sick: American Physicians and Nervous Patients, 1885–1910,' *Journal of Social History* 20, 2 (winter 1986): 260

49 *Canada Lancet* 15 (April 1883): 238–9

50 David Hart and A.H. Freeland Barbour, *Manual of Gynecology*, vols. 1 and 2 (New York 1883), app., 615; Edis, *Diseases of Women*, 530–2

51 See Ann Douglas Wood, '"The Fashionable Diseases": Women's Complaints and Their Treatment in Nineteenth-Century America,' in Judith Walzer Leavitt, ed., *Women and Health in America* (Madison: University of Wisconsin Press 1984), 222–38

52 George Napheys, *The Physical Life of Women* (Toronto 1890): 34

53 *Maritime Medical News* 6 (Jan. 1894): 212–14

54 The term 'moral-pastoral' was coined by Clark in 'Rejection of Psychological Approaches,' 297.

55 *Canada Medical and Surgical Journal* 6 (April 1878): 443–4

56 *Annual Report of the Medical Superintendent* (ARMS), Saint John 1900, Journals of the House of Assembly, New Brunswick, 1901, 32

57 AO, Toronto Asylum Papers, Patient Register and Case Files, patient SB, admitted 24 April 1888

58 *Canada Medical Journal* 18 (Feb. 1865): 405

59 See Annual Report of the Inspector of Asylums (ARIA) 1877, *Ontario Sessional Papers* (*OSP*) no. 4, 1878, 12, for an example of the complete breakdown of causes. This kind of chart was part of the inspector's annual report.

60 *American Journal of Insanity* 26, 1 (July 1869): 35 (my emphasis)

61 Every tenth patient record was studied, or 862 cases. Of those examined, 92 men were labelled insane through heredity, and 121 women. Thus, 43.2 per cent of the heredity patients were male and 56.8 per cent were female – despite the even numbers of men and women in the asylum.

62 Annual Report of the Medical Superintendent, Toronto Asylum (ARMS) 1859, *Sessional Papers* (*SP*), app. 32, Journals of the Legislature Assembly of Canada (JLA) 1860, 51; *Canada Medical and Surgical Journal* 3, 5 (Nov. 1875): 248; ARMS 1879, *OSP* no. 8, 1880, 300, 305; ARMS Hamilton 1898, *OSP* no. 11, 1899, 152; ARMS Kingston, 1893, *OSP* no. 26, 1894, 94; ARMS Toronto 1897, *OSP* no. 10, 1897–8, 5; Alexander Reid of the Mount Hope Asylum in Nova Scotia advocated marriage control. Colin Howell, 'Alexander Peter Reid and the Medicalization of Canadian Society,' unpublished paper, 1983, 12

63 AO, Toronto Asylum Papers, Patient Files, patient number 8450 in the Toronto Asylum, FW, admitted 6 July 1899 and discharged 26 July 1900

64 The one comment I have discovered that suggested that insanity was more transferrable from the father to the child than from the mother is in *Canadian Practitioner* 22, 2 (Feb. 1897): 130.

65 ARMS 1879, *OSP* no. 8, 1880, 301

66 ARMS 1859, *SP*, app. 32, JLA 1860, 54; ARMS 1872, *OSP* no. 2, 1873, 145

67 Lyman, *The Practical Home Physician*, 305

68 William Tyler Smith, *Parturition and the Principles and Practice of Obstetrics* (Philadelphia 1849), 102–3; ARMS 1877, *OSP* no. 4, 1878, 255; *Canadian Medical Times* 1, 5 (Aug. 1878) 38

69 In 1901, 149 men died from epilepsy, and 121 women. *Fourth Census of Canada*, 1901 table v

70 *Canada Medical and Surgical Journal* 5, 1 (July 1876), 3; ARMS 1858, *SP*, app. 11, JLA 1859; *Canada Lancet* 9, 3 (Nov. 1876): 96; *Canada Medical Record* 11, 6 (March 1883): 125

71 ARMS 1858, *SP*, app. 11, JLA 1859

72 *Dominion Medical Monthly* 1 (Sept. 1893): 69; AO, Toronto Asylum Papers, Patient Files, patient 7920, ER, in the Toronto Asylum had problems with opium addiction.

73 ARMS 1858, SP, app. 11, JLA 1859

74 Of the patients whose habits of life were known, 21.1 per cent of the men were viewed as intemperate and only 4.7 per cent of the women.

75 AO, Toronto Asylum Papers, Patient Register and Case Files, patient MT, admitted 25 Feb. 1841

76 E. Hare, 'Masturbation Insanity: The History of an Idea,' *Journal of Mental Science* 108, 452 (Jan. 1962): 1–25; Skultans, *English Madness: Ideas on Insanity*, 71

77 ARMS 1862, *SP* no. 66, JLA 1863; ARMS 1863, SP no. 39, JLA 1864

78 *Canada Medical Journal and Monthly Record of Medical and Surgical Science* 1, 8 (Feb. 1865): 405–6; ARMS 1865, SP no. 6, JLA 1866, 35

79 ARMS 1877, *OSP* no. 4, 1878, 240–1

80 *American Journal of Insanity* 13 (July 1856): 17

81 AO, Toronto Asylum Papers, Patient Register and Case Files, patient SB, admitted 24 April 1888; patient AH, admitted 27 Jan. 1880; patient MH, admitted 17 Dec. 1893 and died 13 Nov. 1898

82 Henry MacNaughton-Jones, *Points of Practical Interest in Gynaecology* (London 1901), 81

83 *Quebec Medical Journal* 1 (April 1827): 142

84 *Canadian Practitioner* 23, 9 (Sept. 1898): 523

85 Tyler Smith, *Parturition and the Principles and Practice of Obstetrics*, 103. In recent years women's groups, psychologists, and therapists have convinced the American Psychiatric Association not to recognize pre-menstrual tension as a category of mental illness. As Toronto psychologist Paula Caplan said, it would give credence to the idea that 'women still go insane once a month.' *Healthsharing* (fall 1986): 4

86 William Goodell, *Lessons in Gynaecology* (Philadelphia 1890), 394; *Canada Lancet* 35, 2 (Oct. 1901): 67; *Canadian Practitioner* 23, 9 (Sept. 1898): 523

87 *American Medico-Psychological Association Proceedings* 5 (1898): 88; *American Journal of Insanity* 49, 1 (July 1892): 62

88 *Dominion Medical Monthly* 4, 2 (Feb. 1895): 83

89 AO, Toronto Asylum Papers, Patient Register and Case Files, patient EC,

admitted 13 Dec. 1870; patient CF, admitted 11 July 1877; patient JM, admitted 12 June 1850

90 *Canada Medical Journal* 1, 8 (Feb. 1865): 405; ARMS 1863, *SP* no. 39, JLA 1864; ARMS 1867, JLA of Ontario, vol. 1867–8

91 *Canadian Medical Times* 1, 12 (Sept. 1873): 91; William Dakin, *A Handbook of Midwifery (London* 1897), 54

92 Kenneth Neader Fenwick, *Manual of Obstetrics, Gynaecology and Pediatrics* (Kingston 1889), 124

93 Elaine Showalter, 'Victorian Women and Insanity,' in Scull, ed., *Madhouses, Mad-Doctors, and Madman,* 330

94 PANS, Nova Scotia Hospital Papers, patient no. 720, Mrs R, admitted June 1871

95 Letitia Youmans, *Campaign Echoes: The Autobiography of Letitia Youmans* (Toronto 1893), 81

96 *Christian Guardian,* 21 Feb. 1872, 59

97 Skene, *Medical Gynecology,* 933

98 *American Journal of Insanity* 15, 1 (July 1858): 22

99 ARMS 1861, *SP* no. 19, JLA 1862

100 *Canada Medical and Surgical Journal* 10, 7 (Jan. 1882): 343; 11 (Feb. 1883): 437; Skene, *Diseases of Women,* 930–1; *Canadian Practitioner* 21 (May 1896): 330; MacNaughton-Jones, *Points of Interest,* 85–7

101 Skene, *Diseases of Women,* 932–3

102 *American Journal of Insanity* 49, 1 (July 1892): 62; *American Medico-Psychological Association Proceedings* 5 (1898): 88; Bucke Collection, 'The Functions of the Great Sympathetic Nervous System' (1877), 15, 20, 27; R.M. Bucke, *The Moral Nature of the Great Sympathetic* (Utica, NY 1878), 24; Skene, *Medical Gynecology,* 77, *Canadian Practitioner* 21 (May 1896): 321

103 *Canadian Practitioner* 23, 10 (Oct. 1898): 579–80; 22, 3 (March 1897): 201; *Canada Lancet* 30, 6 (Feb. 1898): 286; *Canadian Journal of Medicine and Surgery* 4, 5 (1898): 291–2

104 MacNaughton-Jones, *Points of Practical Interest in Gynaecology,* 84

105 *Canadian Journal of Medicine and Surgery* 4, 5 (Nov. 1898): 291–3

106 AO, Toronto Asylum Papers, Patient Register and Files, patient IL, admitted 10 Jan. 1889

107 The equal number of men and women in nineteenth-century asylums in Ontario is quite different from in present-day United States and Canada. In the United States over 70 per cent of the asylum population are women, whereas in Canada men predominate. Janice Raymond, 'Medicine as Patriarchal Religion,' *Journal of Medicine and Philosophy* 7, 2 (May 1982): 198; Statistics Canada, *Women in Canada: A Statistical Report* (Ottawa: Statistics Canada 1985), 99. The situation in nineteenth-century England was also quite different. For every 1000 male lunatics in English asylums in 1871, there were 1182 female. Elaine Showalter has accounted for this in three ways. First, once committed, women stayed in asylums longer than men so that authorities had to allocate more space and beds to them. Second, asylums had ben designed to take care of the poor insane and more women than men were poor. Third, as asylums improved the quality of care they provided, families became less reluctant to commit their female relatives. Reluctance continued for men, however, since families feared that men's future earning power would be limited if it became known they had been insane. Showalter, 'Victorian Women and Insanity,' 162–3

108 *Canada Medical Journal* 1, 8 (Feb. 1865): 401

109 ARMS 1861, *SP*, app. 19, JLA 1862

110 In 1891 there were 13,355 insane in Canada, 7162 men and 6193 women or 29.1 men per 10,000 population and 26.1 women per 10,000 population. *Statistical Year Book of Canada* 1906, 411

111 D. Tuke and H.K. Lewis, *The Insane in the United States and Canada* (London 1885), 210

112 ARIA 1876, *OSP* no. 2, 1877, 26; ARIA 1880, *OSP* no. 8, 1881, 25–6

113 AO, Toronto Asylum Papers, Patient Register and Case Files, patient AS, no. 6090

114 ARMS 1875, *OSP* no. 4, 1875–6, 216

115 ARMS 1899, *OSP* no. 34, 1899, 53

116 ARIA 1888, *OSP* no. 1, 1889, 35

117 The number of elderly in the sample were small, twenty-nine women and twenty-one men. In the 1890s, 44.8 per cent of old women entered and made up 14.6 per cent of those who entered in that decade.

118 OA, Toronto Asylum Papers, Patient Register and Case Files, patient AK, no. 7590, admitted 30 Nov. 1893

119 Only five cases of the sample had marital status undesignated. The numbers for married, single, and widowed or deserted are 398, 402, and 57, respectively. The number for men were 172, 225, and 18, respectively, and for women 226, 177, and 39. This is out of a sample of 415 male patients and 442 female patients.

120 ARMS 1864, *SP* no. 14, JLA 1865, 108–9; the figures for the asylum in Saint John are different. Between 1875 and 1900 there were 1448 women admitted – 705 single, 550 married, and 193 widowed. For men the figures were 1073, 687, and 116. While this meant single people dominated, women were under-represented among them at 39 per cent, although women comprised 44 per cent of the asylum population. Annual Report of the Medical Superintendent, Saint John, 1876, Journals of the House of Assembly 1877, 4

121 See ARMS, London, 1877, *OSP* no. 4, 1878, 289.

122 In general, elderly women were likely to be taken in by their families and elderly men more likely to be institutionalized. However, families may not have been willing to take in elderly female relatives if they were insane. This is a significant finding and is not accounted for by the difference in widowhood. If widowhood is eliminated from the cross-tabulation of sex by marital status, it still results in 43.5 per cent of the men being married and 56.4 per cent of the women. For this cross-tabulation $x = .0006$ with Cramer's $v = .13581$. Thus the significance is there, although it is not strong.

123 ARMS 1858, *SP*, app. 11, JLA 1859

124 ARMS 1859, *SP*, app. 32, JLA 1860

125 ARMS 1860, *SP*, app. 24, JLA 1861

126 ARMS 1862, *SP* no. 66, JLA 1863

127 Ibid. Not all physicians were convinced. Indeed, the *Montreal Medical Journal* of 1890 quoted a British physician who warned gynaecologists to look to the mental and hysterical state of the unmarried female over the age of thirty. *Montreal Medical Journal* 19, 6 (Dec. 1890): 435

128 *Canada Medical Journal* 18 (Feb. 1865): 406–7

129 The Upper Canada census figures for 1860–1 indicate there were 65,813 married men in the population and 61,403 married women between the ages of thirty and forty. In the asylum there had been 731 married men. Based on these figures there would be a predictive 682 married women. However, the actual figure was 950. Using Workman's figures does

indicate an over-representation of single women, but using the correct figures does not.

130 In the asylum from its opening to the end of the century the age composition of the married male population was as follows: under 19, 0.6 per cent; 20 to 30, 15.3 per cent; 30 to 40, 30 per cent; 40 to 50, 25.9 per cent; 50 to 60, 18.2 per cent; and over 60, 10 per cent. This represents 1, 26, 51, 44, 31, and 17 men, respectively. For women it was 1.3 per cent, 22.7 per cent, 39.1 per cent, 8 per cent, and 5.3 per cent; this represents 3, 51, 88, 18, and 12 women, respectively.

131 ARMS 1873, *OSP* no. 2, 1874, 160

132 University of Western Ontario, Richard Maurice Bucke Collection, A9, 'Surgery at the Asylum' (1897): 2

133 *Dominion Medical Monthly* 13, 4 (Oct. 1899): 179

134 *Canada Lancet* 37, 4 (Dec. 1903): 306

135 AO, Toronto Asylum Papers, Patient Register and Case Files, patient EH, no. 3270, admitted 22 Nov. 1866

CHAPTER 11 Insane Women: Their Symptoms and Treatment

1 Archives of Ontario (AO), Toronto Asylum Papers, Patient Register and Case Files, patient MB, no. 5000, entered 4 April 1878; patient AB, no. 5920, entered 20 Sept. 1886; and patient AR, no. 5120, entered 4 Oct. 1879

2 Every tenth patient record was examined. Of the 749 cases whose classification was known, 70.2 (526) per cent were manic, 15.9 (119) were melancholic, and 7.6 (57) were demented. The remaining cases had other designations. When cross-tabulated by sex, the three classifications resulted in 251 male and 275 female manic, 52 and 67 melancholics, and 28 and 29 demented.

3 Only 109 valid cases existed, 68 women and 41 men.

4 AO, Toronto Asylum Papers, Patient Register and Case Files, patient SC, no. 4060, entered 5 June 1873

5 The records show 223 cases were excited and 120 were incoherent.

6 AO, Toronto Asylum Papers, Patient Register and Case Files, patient SB, no. 5730, entered 26 Feb. 1884

7 Annual Report of the Medical Superintendent, Toronto Asylum (ARMS) 1856, *Sessional Papers (SP)*, app. 2, Journals of the Legislative Assembly of Canada (JLA) 1856; Annual Report of the Inspector of Asylums (ARIA)

1868, *Ontario Sessional Papers* (*OSP*) no. 4, 1869, 29; ARIA 1878, *OSP* no. 8, 1879, 30

8 Phyllis Chesler, *Women and Madness* (New York: Avon Books 1972), 55

9 Fifty-one men were deemed incoherent, and 69 women.

10 These represented 327 cases.

11 *American Journal of Insantity* 26, 1 (July 1869): 34–6

12 See patient 4060, 4590, 4610, 4890, 7460. Almost 12 per cent of the women whose actions appeared deviant refused to work, whereas for men it was just under 8 per cent.

13 AO, Toronto Asylum Papers, Patient Register and Case Files, patient 4590, entered 10 June 1876

14 Ibid., patient MY, no. 7460, entered 11 April 1893

15 Elaine Showalter, *The Female Malady: Women, Madness, and English Culture, 1830–1980* (New York: Pantheon Books 1985), 74

16 The number of patients exhibiting unsocial actions were 46, 17 men and 29 women; sexual actions were 48, 33 and 15, respectively; food-related actions, 44, equally divided between the sexes; restless activity, 141, 60 and 81, respectively; and other, 48, with 26 men and 22 women.

17 AO, Toronto Asylum Papers, Patient Register and Case Files, patient MT, no. 1430, admitted 13 Sept. 1853; AB, no. 1480, admitted 2 Dec. 1853; MC, no. 3110, admitted 5 Dec. 1864

18 Those exhibiting delusions numbered 290: 9 had sexual, 81 had spiritual, 73 had grandiose, 17 had domestic, and 27 had seeing and hearing delusions. Eighty-three patients had delusions, but no details of them were provided.

19 AO, Toronto Asylum Papers, Patient Register and Case Files, patient FW, no. 8270, entered 7 Jan. 1898

20 Ibid., patient MB, no. 3540, entered 11 Oct. 1869

21 This represented 268 cases.

22 One hundred cases were violent against property, 36 males and 64 women.

23 AO, Toronto Asylum Papers, Patient Register and Case Files, patient AR, no. 4890, entered 27 July 1877

24 A total of 346 cases were violent, 205 men and 141 women. Of these, 48 were violent towards others (13.9 per cent), 30 men and 18 women, 121 were violent towards family members (35 per cent), 67 men and 54 women.

25 AO, Toronto Asylum Papers, Patient Register and Case Files, patient AG, no. 3140, entered 5 May 1865; patient EB, no. 3830, entered 21 Sept. 1871; patient JD, no. 4140, entered 23 Dec. 1873; patient ED, no. 3230, entered 6 May 1866; patient MK, no. 6720, entered 8 Aug. 1890

26 Almost 23 per cent of the patients examined were suicidal, with approximately 36 per cent having actually tried to commit suicide and 64 per cent having threatened to do so. There was no gender difference between those who attempted and those who simply threatened to do so.

27 In the sampling, 73 men patients and 96 women patients had been previously admitted. In the 1870s it was 13 men and 10 women, whereas in the 1890s it was 15 men and 24 women. Previous admissions will be a very conservative figure.

28 AO, Toronto Asylum Papers, Patient Register and Case Files, patient MM, no. 1180, entered 30 April 1852; patient AS, no. 3950, entered 18 July 1872; patient MH, no. 5300, entered 24 Nov. 1881; patient ET, no. 6400, entered 22 Dec. 1889.

29 Ibid., patient RP, no. 7130, entered 20 Nov. 1891

30 ARMS 1851, *SP*, app. J, JLA 1852–3

31 Annual Report of the Board of Directors (ARD) 1852, JLA 1852–3; ARMS 1854, *SP*, app. H, JLA 1854–5

32 ARBI 1865, *SP* no 6, JLA 1866, 7

33 ARBI 1883, *OSP* no. 8, 1884, 52, 54. S.E.D. Shortt has suggested that eventually the use of female attendants on the male wards failed. S.E.D. Shortt, *Victorian Lunacy: Richard M. Bucke and the Practice of Late 19th-Century Psychiatry* (London: Cambridge University Press 1986), 44

34 D. Tuke and H.K. Lewis, *The Insane in the United States and Canada* (London 1885), 223

35 ARIA 1881, *OSP* no. 8, 1882, 24

36 Tuke and Lewis, *The Insane in the United States and Canada*, 222–3

37 ARD 1850, *SP*, app. C, JLA 1851

38 ARMS 1870, *OSP* no. 6, 1870–1, 87

39 In 1887 the provincial government determined that no married attendants should be hired. Shortt, *Victorian Lunacy*, 45–6

40 ARIA 1881, *OSP* no. 8, 1882, 26

41 ARMS 1896, *OSP* no. 10, 1897, 41–2; ARMS 1898, *OSP* no. 11, 1898–9, 42

42 ARIA 1881, *OSP* no. 8, 1882, 26. In the United States Constance McGovern noted that women received more sedatives than men and less restraint, the latter not seeming to be as appropriate for women. Constance McGovern, 'The Myths of Social Control and Custodial Oppression: Patterns of Psychiatric Medicine in late Nineteenth-Century Institutions,' *Journal of Social History* 20, 1 (fall 1986): 13

43 ARMS, London, 1880, *OSP* no. 8, 1881, 313

44 ARMS 1884, *OSP* no. 11, 1885, 97–8

45 ARMS 1868, *OSP* no. 4, 1869, 52

46 Tuke and Lewis, *The Insane in the United States and Canada*, 222

47 ARMS 1884, *OSP* no. 11, 1885, 114

48 ARIA 1879, *OSP* no. 8, 1880, 20

49 AO, Toronto Asylum Papers, Patient Register and Case Files, patient SC, no. 6990, entered 2 April 1891; patient MA, no. 7630, entered 21 Feb. 1894. It is unclear whether patients were actually paid for their work. There is certainly no evidence of it in the nineteenth century.

50 ARIA 1879, *OSP* no. 8, 1880, 22

51 ARMS 1899, *OSP* no. 34, 1899, 38

52 ARMS 1880, *OSP* no. 8, 1881, 284

53 Return to an Address, JLA 1857

54 ARMS 1878, *OSP* no. 8, 1879, 267

55 ARMS 1876, *OSP* no. 2, 1877, 213

56 AO, London Insane Asylum Papers, Patient Casebook, patient MS, no. 775

57 Thomas Brown, 'Living with God's Afflicted: A History of the Provincial Lunatic Asylum at Toronto, 1830–1911' (PHD thesis, Queen's University, 1982), 275

58 Elaine Showalter, 'Victorian Women and Insanity,' in Adrew Scull, ed., *Madhouses, Mad-Doctors, and Madmen: The Social History of Psychiatry in the Victorian Era* (Philadelphia: University of Pennsylvania Press 1981), 321

59 *Canada Medical Journal* 1, 8 (Feb. 1865): 402

60 ARMS 1874, *OSP* no. 2, 1874 (2), 156

61 ARIA 1875, *OSP* no. 4 1875–6, 16. If true this would be quite different from in the United States where men tended to stay longer because they were not committed as quickly. McGovern, 'The Myths of Social Control,' 8

62 The exact figure for women was 54.7 per cent. This represented 249 men and 238 women.

63 ARIA 1879, *OSP* no. 8, 1880, 14. See David Rothman, *Conscience and Convenience: The Asylum and Its Alternatives in Progressive America* (Boston and Toronto: Little, Brown and Co. 1980), 61–8, for an interesting discussion of probation for criminals as a form of social control.

64 ARMS 1877, *OSP* no. 4, 1878, 258

65 Valid cases were 845.

66 ARMS 1858, *SP*, app. 11, JLA 1859

67 Altogether 27 patients of the sample were discharged improved, 12 men and 15 women, but in the 1890s the division was 4 men and 11 women.

68 Of the 862 records examined, 13 men escaped and 2 women.

69 ARMS 1864, *SP* no. 14, JLA 1865, 121, 124–5

70 ARMS 1870–1, *OSP* no. 4, 1871–2, 135

71 ARMS 1861, *SP* no. 19, JLA 1862

72 ARMS 1882, *OSP* no. 8, 1882–3, 47

73 ARMS 1860, *SP*, app. 24, JLA 1861

74 ARMS 1873, *OSP* no. 2, 1874 (1), 160

75 Showalter, 'Victorian Women and Insanity,' 315; Andrew Scull, 'The Domestication of Madness,' *Medical History* 27 (1983): 233–48

76 Chesler, *Women and Madness*, 35

77 AO, London Insane Asylum Papers, Patient Register and Casebook, patient ES, no. 3080

78 Bucke was not the only asylum officer who was sensitive to how disorders of women's bodies affected both their physical and mental health. At the end of the century, staff at the Kingston Asylum kept a close watch on whether women patients menstruated and, if not, provided treatment accordingly. At times doctors felt obligated to do a complete internal examination. Briget Fennell entered the asylum on 4 April 1898. On 23 April the doctors examined her and discovered she had a marked retroversion in addition to laceration of the cervix. The uterus was moveable and the fundus uteri was pressing against the rectum. Treatment consisted of replacing the uterus by manipulation and inserting a tampon saturated in glycerine. Briget received daily douches, a full diet, and exercise. The doctors at Kingston also seemed to favour ovarian tissue extract, but whether for physical or mental

disorders is unclear. Nonetheless, they were never as adventuresome as Bucke was at the London Asylum. AO, Kingston Asylum Papers, Patient Casebook, see patients HS (2999), admitted 5 Sept. 1895, and NM, admitted 30 May 1896, for general focus on menstruation. Patient BF, no. 3200, entered 4 April 1898. For use of ovarian tissue extract see patients AM, no. 3124, MR, no. 3145 and HA, no. 3128.

79 ARMS 1896, London, *OSP* no. 10, 1897, 80. Bucke was a man who was ambitious and interested in doing well in his profession. Receiving his medical degree from the McGill Medical School, Bucke went on to become superintendent of the Provincial Asylum for the Insane in Hamilton in 1876 and the next year the superintendent of the newly built asylum in London. Brian Lauder, 'Two Radicals: Richard Maurice Bucke and Lauren Harris,' *Dalhousie Review* 56, 2 (summer 1976): 307. An early indication that Bucke was not going to be satisfied providing custodial care to his patients came shortly after he came to London. It was part of medical wisdom at the time that masturbation could cause insanity. If Bucke could get those patients who masturbated (mostly men) to stop, they might have a chance at recovery. He did this by wiring fifteen male patients – that is, piercing the prepuce of the penis with a silver needle. The procedure was not particularly successful. When next Bucke decided to intervene, it would be on female patients.

80 AO, Inspector of Asylum Papers, Correspondence between London Asylum and the inspector of asylums, Bucke to Christie, 15 April 1895, file 6460

81 University of Western Ontario, Richard Maurice Bucke Papers, A12, 'Operations Initiated at the London Asylum for the Insane' (1899): A11, 'Surgery at the London Asylum for the Insane' (1898), 1–2; ARMS, 1895, London, *OSP* no. 11, 1896, 42–5

82 *Canadian Practitioner and Medical Review* 24 (7 July 1899): 379; *Canada Medical Record* 26, 8 (May 1898): 108

83 ARMS 1896, London, *OSP* no. 10, 1897, 79–80

84 *Canadian Practitioner* 23 (Sept. 1898), 517; see also *Canadian Practitioner and Medical Review* 22 (July 1899): 383–4; R.M. Bucke, 'Operations Initiated at the London Asylum'; Richard Bucke, 'Two Hundred Operative Cases,' *American Medico-Psychological Association Proceedings* 7 (1900): 99.

85 ARMS 1896, London, *OSP* no. 10, 1897, 79–80

86 *Canadian Practitioner* 23 (Sept. 1898): 520; *Dominion Medical Monthly and Ontario Medical Journal* 13 (Oct. 1899): 175; *Canadian Practitioner and Medical Review* 24 (7 July 1899): 380

87 AO, London Insane Asylum Papers, Patient Register and Case Files, patient GP, no. 3503

88 R.M. Bucke 'Gynecological Notes,' *American Medico-Psychological Association Proceedings* 3 (1896): 139

89 R.M. Bucke, 'Surgery among the Insane in Canada,' *American Medico-Psychological Association Proceedings* 5 (1898): 74

90 *Canadian Practitioner and Review* 22 (July 1899): 383–4

91 ARMS 1898–9, London, *OSP* no. 34, 1900, 72

92 Bucke, 'Two Hundred Operatives Cases,' 100–1

93 Bucke, 'Surgery among the Insane in Canada,' 87

94 AO, London Insane Asylum Papers, Patient Register and Case Files, patient JM, entered 16 April 1884

95 ARMS 1896, London, *OSP* no. 10, 1897, 81

96 AO, Correspondence between the London Asylum and the inspector of asylums, box 223, no. 6511, letter from Bucke asking permission for Hobbs to go to New York, 23 March 1900

97 Ibid., file 6460, Bucke to Stratton, 30 Nov. 1900

98 *Canadian Practitioner* 22, 6 (June 1897): 416

99 *Canadian Medical Review* 8, 4 (Oct. 1898): 106–7

100 *Dominion Medical Monthly and Ontario Medical Journal* 12, 1 (Jan. 1899): 2, 12–13; *Canada Lancet* 34, 4 (Dec. 1900): 172

101 Henry MacNaughton-Jones, *Points of Practical Interest in Gynaecology* (London 1901), 91

102 Bucke, 'Two Hundred Operatives Cases,' 104

103 *Canadian Journal of Medicine and Surgery* 4, 5 (Nov. 1898): 291

104 See cases in *Canadian Medical Review* 8, 4 (Oct. 1898): 108–10.

105 *Canada Medical and Surgical Journal* 13, 4 (Nov. 1885): 229

106 Buck, 'Gynecological Notes,' 155

107 *Dominion Medical Monthly and Ontario Medical Journal* 12, 1 (Jan. 1899): 15. Bucke seldom referred to his wiring of male patients when accused of focusing sexual therapeutics on women. Of course, wiring was not as extreme in its consequences as some of the surgery Hobbs was performing on women.

108 University of Western Ontario, Bucke Papers, B5. 'The Functions of the Great Sympathetic System.' 26

109 *Canadian Medical Review* 8, 4 (Oct. 1898): 110

110 Bucke, 'Gynecological Notes,' 160

111 Ibid., 156

112 While the focus on individualized nursing was not new and made sense, according to S.E.D. Shortt, for patients undergoing non-gynaecological surgery, there appeared to be few if any recoveries as a result. It is difficult to know how to interpret this result. Shortt is not clear whether he accepted Bucke's evaluation, or whether he based his conclusions on the patients' case histories. Shortt, *Victorian Lunacy*, 152

113 *Canadian Practitioner* 23, 10 (Oct. 1898): 587–9, 580, 584

114 AO, Kingston Asylum Papers, Patient Casebook, patient AM, no. 3124, entered 3 April 1897

115 ARMS 1897, *OSP* no. 10, 1897–8, 9

116 ARMS 1898, *OSP* no. 11, 1898–9, 39

117 Andrew Scull and Diane Favreau, 'A Chance to Cut is a Chance to Cure: Sexual Surgery for Psychosis in Three Nineteenth Century Societies,' *Research in Law, Deviance and Social Control* 8 (1986): 16–17

118 ARMS Kingston, 1895, *OSP* no. 11, 1896, 88

119 AO, Inspector of Asylum Files, Clarke to Christie, 1 Feb. 1899; Christie to Russell, 2 Feb. 1899; Christie to Clarke, 2 Feb. 1899

120 AO, Inspector of Asylum Papers, box 223, file 6511, Correspondence between the London Asylum and the inspector of asylums

121 Ibid., Bucke to Christie, 15 Feb. 1897

122 ARMS 1898, London, *OSP* no. 11, 1898–9, 74–5

123 AO, London Insane Asylum Papers, Patient Casebook, patient HC, no. 431, entered 11 May 1877

124 Ibid., patient MC, no. 2946; see also patients EF, no. 2838, EM, no. 4106, and EP, no. 3120, for similar examples of some short-term gain but no permanent improvement.

125 Ibid., patients AC, no. 2848, MB, no. 2036, and CH, no. 4193; see AS, no. 3528 (2462), KH, no. 3763, EP, no 3769 (3607, 3356), and AN, no. 3791.

126 Scull and Favreau, 'A Chance to Cut,' 32

127 AO, London Insane Asylum Papers, Patient Casebook, patient VS, no. 3648 (4171)

128 Ibid., patients EM, no. 4106 (5213), EW, no. 2970, EF, no. 2594, GT, no. 4539 (5088). Sexual surgery on insane women continued elsewhere. In the 1920s Dr Henry Cotton of the New Jersey State Hospital performed 758 hysterectomies, only 38 of which were necessary. Eliot Valenstein, *Great and Desperate Cures* (New York: Basic Books 1986), 37–9

129 AO, London Insane Asylum Papers, Patient Casebook, patients SL, no. 3449 (3981), and EM, no. 4106 (3213)

130 AO, Inspector of Asylums Papers, file 6460, Bucke to Christie, 14 May 1901

131 ARMS, London, 1900, *OPS* no. 35, 1901

132 The above comes from ARMS, London, 1895–9. Elsbeth Webster is casebook no. 4008.

133 University of Western Ontario, Bucke Papers, A11, 'Surgery at the London Asylum for the Insane,' 3

134 Based on 225 cases.

135 Constance McGovern, 'The Myths of Social Control,' 13

NOTES ON SOURCES AND METHODOLOGY

1 Charles G. Roland and Paul Potter, *An Annotated Bibliography of Canadian Medical Periodicals 1826–1975* (Toronto: Hannah Institute for the History of Medicine 1979). For a description of the sometimes ephemeral nature of these journals see Charles G. Roland, 'Ontario Medical Periodicals as Mirrors of Change,' *Ontario History* 72, 1 (March 1980): 3–15.

2 David Flaherty has discussed the need to be concerned about this issue when dealing with the records of living people. Surely the same concerns should exist for those no longer living as well. David Flaherty, 'Privacy and Confidentiality: The Responsibilities of Historians,' *Reviews in American History* (Sept. 1980): 419

3 Nancy Cott, *The Bonds of Womanhood: 'Women's Sphere' in New England, 1780–1835* (New Haven: Yale University Press 1977), 2

4 Thomas Szasz, *Sex: Fact, Frauds, and Follies* (Oxford: Basil Blackwell 1981), 18

Medical Glossary

abortifacient an agent that induces abortion.

allopathy the practice of what has become the dominant form of
medicine; the curing of a diseased action by the inducing of another of a
different kind, yet not necessarily diseased.

amaurosis loss of sight without apparent lesion of the eye, as from
disease of the optic nerve, spine, or brain.

amenorrhoea absence of the menses, cessation of the menstrual flow.

anaemia reduction below normal of the number of red blood cells, the
quantity of haemoglobin, or the volume of packed red cells in the blood.

anteflexion the bending of an organ so that its top is thrust forward.

anteversion the tipping forward of an entire organ.

antero position in front, directed towards the front.

antiseptic preventing sepsis; any substance that inhibits the growth of
bacteria.

aseptic adjective describing the absence of septic matter; freedom from
infection or infectious material.

asthenopia weakness or easy fatigue of the eye, with pain in the eyes,
headache, dimness of vision and the like.

biliary colic abdominal pain due to passage of gallstones along the bile
duct.

Bright's disease a broad descriptive term once used for kidney disease;
derived from a description of the diseases published in 1827 by Richard
Bright, an English physician.

broad ligament of the uterus a broad fold of peritoneum supporting the
uterus.

bronchi   passages conveying air to and within the lungs.

bronchitis   acute or chronic inflammation of one or more bronchi.

Caesarian section   delivery of a fetus by incision through the abdominal wall and uterus.

catarrh   inflammation with persistent discharge.

cellulitis   inflammation within solid tissues, characterized by edema, redness, pain. Pelvic cellulitis involves the tissues surrounding the uterus and is now called parametritis.

cerebro-spinal   pertaining to the brain and the spinal cord.

cervix uteri   neck of the uterus.

chlorosis   a disorder, generally of pubescent females, characterized by greenish yellow discoloration of the skin; believed to be related to iron deficiency.

chorea   the ceaseless occurrence of rapid, jerky, involuntary movements.

climacteric   the changes occurring at the end of the female reproductive period; menopause.

clavicle   collar bone.

clitoridectomy   excision of the clitoris.

coitus interruptus   sexual intercourse during which the penis is withdrawn from the vagina before ejaculation.

coitus obstructus   a contraceptive technique in which pressure is applied to the testicles and penis in order to block the passage of semen from the urethra by forcing the semen to pass into the bladder.

coitus reservatus   sexual intercourse in which ejaculation of semen is intentionally suppressed.

congestion   abnormal accumulation of blood in a body part.

craniotomy   puncture of the skull and removal of its contents to decrease the size of the head of a dead fetus and facilitate delivery; any operation on the cranium.

curette   a spoon shaped instrument for cleansing a diseased surface.

cyst   a closed sac or capsule containing a liquid or semisolid substance, usually benign.

cystic   containing cysts.

degeneration   deterioration, change of tissue to a less functionally active form; often accompanied by the deposit of abnormal matter in the tissue.

dementia   organic loss of intellectual function.

dilator   an instrument used to dilate the cervix.

delirium tremens   DTS; a form of alcoholic psychosis ordinarily seen after withdrawal from heavy alcohol intake.

dorsal   directed towards or situated on the back surface.

dropsy   abnormal accumulation of fluid in a body cavity.

dysmenorrhoea   painful menstruation, cramps often accompanied by headache, depression, and fatigue.

dyspepsia   impaired digestion, sometimes associated with excessive acidity of the stomach.

eclampsia   convulsions and coma occurring in pregnant or puerperal women, associated with hypertension, edema. The maternal and infant mortality rate are high. Recovery is rapid after delivery of the child.

electro-galvanism   use of electricity as a form of treatment.

embryotomy   dismemberment of the fetus in difficult labour in which a normal delivery is impossible.

endometritis   inflammation of the endometrium (the mucous membrane lining the uterus).

enteroptosis   abnormal downward displacement of the intestine.

erethism   excessive irritability or sensitivity to stimulation.

erotomania   morbidly exaggerated sexual behaviour or reaction; preoccupation with sexuality.

fibroid tumours   benign tumours derived from smooth muscle, found in the uterus.

fibroma   a tumour composed of fibrous or fully developed connective tissue.

fistula   any abnormal, tube-like passage within body tissue, usually between two internal organs, or leading from an internal organ to the body service. In women, difficult labour in childbirth may result in the formation of a vesico-vaginal fistula between the bladder and the vagina, or a recto-vaginal fistula between the rectum and the vagina.

fundus   the bottom or base of an organ.

Galen   Greek physician to the Roman emperor Marcus Aurelius. His writings influenced medical practitioners until the late nineteenth century.

gallstone   stonelike mass that forms in the gallbladder.

gastritis   inflammation of the lining of the stomach.

general paresis   chronic syphilitic menigoencephalitis; also known as Dementia Paralytica; one form of tertiary stage syphilis.

genito-urinary system   the organs of reproduction, together with the organs concerned with production and excretion of urine.

gestation   the duration of pregnancy.

gonorrhoea   highly contagious bacterial infection transmitted sexually.

haematocele of the broad ligament   effusion of blood into the fold of peritoneum supporting the uterus.

homeopathy   a medical system in which diseases are treated by minute doses of drugs that are capable of producing in healthy persons symptoms similar to those of the disease to be treated.

humerus   the bone of the upper arm, extending from shoulder to elbow.

hydrocephalic   adjective describing enlargement of the cranium caused by abnormal fluid accumulation.

hypertrophy   increase in volume of a tissue or organ produced entirely by enlargement of existing cells.

hysteria   a state of tension or excitement in which there is a loss of control over emotions; anxiety may be converted into physical symptoms.

hysterectomy   surgical removal of the uterus.

hystero-epilepsy   severe hysteria with epileptic convulsions.

hystero-neurosis   see hysteria.

idiotism   severe mental retardation.

iliac region   region surrounding the lateral portion of the hip bone.

imperforate hymen   abnormally closed membrous fold which closes the vaginal orifice.

intercostal neuralgia   sharp, spasm-like pain occurring between two ribs.

labia minora   small folds of skin near opening of the vagina.

leucorrhoea   a whitish or yellowish discharge from the vagina or uterine cavity, which may be a symptom of a disorder either in the reproductive organs or elsewhere in the body.

lumbar   pertaining to loins.

mania   a disordered mental state of extreme excitement. Also used as a word to denote obsessive preoccupation with something.

marasmus   a form of protein-calorie malnutrition.

materia medica   pharmacology.

melancholia   a mental state characterized by extreme sadness or depression, with inhibition of mental and physical activity.

menarche   establishment or beginning of the menstrual function.

menorrhagia   excessive menstruation.

mesmerism   hypnotism.

metritis   inflammation of the uterus.

metrorrhagia   irregular uterine bleeding.

monomania   psychosis on a single subject or class of subjects.

morbidity patterns   the ratio of sick to well persons in an area.

myoma   a tumour formed of muscle tissue; myoma uteri: a benign tumour of the smooth muscle fibres of the uterus.

neuralgia   sharp pain in a nerve or along the course of one or more nerves.

neurasthenia   neurosis marked by chronic fatigue, lack of energy, feelings of inadequacy, depression, inability to concentrate, insomnia; popularly called nervous prostration.

nulliparous   adjective describing a woman who has not produced a viable offspring.

oestruation   the recurrent, restricted period of sexual receptivity in female mammals other than human females.

oophorectomy   excision of one or both ovaries.

ophthalmia   severe inflammation of the eye, sometimes due to gonorrhoeal infection.

os uteri   the mouth or opening to the uterus.

ovarian follicle   the ovum and its encasing cells.

ovariotomy   removal of an ovary or ovaries; also known as oophorectomy.

ovaritis   inflammation of any ovary; also called oophoritis.

perimetritis   inflammation of the membrane surrounding the uterus.

perineum   the pelvic floor and associated structures occupying the pelvic outlet.

peritoneum   the serous membrane lining the walls of the abdominal and pelvic cavities.

peritonitis   inflammation of the peritoneum; can be fatal if neglected.

pessary   an object placed in the vagina to support the uterus or rectum or used as a contraceptive device; a medicated vaginal suppository.

placenta praevia   where the placenta is located so that it covers the mouth of the uterus. Any expansion of the cervix may cause tearing of placental tissue and bleeding. The condition is life threatening to mother and fetus and may require delivery by Caesarean section.

podalic version   the manual turning of the fetus in delivery into a footling presentation.

polyp any growth or mass protruding from a mucous membrane; usually an overgrowth of normal tissue although sometimes consists of new tissue; usually benign.

post-partum occurring after childbirth.

primipara a woman who is bearing a child for the first time.

prolapse of the uterus also known as falling of the womb; downward displacement of the uterus so that the cervix is within the vaginal orifice.

prophylactic an agent that tends to ward off disease.

prophylaxis prevention of disease; preventative treatment.

puerperal fever an infectious disease of childbirth; called also puerperal sepsis and childbed fever.

puerperal mania a disordered mental state associated with childbirth.

puerperal septicaemia blood poisoning in which the focus of the infection is a lesion of the mucous membrane received during childbirth.

retroflexion the bending backward of the body of the uterus upon the cervix.

retroversion the tipping backward of an entire organ.

rheumatism any of a variety of disorders marked by inflammation, degeneration, or metabolic derangement of the connective tissue structures, especially the joints and related structures.

rickets a Vitamin D deficiency leading to disturbance or ossification of bone; various degrees of deformity are produced.

round ligament of the uterus a fibromuscular band attached to the uterus near the uterine tube.

salpingectomy excision of a uterine tube.

scrofula primary tuberculosis of the cervical lymph nodes.

sepsis presence in the blood or other tissues of pathogenic micro-organisms or their toxins.

septicaemia blood poisoning; systemic disease associated with the presence and persistence of pathogenic micro-organisms or their toxins in the blood.

septicaemic fever see septicaemia or puerperal septicaemia.

sound a slender instrument to be introduced into body passages or cavities, especially for the dilation of strictures or detection of foreign bodies.

speculum instrument for opening or distending a body orifice or cavity to allow visual inspection.

spermatorrhoea involuntary escape of semen, without orgasm.

subinvolution failure of a part to return to its normal size and condition after enlargement from functional activity.

supra-renal glands above a kidney; adrenal glands.

sympathetic nervous system the cerebro-spinal and sympathetic systems form what is commonly called the central nervous system; consists of a double chain of ganglia, with connecting fibres, along the vertebral column, giving off branches and plexuses that supply the viscera and blood vessels and maintain relations between their various activities.

symphysiotomy division of the symphysis pubis to facilitate delivery.

symphysis pubis the line of union of the bodies of the pubic bones in the median plane; the bones are united by a plate of fibro-cartilage.

tent a conical, expansible plug of soft material using to dilate an orifice or to keep a wound open.

tetanus also known as lockjaw; a highly fatal disease, characterized by muscle spasm and convulsions.

trachelorrhaphy suture of the uterine cervix.

vaginismus painful spasms of the muscles of the vagina.

vaginitis inflammation of the vagina.

venesection phlebotomy; incision of a vein.

ventrofixation fixation of a viscus, e.g., the uterus, to the abdominal wall.

version the act of turning; especially the manual turning of the fetus in delivery.

vertigo a sensation of rotation or movement of one's self or of one's surroundings; may result from diseases of the inner ear or disturbances of the central nervous system.

vesico-vaginal fistula fistula between the bladder and vagina with resulting leakage of urine into the vagina; often the result of difficult labour in childbirth.

vulva the external genital organs in the female.

vulvitis inflammation of the vulva.

Picture Credits

Academy of Medicine, History of Medicine Museum (photographs by Rex Lingwood): obstetrical forceps, vectis (x943.2), Smellie's forceps (x969.28); gynaecological instruments, uterine sound (x969.306), bivalve vaginal speculum (x930.12), Ferguson vaginal speculum (988.15.2), pessary (979.7.6–10)

John Baldy *An American Text-book of Gynaecology* (Philadelphia 1894): nineteenth-century menstrual pad

B.G. Jeffris and J.L. Nichols *Search Lights on Health: Light on Dark Corners* (Toronto 1897): the effects of tight lacing, title page

National Archives of Canada: unidentified woman with churn (PA 126654, photography by W.B. Bayley); Isobel Cameron (C 22934, photograph by C.W. Parker); Mrs Albert Campbell (PA 130015, photograph by James Ballantyne)

Archives of Ontario: Katie Welsh (9491 S14900); Toronto Hospital for Consumptives (14662–14)

McGill University Archives: women faced severe medical problems

Index